THE Earthwise
H E R B A L

Other books by Matthew Wood

The Earthwise Herbal:
A Complete Guide to Medicinal Plants of the Old World

The Practice of Traditional Western Herbalism:
Basic Doctrine, Energetics, and Classification

The Book of Herbal Wisdom: Using Plants as Medicines

Seven Herbs: Plants as Teachers

Vitalism: The History of Herbalism, Homeopathy,
and Flower Essences

THE Earthwise
H E R B A L

A Complete Guide to New World Medicinal Plants

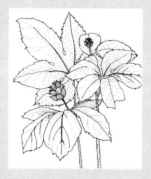

MATTHEW WOOD
MS (Herbal Medicine)

Registered Herbalist (American Herbalists Guild)

North Atlantic Books
Berkeley, California

Illustration on page 158 from *A Guide to Health*, 3rd ed., by Benjamin Colby. Originally published in 1846 by John Burns, Milford, NH.

Published by   Cover art by Matthew Wood
North Atlantic Books   Cover and book design by Suzanne Albertson
P.O. Box 12327
Berkeley, California 94712   Printed in the United States of America

The Earthwise Herbal: A Complete Guide to New World Medicinal Plants is sponsored by the Society for the Study of Native Arts and Sciences, a nonprofit educational corporation whose goals are to develop an educational and cross-cultural perspective linking various scientific, social, and artistic fields; to nurture a holistic view of arts, sciences, humanities, and healing; and to publish and distribute literature on the relationship of mind, body, and nature.

North Atlantic Books' publications are available through most bookstores. For further information, call 800-733-3000 or visit our website at www.northatlanticbooks.com.

MEDICAL DISCLAIMER: The following information is intended for general information purposes only. Individuals should always see their health care provider before administering any suggestions made in this book. Any application of the material set forth in the following pages is at the reader's discretion and is his or her sole responsibility.

Library of Congress Cataloging-in-Publication Data

Wood, Matthew, 1954–
    The earthwise herbal. A complete guide to New World medicinal plants /
Matthew Wood.
        p. ; cm.
    Complete guide to New World medicinal plants
    Companion volume to: The earthwise herbal : a complete guide to Old World medicinal plants / Matthew Wood. 2008.
        Includes bibliographical references and index.
    ISBN 978-1-55643-779-3
    1. Herbs—Therapeutic use. 2. Medicinal plants. 3. Materia medica, Vegetable. I. Title. II. Title: Complete guide to New World medicinal plants.
    [DNLM: 1. Medicine, Herbal—North America. 2. Plants, Medicinal—North America. 3. Phytotherapy—North America. WB 925 W877E 2009]
    RM666.H33W6556 2009
    615'.321—dc22   2008041429
        CIP

1 2 3 4 5 6 7 8 9 VERSA 14 13 12 11 10 09

To My Many North American Herbal Friends, but especially

Phyllis Light
Arab, Alabama

Margi Flint
Marblehead, Massachusetts

Rosemary Gladstar
Sage Mountain, Vermont

Will Winter, DVM
Minneapolis, Minnesota

ACKNOWLEDGMENTS

In addition to the many sources quoted in the following text, I have been greatly assisted by my dear friend Julia Graves, a perceptive herbalist living in Normandy, France. Julia alone took the trouble to read the entire manuscript from beginning to end. She has also contributed many fine discoveries of her own, and some important facts from literature that I had overlooked. I have appreciated our many conversations scattered over the years, occurring when we were fortunate enough to be on the same continent. Second, I wish to thank another dear friend, Phyllis Light. A gifted and experienced herbalist living in Arab, Alabama, Phyllis and I have had the opportunity to live on the same continent and communicate hundreds of times, during which we have educated each other on the intricacies of herbalism, North and South, and of holistic medicine. Third, I must thank my deceased friend, William LeSassier, herbalist, acupuncturist, and healer extraordinaire, whose spirit touched the depths of humanity, the plant world, and so many of us in the herb world. Fourth, I wish to acknowledge the deep conceptual debt I have to David Winston, herbalist (AHG), of Broadway, New Jersey, who first taught me how to link pharmacology and energetic thinking.

TABLE OF CONTENTS

Introduction ix

PART I

Specificity in Herbal Medicine 1

PART II

Materia Medica 45

INTRODUCTION

I have not thought it beneath me to converse with
Root and Indian Doctors, and everyone who has
professed to possess any valuable remedy.

—WOOSTER BEACH (*THE AMERICAN PRACTICE*, 1833, 10)

The *Earthwise Herbal* has been published in two books: not volumes one and two, but two companions that supplement one another. The first to appear was a volume on medicinal plants of the Old World used in traditional Western herbalism. The second complements and completes the set by covering herbs of North American origin.

In the introductory chapters of each volume, I have supplied an account of the practice of traditional Western herbalism from the European and American perspectives, respectively. *Earthwise* the first includes material on Greek medicine, while *Earthwise* the second includes medical traditions originating in North America. More in-depth discussions of these theories and practices are offered in my earlier works, *Vitalism* (1992) and *The Practice of Traditional Western Herbalism* (2004).

In what way can I claim that these two books are "complete guides"? As one of my teachers, Bob Gallagher, of Present Moment Herbs, in Minneapolis, said: "One of the neat things about herbalism is that there is no limit to the subject." There is always more to learn. Herbalism is an ongoing empirical art, not a fixed, fully explored, "complete" field. Practically speaking, it would be impossible to cover all herbal medicines used in the Western tradition. *The Earthwise Herbal* is also incomplete in terms of modern knowledge of pharmacology, herb/drug interactions, clinical studies, and so forth. For these the reader/user must turn elsewhere. However, there is one area where these two books do attempt completion.

Plants are not just slurries of chemicals casually operating together to keep an organism alive. Rather, they are a unity of constituents and functions drawn together under a presiding drive or arch-function that can be described as a primal essence or personality. The plant lives in a certain environment and has undergone stresses in the crucible of natural selection. All its constituents, colors, shapes, and adaptations are the expression of a ruthlessly honed individuality. Plants may not be conscious, as we are, but their chemistry, appearance, and uses reflect an innate personality as much as they reflect physiology. Herbs have long been used for their physiological applications in the human organism; now we must learn to appreciate them as entities expressing on psychological and physiological levels in an integrated, complete, person-like fashion. This has been the direction of developments in homeopathy, flower essences, and herbalism as taught by John Scudder (1829–94), the Australian herbalist Dorothy Hall, now retired, and myself.

The special emphasis of this book is therefore on understanding the plant as a sort of "individual," then tracing this plant essence as it translates or incarnates into the numerous medicinal functions and symptoms for which it is used. When we understand a plant from "top" to "bottom," from its most inward character to its outward appearance, throughout its diverse medicinal influences, we understand it in a "complete" fashion, and it is only in this way that *The Earthwise Herbal* claims to live up to its subtitle.

The two volumes of *The Earthwise Herbal* constitute a materia medica, or herbal, describing a very large selection of the nontoxic herbs used in traditional Western herbal medicine. No attempt has been made to include toxic medicine plants. I leave this to my homeopathic friends, who have long understood the inwardness or personality aspect of their remedial agents, most of which are poisons.

The present volume covers the medicine plants, as the Indian people would describe them, native to North America. The introductory chapters are devoted to coverage of North American perspectives on herbal medicine. The companion volume chronicles both the materia medica and the philosophy of European herbalism. However, I have already discussed much of the American contribution to plant medicine in *Vitalism* and *The Practice of Traditional Western Herbalism*. Therefore, I have limited my discussion here to the six tissue states, specific medicine, and Southern blood typology. The first two of these methods represent the work of the physiomedical and eclectic schools of botanical medicine, which flourished in the nineteenth century. The latter is currently associated with Appalachian and African American herbalists and healers. Coverage would be complete if I included a discussion of American Indian herbalism, but this subject is vast and, in *Vitalism*, I have already posited a relationship between Native medicine and Samuel Thomson's concept of cure by diaphoresis and warming the organism.

The Decline and Revival of Western Herbal Medicine

At the beginning of the twentieth century, herbalism was still widely practiced in the United States. At the end of the twentieth century it was only
used in poor populations scattered around the world that were unable
to afford modern medicine, or by people who had broken away from
conventional medicine to become "alternative." What caused these
changes?

Beginning in the 1930s drug companies began to introduce expensive,
synthetic drugs. They saw cheap, readily available herbs as competition.
A marketing campaign was developed that emphasized that herbs were
old-fashioned products used by old, poor, and uneducated people, whereas
drugs were used by educated, sophisticated people. A similar campaign
was waged against traditional foods. I remember looking at a cookbook
that showed the young housewife correcting her old mother. No, she was
pointing out. Lard is old-fashioned, now we use cottonseed oil. Vast quantities of government money went into research and development of drugs
and food founded on chemistry and mass production. Regulations changed
to support corporations and eliminate herbs. At the same time, there was
a fundamental change in medicine. Drugs became molecularly specific
weapons directed against germs or specific molecular lesions. Herbs,
suited to general physiological imbalances, no longer fit the prevailing
view of the human body.

The change from herbalism to commercial drugs is not founded upon
"science," but upon a complex commercial and political plaform supporting a materialistic vision of human life. There is no proof that "herbs
do not work." They are simply ignored and ridiculed. Studies are invented,
not to try to show that they work, but designed to demonstrate that they
do not. Modern people live a luxurious lifestyle that allows them to use
expensive drugs and to ignore basic principles of nature and right living.
Average life expectancy has increased, but the number of centenarians
has decreased. Public health measures have lengthened life expectancy,
but medical treatment has shortened the life of those who are living longer.

The change from old-time herbal medicine to modern drug medicine
is described by one herbalist who lived through this period (Willa Shaffer,
1986, i):

> *Throughout her childhood Willa suffered from bronchial disorders
> and pneumonia. The herb Lobelia was introduced to Willa by her*

grandmother. The Lobelia always worked to break up the conges-
tion caused by these illnesses. Herbs continued to be her main source
of "cure" for illness until she was sixteen. At this time herbs become
extremely difficult to buy. Between 1931 and 1935 the pharmacies
converted their stock from mainly herbs to drugs. The pharmacies
then became known as "Drug Stores" and the herb market was
completely forgotten.

The disappearance of both herbs and natural foods was largely the
product of a well-financed marketing campaign that included making
the practice of herbal medicine illegal in most jurisdictions. It became virtually impossible to use herbs, even if one wanted to. However, the antidote to this poison was built into the situation, and Willa Shaffer puts
her finger on this solution. Instead of accepting information derived from
marketing and politically empowered corporations and collective opin-
ions, she took responsibility for her own health and learned from personal experience (Willa Shaffer, 1986, i):

Willa spent the next thirty-two years in poor health. Turning back
to herbs, the light finally dawned on a new era of herbs in her life.
Her interest drove her to educate herself on the subject of herbs. She
acquired her knowledge through seminars, research and more
research and most importantly, through EXPERIENCE.

The revival of herbal medicine is, ultimately, based on the *experi-*
ence of people like Willa, who found conventional answers lacking and
returned to old, time-tested methods that worked. Too many people
trustingly follow the dictates of conventional marketing, politics, and
science. This leads to debacles like hormone replacement therapy. When
it was discontinued, breast cancer levels declined precipitously. Yet, it
is impossible either to prove that herbs work or that HRT causes cancer.
Clinical trials are not subtle tools, but clumsy ones. There is no replacement for experience.

The Earthwise Herbal is thus based on the hardwrought experiences
of practicing herbalists. It appeals to experience and attempts to develop
hands-on knowledge of the healing art. In this it departs from the popular method, which imposes biomedical standards on herbalism through
emphasis on pharmacology and clinical trials, while ignoring the experiences and literature of actual, practicing herbalists.

PART I

Specificity in Herbal Medicine

CHAPTER ONE

The Six Tissue States:
Patterns of Disharmony

Diseases, except where they are very dangerous, should not be irritated by drugs. For every disease has a structure that resembles in a certain manner the nature of living creatures. For the composition of these living creatures has prescribed periods of life for the species as a whole. . . . It is the same with the constitutions of diseases: whenever anyone destroys this by drugs, contrary to the allotted period of time, many serious diseases are wont to arise from those that are few and slight. Consequently, so far as leisure permits, one should control all such diseases by regimen, instead of irritating a troublesome evil by administering a drug.

—PLATO (*TIMAEUS*, 89B–D)

Modern science and medicine are reductionist; that is to say, they reduce all phenomena to their smallest pieces to gain understanding. This perspective ignores the possibility that there is a unified being, consciousness, identity pattern, or functional whole at the base of a human, animal, plant, or disease organism. Holism, in contrast, concerns itself with this underlying, unifying entity. Traditional science and medicine, as exemplified in the quote from Plato, has always held such a view.

The whole is not only a unified entity, but possesses a pattern or characteristic manner of expression. Each human can be said to have a personal identity and an individual constitution, with innate and acquired characteristics. Animals, plants, and microbes lack a self-conscious personality but possess an innate constitution. The holistic practitioner, in almost every field of holistic medicine, attempts to establish the individual identity and pattern of the sick person, the disease, and the therapeutic tool. This is one of the most important and characteristic differences between conventional and alternative medicine.

In alternative practice the study of the individual constitution and pattern is called "energetics." The constitution is looked upon as a pattern of energy, unique to the individual (in humans) or the species (in animals, plants, and microbes). The "energy" involved is usually visualized as some kind of life force, like *qi, prana,* or *vital force.* However, even this tip of the hat to vitalism is not necessary; without proving the existence of a vital force we still see the pattern or "energetic" in the individual.

The term "energetics" is of recent origin. It is usually used by people within the holistic movement and seldom by those without. As far as I know, the term was introduced by Dr. Randolph Stone, the famous osteopath and naturopath who incorporated Ayurvedic concepts into bodywork. He used it to refer to differences in patterns of energy. In the early 1970s the term became more widely used (Arroyo, 1975).

Different cultures have different systems of energetics. Yin and yang provide a simple dual energetic system. The four or five elements are used in Greek, East Indian, and Chinese philosophy, science, and medicine to discuss basic polarities and types of energy expression and pattern. The four directions and animal totems are used in Native American medicine.

It is sometimes said that Western herbalism lacks a system of energetics. However, as I have shown in *The Practice of Traditional Western Herbalism* (2004), nineteenth-century physiomedicalism used a system of six energetics (excitation and depression, tension and relaxation, atrophy and stagnation) analogous to the old Greek use of hot and cold, tense and relaxed, dry and damp. This system is still used by physiomedicalists in Great Britain, as exemplified in *Herbal Medication* by A. W. and L. R. Priest (1982).

In *The Practice of Traditional Western Herbalism* (2004) I reintroduced this system, which I called "the forgotten energetics of Western herbalism." This method has great appeal because it links the old system of energetics in Greek medicine with the system used in nineteenth- and twentieth-century herbalism with contemporary language, including terminology used in biomedicine. Both in *The Practice* and in the accompanying volume of *The Earthwise Herbal* I traced the relationship between the six tissue states and Greek energetics.

The Six Tissue States

A perusal of nineteenth- and early-twentieth-century medical literature of all schools shows that these were common terms. Indeed, they are still used in neurology and medicine to describe general tissue conditions in the organism. The six tissue states may therefore be described either as a system of energetics or as descriptions of general physiology and patho-physiology.

At any rate, it is necessary to describe the six tissue states as they are used to define the properties of plant medicines in *The Earthwise Herbal.*

HEAT/EXCITATION

If we start with our own experience of food we can easily demonstrate to ourselves which are the cooling and which are the heating remedies. In the middle of the summer, when it is hot, we like to consume fruit. Not surprisingly, many of our cooling remedies come from the fruit-laden rose family. There is a reason for this. Flowers and fruits are especially rich in flavonoids, substances that contribute to the development of color. In medicine, flavonoids are known as antioxidants and capillary healers. Oxidation is the scientific word for heat or weathering processes, so antioxidants are cooling, while substances that soothe and heal the capillaries also cool by helping the blood to not get congested in the peripheral vessels. Some of the flavonoids produce cyanide as they break down, a substance that kills by throwing a monkey wrench into the Krebs cycle, the energy-generating cycle in the mitochondria of the cell. In small doses cyanide cools by slowing down the Krebs cycle, instead of stopping it altogether. The cyanogenic glycosides, as they are called, give rise to the bitter almond flavor found in some of the seeds, bark, and leaves of some of the fruity members of the rose family—**almond, peach, apple, wild cherry.**

The flavor of fruit is sour and this is also a good guide to cooling remedies. Thus, members of the rhubarb family, which have an acid taste but no particular flavonoids, are also cooling. The citrus family gives us many acidic fruits but here the antioxidant cooling agent is limonene, one of the few essential oils that is cooling. This compound is also found in **lemon balm,** one of the few sour and cooling members of the mint family. All told, the rose, citrus, rhubarb, heath, and honeysuckle families provide us with many cooling remedies, including **rose hips, hawthorn, wild cherry, peach, lemon, lime, yellow dock root, rhubarb root, sheep sorrel, garden sorrel, cranberry, blueberry, bilberry, honeysuckle,** and **elderberry.** In addition, some oddball plants contain high levels of flavonoids, which make them cooling, even if they do not have prominent fruits or the "right sort" of families. This includes **yarrow, hibiscus,** and **lemon balm.**

Although experience proves that the sweet and sour taste of fruit is cooling, theory, in the form of Ayurvedic medicine, claims that the sour flavor is warming. This is evidently because large doses of acids are burning. However, in Ayurvedic medicine we usually find that fruits are classified as cooling. This demonstrates that experience is often more accurate than theory.

COLD/DEPRESSION

Just as we know cooling foods such as fruits and lemon juice from experience, we can identify the warming and stimulating foods and spices such as **curry, cayenne, turmeric, cinnamon,** and **nutmeg.** These foods tend to be aromatic and pungent or spicy. There is a connection between the aroma and the spiciness, because it turns out that the pungent or spicy flavor is actually due to aromatic oils that stimulate the nasal scent receptor to mimic a taste-like reaction. In other words, the pungent or spicy flavor is not felt on the tongue but is due to volatile oils stimulating the nose. Thus, the great majority of our stimulants are pungent, spicy, and aromatic, and contain volatile or essential oils. The stimulants are also largely equivalent to the "aromatics" or herbs high in volatile oils. Think here of **rosemary, thyme, dill, fennel, angelica, osha, savory, ginger,** and **oregano.**

Stimulants are remedies that increase activity, function, and energy in the tissues and cells of the body. They may irritate the tissues, thereby increasing reaction, or they may enhance depressed functions in the cells. For this reason stimulants are largely warming—think of **rosemary, thyme, mustard, cabbage, cayenne, turmeric,** etc.—but paradoxically some of them are cooling—**lavender, echinacea, coriander,** and **yarrow.** That is because some of them stimulate functions that have an overall cooling effect. For instance, both lavender and yarrow stimulate circulation, which moves overheated blood out of inflamed areas more quickly. Also, some aromatics—**lavender, lemon, lemon balm**—are cooling because a few volatile oils (such as limonene) are cooling. Some plants, like **yarrow** and **elder,** contain both flavonoids and volatile oils, so they are cooling and warming simultaneously.

Members of the cabbage family *(Brassicaceae)* contain aromatic thiol compounds that are highly stimulating. Thiols contain sulfur, which acts like a metabolic match, starting up fires to remove toxins and stimulating waste removal. Alliin, in some onions *(Alliaceae),* contains sulfur as well. Here we think of **mustard, cabbage, shepherd's purse, onion,** and **garlic.**

The Greeks observed that the cold organism could start generating heat. This was not due to overactivity or overbuilding, as in the true heat of overstimulation, but due to "putrefaction" or the breakdown of tissue that releases heat as it is metabolized. The Greeks considered putrefaction to be the result of poison, which is pretty accurate. Antiseptics include **baptisia, isatis, echinacea, helianthemum,** and **calendula.**

In this case the cell life has become so depressed that it cannot break down waste products, or even food (which therefore become waste). Bacteria come in and live off the waste products, generating a foreign heat. But bacteria and parasites also put out toxins (poisons) that suppress the life of the cells, so that they can live and not the cells. (This is why many people still feel like they are infected with parasites after stool samples show that they are clear—the organisms are gone but the toxins remain.) Thus, the depressed tissue state is (1) likely to invite bacterial and parasitic invasion and (2) likely to be encouraged by that invasion. Actual poisons, bug and snake venoms, and unhealthy foods and drinks can also cause putrefaction.

Putrefaction or "heat from cold" is therefore a kind of heat that needs to be treated by stimulants—here the cooling stimulants such as **lavender, echinacea,** and **yarrow** have a long history of use. However, there is another category of medicines that need to be mentioned here, the antiseptics. These are especially geared to fight sepsis or putrefaction. Some of them are stimulants, but they also possess unique compounds such as pine oil (pinene) or thyme oil that kill low forms of life. These too are heavily scented, like the pungent aromatic herbs mentioned above. This category includes **balsam fir, pine, cedar, juniper,** and **thyme.**

An interesting category that David Winston has introduced is that of the "fragrant bitters." This simplifies a lot of complex pharmacology down to a basic sensory test. Bitters that are fragrant (**wormwood, wormseed, sweet Annie, elecampane, black walnut**) are usually vermifuges or parasiticide. As mentioned above, the presence of parasites is a characteristic of depressed tissue life.

It is interesting to observe that throughout the world smudges, fumigants, and incense are used to drive away bad, dead, depressed, and negative energies and bring in new, healthy, refreshing, and positive ones. Thus, the relationship between aromatics and warming and stimulating properties is demonstrated by worldwide practices.

DRY/ATROPHY

The dry organism needs fluid, of which there are two kinds, water and oil. When the organism is dry, however, it also can easily become under-nourished or atrophic because it takes water and oil to move food from the inlets in the small intestine to the cells. Thus, dryness and atrophy represent two sides of the same coin.

In addition to water and dietary oils (these are the fixed oils, distinct from the volatile oils, because they do not evaporate easily), the dry/atrophic condition may need lubricating or moistening of surfaces, softening of hard spots, and deep feeding with nutrients or micronutrients. Thus, almost any kind of healthy food or beverage addresses the dry/atrophic state, as well as a certain number of agents that improve digestion and assimilation. For this reason, dry/atrophy is addressed by a great number of different tastes. The most basic remedial agent for this category is the mucilage. These polysaccharides produce a sensation of filminess and are bland or sweet. They coat and soothe mucosa, replacing mucus secretion that is deficient. The most important ones in Western herbalism are **marshmallow root, flower,** and **leaf, fenugreek, slippery elm,** and **comfrey.** Western herbalism has recently adopted from Chinese medicine the category called the "sweet tonics." These contain carbohydrates and increase tissue nutrition. A Western "sweet tonic" would be **slippery elm** or **milky oatseed.** Some bitter tonics increase salivation, appetite, digestion, and bile flow, to promote nutrition. Here we would think of **burdock, Oregon grape root,** and **angelica.** Some of the best aperients or appetite-enhancers are bitter and sweet—like **burdock, American ginseng,** and **goldenseal.** Salty remedies soften hard spots, because water follows salt. These are usually combined with mucilage. This group is called the emollient, and includes **fenugreek, marshmallow root,** and **mullein.** The starved organism often needs oil as much as water, so we use the fixed oils, as in **flaxseed, pumpkin seed,** and **sesame.** A number of oily substances remove constipation by stimulating the gallbladder and lubricating the colon—**butternut, wild bergamot,** and **poppy seed.** After the use of opiates, **poppy seed** is excellent for the constipation. A number of plants contain small amounts of oil that act on the "oil pathways" of the liver and cells, increasing lipid metabolism and nutrition. These oily or nutty tonics include **burdock, angelica, fenugreek,** and **sage.** A few herbs are proteinaceous or meaty—**nettles** and some **mushrooms.** The latter contain many curious immune-stimulating properties.

General constitutional weakness is sometimes accompanied by immune weakness. The immune system does not only fight off invaders that penetrate the perimeter, but helps to break down proteins in the digestive tract (which are a form of invader). If the immune system is weak there will be poor tissue nutrition. The weakness may also be in the bone marrow, where stem cells manufacture red and white blood cells and replacement parts, or it may be particular to the immune system. It is now known that some polysaccharides (large, complex sugar molecules) stimulate the immune system. These include mucopolysaccharides in mushrooms like ling zhi (*Ganoderma* spp.). Another group that acts on the immune system is the essential fatty acids (**borage, black currant, evening primrose, black cumin**). They also seem to be building, hence, suited to the atrophic category.

There are polysaccharides in **echinacea**—hence the sweet taste. Unfortunately, echinacea has been wrongly marketed as an immune tonic to help protect against colds and flus; its traditional use is in a different kind of immune problem, defending the body when there is sepsis and tissue destruction. Here we see that its sweetness would be pertinent; it has been used for tissue wasting.

Saponins have many properties, including lubricating, cleansing, expectoration, and (steroidal saponins) endocrine building. They combine dry/atrophy with other categories. **Senega snake root** is an important expectorant in debilitated cases with deep bronchopneumonia.

DAMP/STAGNATION

There are actually two damp tissue conditions, relaxation and stagnation. The former refers to clear, runny fluids leaving the surfaces of the body, the latter to stuck fluids bloating the tissues and, especially, thickening into catarrh, phlegm, or mucus.

Damp/stagnation corresponds to conditions where the metabolism and the transportation of metabolites in the body are sluggish so that there is a buildup of toxins and a stagnation of fluids and movement. This was called "humors in the blood," "impure blood," "bad blood," and (nowadays) "toxins in the blood." This condition is treated with "blood purifiers" or "alteratives."

The Greek term for the process that occurs between digestion and assimilation of food into the body was "alteration"—that is, metabolism. Hence the alteratives are those agents that promote metabolism. In folk medicine these were traditionally called "blood purifiers" because a poorly burning metabolism often causes toxins that work their way to the surface to cause skin lesions. This is the tissue state that responds to alteratives, or blood purifiers. Most of these are bitters, because many bitters stimulate the liver and, hence, blood cleansing. However, some act on the lymph or generally on the organism.

As Dr. Broda Barnes (1976) showed, the old symptoms of "bad blood" are often the same as those of low thyroid function. When the thyroid is low there will be low metabolism in the cells. However, it is also possible to have "bad blood" due to low activity in the liver, poor transportation by congested lymphatic ducts and stagnant fluids, or congestion in the channels of elimination (skin, kidneys, bowels, lungs). Sometimes, backup of toxins from the large intestine causes this tissue state.

Because of the many origins of damp/stagnation, or torpor, or toxemia, or bad blood, or impure blood, there are many remedies. By and large, the largest number of these are the bitter tonics, which were traditionally used to "clean the blood." These usually increase secretion in the liver and gastrointestinal tract (hence their use also in dry/atrophy) and this stimulates metabolism and waste removal. However, some alteratives are not bitter (**red clover, chickweed, cleavers, scrophularia**). They often work on the glands—thyroid or lymphatic. Some agents work on the skin or kidneys. Thus, alteratives are a mixed bunch of herbs: **nettles** (earthen, "meaty," bitter), **red clover** (sweet), **burdock root** (oily, bitter, sweet), **dandelion root** (bitter, sweet, oily), **yellow dock root** (bitter, astringent, sour), **scrophularia** (pungent, aromatic, bitter), **Oregon grape root** (bitter), **phytolacca** (bitter, pungent), **barberry root** (bitter), **black walnut** (acrid, oily, bitter).

Allied to the alteratives are the laxatives and cathartics, which also depend on bitter principles, to stimulate either the gall, or the peristaltic action of the gut (bitter anthraquinones): **senna, yellow dock root, rhubarb root, cascara sagrada.**

WIND/CONSTRICTION

There are two sets of remedies that act on tissue constriction or tension. These are the acrid-tasting remedies (**lobelia, catnip, valerian, cramp bark, hops**) and the bitter nauseants (**lobelia, blue vervain, boneset, blessed thistle, quinine, hops**). Both of these groups reduce excessive sympathetic activity or sympatheticotonus, when the autonomic nervous system gets stuck in the "awake, alert, run, attack" mode and cannot get back into the parasympathetic relaxation mode.

The term "acrid" is often used to designate the pungent or spicy flavor, but here it has a different meaning. Pungent, spicy herbs stimulate a response through the nasal scent glands that mimics a taste reaction. True acridity, on the other hand, is the sensation caused by bile in the back of the throat. *It is the only completely unpleasant taste.* There is no way to "fix it up" by the addition of other flavors, though sugars dilute it. Thus, for example, the very sweet taste of Solomon's seal is ruined by a pinch of acridity, though the latter is largely lost on drying. (Solomon's seal is a good remedy for tension and debility in tendons.)

In traditional Chinese medicine the acrid flavor is associated with herbs that "open the periphery"—that is, diaphoretics that get sweating going in the skin. Generally, also, these agents act upon the peripheral circulation to open the capillaries. Thus, they bring perspiration and toxins out of the body and relax the organism. The capillaries and sweat glands are under the influence of the sympathetic branch of the autonomic, so in fact this influence extends through the periphery into the nerves and muscles.

The nauseant bitters are recognized, both in biomedicine and in herbalism, to induce expectoration. They stimulate the vagus nerve, which causes a contraction to run through both the lungs and the stomach. Nauseant bitters can provoke vomiting, as well as expectoration. Another thing that happens is that they send a shiver or shudder through the frame. Since the shivering mechanism is under the control of the sympathetic, this penetrates into the autonomic again. These remedies treat chills and fever.

DAMP/RELAXATION

In this state the tissues are relaxed so that they lose their tone and sag or prolapse. The pores in them also lose tone, hence fluids run out of them to produce diarrhea, urinary frequency, excessive sweating, clear, free expectoration, and bleeding. With this there is often a loss of electrolytes and minerals, leading to prolapse of tissues and softening of bones and cartilage. The minerals sometimes deposit out of the circulation, causing stiff, hard tissue.

This is the tissue state that responds to astringents. They "pucker" up collapsed or prolapsed membranes that have lost their tone or are losing fluids. Astringents depend on the presence of tannins, which coat mucosa and other membranes, preventing the loss of fluids and loss of tone. This also preserves potassium ions, which prevent the loss of too much water through the kidneys. Thus, astringents are indicated when there is a loss of fluids through any of the channels of elimination (skin, kidneys, colon, lungs, menses). Strong astringents include **raspberry leaf, blackberry leaf** or **root bark, wild geranium, sumach, oak bark, horse chestnut,** and **collinsonia.**

The tissue state model explains the actions of herbs very well and even correlates nicely with the tastes and pharmacology, as described in Chapter 2 and Chapter 4. The tissue states are eminently well suited to bringing forward the intrinsic properties of medicinal plants. In contrast, Southern blood typology is an energetic system that arises from examination of patterns in the organism.

CHAPTER TWO

Southern Blood Typology:
An Indigenous American System
of Folk Medicine

*In the spring collect the spicy, warm sassafras root bark
to thin the blood; in the fall collect the mucilaginous
bark to thicken the blood.*

—ANONYMOUS

T he blood has always been a source of important information for the medical practitioner, both traditional and biomedical. The four humors of Greek medicine are components of the blood that separate out and cause pathology when they are not completely "cooked" or incorporated into the body. Greek medicine was still the model of practice when the first Spanish, French, and British settlers arrived on the eastern coast of North America. Among them were North African Moors and West Africans who either practiced the same Greek-Arabic system or had their own traditions in which, most likely, the blood played an important part. The American Indians, whom they met on the thickly wooded shores of the New World, also considered the blood an important medical substance.

The settlement of the South presented particular problems for the first emigrants. The Anglo-Celts, with their fair skin and hair, coming from a cool, damp, northern climate, were not well suited to the area. Blacks and whites from southern Europe had some advantages—genes suited to malaria and greater familiarity with heat and humidity. However, some of them ended up in climates where unfamiliar cold settled over the land. All were moving from areas where their ancestors had been settled—for hundreds or thousands of years—into new and challenging territory.

It was at this time that a theory of "seasoning" developed among the new settlers. It was believed that people needed to be "seasoned," or slowly and carefully exposed to new environments. People with "thin" blood were thought better suited to the hot South because their blood was waterier, and therefore cooler and more inclined to produce cooling perspiration. Settlers with "thick" blood were better suited to the cold North. Thick blood is oilier, so it protects against cold and damp, like the oily wool sweater of a Scottish fisherman. In order for the blood to adjust, it was thought necessary to use herbs and foods to thicken or thin the blood and to let people "season" for a year or two, moving slowly from region to region.

We do not know when or how the system of evaluation from the blood developed, but the form in which it has come down to us is an indigenous production of the American South, and has always been identified as such by sociologists and anthropologists. Practitioners, both black and white, refer to the rising and falling of the sap in trees, in summer and winter, to explain the logic behind the system. For this reason, I like to think that it was the trees that taught people the blood type system. And if there was one tree responsible for the concept it was certainly sassafras. The bit of lore quoted at the head of this chapter, handed on from an Ohio herbalist, contains the bare outlines of the entire system.

I must thank my friend Phyllis Light, of Arab, Alabama, for introducing me to Southern blood typology and teaching me much of what I know about it, including most of the herbs suited to the treatment of the different states. Phyllis is one of the most skilled herbalists in the United States. She possesses that sense for tradition that is necessary for the herbalist to be fully grounded in traditional medicine. Adopting "Southern blood typology" can greatly enlarge our ability to track, understand, and treat slow, progressive, chronic changes in pathology corresponding to the most serious chronic illnesses.

The South was an ideal place for a blood-based folk medicine to originate and develop. Here, more than in almost any other culture in the world, blood ruthlessly defined social relationships and civil rights. After the Dred Scott case, in 1857, one drop of African blood was enough to lose one's civil rights. (Up here in Minnesota the case disenfranchised the French-Indian mixed bloods, sending them from their farms to the reservations.) The blood also had important religious connotations. We do not hear serious discussion of the "saving blood of Christ" in European or Northern theology, but in the Old South it made sense that people should be *related to God through their blood,* just as they were related to their kin by blood. In this culture, the blood became a powerful oracle for the inner condition, both spiritual and physical, likewise for medical conditions.

Cycles, Qualities, and Tastes of the Blood

There are three major methods for classifying blood in Southern folk medicine. The yearly cycle of the seasons, correlating with the rise and fall of the sap in the trees, provided the conceptual foundation behind four qualities of the blood. During the summer the sap ran **high, thin,** and **fast,** while in the winter it was **low, thick,** and **slow.** Blood changed the same way. If one or more of these mechanisms were blocked, the blood would become **hot** or **cold.**

Blood actually tastes metallic from the presence of iron. However, in Southern folk medicine, the blood has four "tastes"—**sour, sweet, salty,** and **bitter.** As in Greek medicine, there is no pungent, sharp, or spicy taste in the blood. I have not attempted to chronicle this system.

The concept of **bad** or **impure** blood was widely recognized, in both the North and the South. The former term was preferred by American Indian practitioners; the latter was introduced by German immigrants. This concept is still widely used today; it is more frequently called "toxins in the blood." Bad blood is paired with its opposite quality, the desirable **good** blood. The latter represents the perfect mixture of blood. It indicates a physically balanced condition resulting from right living and thinking.

CYCLES OF THE BLOOD

In spring the sap rises. There is so much of it, and it is so watery and thin, that it rises fast and drips. This can be seen on the leaves and bark of big trees like the elm, ash, maple, and sweet gum. The sap rises so that it is high in the tops of trees. As the sap runs in spring, the new layer of inner bark (cambium) is laid down, so the sap is high in the sense that it is moving to the surface, away from the old cambium layer, which is now becoming wood. Spring sap is also high in terms of nutrients and the pressure needed to drive the sap up the tree. Thus, the sap is high in terms of position, nutrients, and pressure. As the sap rises in spring and summer it is also watery and thin, allowing it to rise faster and higher. Water is cold, so thin sap is cooling. In short, sap in the spring and summer is *high, thin,* and *fast.* It is more likely to be *clean,* or *good.*

In the fall, the sap starts to go down. It is "low" in the sense that it sits low down in the tree and the pressure to move it upward is also low. As it settles, it becomes thicker and slower. It contains more mucilage as the water thickens and condenses. Nutrients are stored for the winter in the sap, while in the summer they are quickly taken up by the sapwood or cambium layer. Thus, in winter the sap is *low, thick,* and *slow.* It is more likely to be *dirty,* or *bad.*

Blood in people goes through the same changes. In spring and summer it is high in terms of position, nutrients, and pressure. It goes to the surface to discharge heat, making the skin red and warm. It rises to the head for the same reason. In hot weather the head feels hot, from congestion to the head. Blood pressure rises and there are more headaches, heart attacks, bleeding, and strokes. To compensate, the body tries to make the blood thin and fast. Thin blood is not only cooling, due to the presence of more water, but moves more readily through the capillaries, so it allows the blood to discharge more heat and cool off.

In a similar manner, the blood in fall and winter is thick, low, and slow. Thick blood slows down and remains deeper in the body. It cannot flow through the small capillaries as efficiently, so the extremities are colder. However, thick blood holds heat better because there is less water, which is cooling, and more oil, which protects against cold and damp. When a person is cold, the blood goes deeper to keep the body from losing heat. The surface is pale because there is less blood in the capillaries. There is low blood in the sense that the blood is deep in the body. There is less pressure to push it up and out, so low blood also has low blood pressure. In old age, the winter of life, the blood stays low down in the legs, sometimes producing a ring of dark skin around the ankles. This is also called low blood. Since there is less food in winter, less blood is manufactured, producing nutrient-poor low blood. This also results in pallor. To retain heat, blood in the winter is low, thick, and slow.

In spring, the blood starts to rise. If blood rises too quickly a person gets "spring fever." Today this expression refers to a person who can't wait for spring to come, but originally it described a type of fever that occurred due to eating too much rich food as it became available in the spring, or remaining on the winter diet too long.

The Yearly Cycle of the Blood

Summer	Winter
High	*Low*
Fast	*Slow*
Thin	*Thick*
Clean	*Dirty*

Hot and cold blood arise when one or more of the mechanisms above is blocked. For instance, if there is a fever and the blood is heated up, the healthy response of the body is to speed up the pulse, push the blood to the periphery, and thin it out. However, if one or more of these mechanisms is blocked, the blood will heat up and produce "hot blood." Usually, however, hot blood refers to conditions where there is a source generating heat within the body—an unresolved focus of infection or toxin. The same kind of background produces "cold blood." If a person gets a chill and the body does not respond appropriately, cold gets stuck in the body, resulting in cold blood. However, cold blood can also be caused by lack of internal heat.

Cycles of the blood are also observed in the cycle of human life. In youth there is an abundance of good, rich blood, making children more vibrant and active. However, they can suffer from symptoms of high, hot, fast, or thin blood, resulting in hyperactivity, headache, allergies, nosebleed, fever, overheating, and recklessness. If this condition persists after puberty they are said to be hot-blooded. The Greeks would have used the word sanguine (full of blood). In old age the blood can become cold, low, slow, and thick. This results in varicose veins, prolapse of tissues, less blood to the head, dizziness, mental vacuity, decline of mental and physical energy, arthritis, diabetes, stroke, vascular disease, or heart attack.

Here's an example of how the cycle of human life was observed. One time when my dad was a little boy he was out fishing with his father and grandfather. The weather was cold and wet. Although his granddad was a confirmed teetotaler, he took along "Southern Comfort Cough Medicine" for "medicinal purposes." My dad wanted to be like his grandfather so naturally he wanted some too. "No," explained his grandfather gravely. "This is for older folks because we get cold more easily. Little kids like you are already warm."

QUALITIES OF THE BLOOD

The blood is like a "scales" and needs to be balanced, explained the late Mr. John Lee (Payne-Jackson, 1993, 23). There are up to five basic categories of the qualities: cleanliness, location, viscosity, speed, and temperature. Much of the following information I learned from Phyllis Light, herbalist (AHG), of Arab, Alabama.

CLEANLINESS

Good Blood. A person with good blood has a strong, balanced, healthy system that can meet and overcome adversity. Not only does he or she have good blood from proper food and exercise, but also by inheritance and living a "clean life." Blood is cleaner in youth and summer.

Bad Blood. This condition is widely recognized in Western folk medicine. It is as frequently encountered in the North as well as the South. The basic idea is that the blood is "unclean" due to the presence of "toxins," as many people would say today. These are picked up from food or the environment. Causes include incomplete metabolism of food or waste products in the body, or poor excretion of waste products through the channels of elimination. The major organ systems involved are the liver (seat of the preparatory metabolism), cells (seat of metabolism), thyroid (metabolic rate), the lymphatics (internal transportation), and the four major channels of elimination—kidneys, skin, colon, and lungs.

In the old days there was also an implication that bad blood could be picked up from sexual or inherited taints. In the nineteenth century, when treatment of syphilis and gonorrhea was not as reliable as today, it was believed that residues of these diseases, or the toxins they created, could remain behind after the main expression of the disease had disappeared. This created "miasms" or "taints" to the blood. These could be passed on to children through the blood.

Originally the symptoms of scurvy were included under "bad blood." Thus, many of the traditional "blood purifiers" or "alteratives" are also denoted as "antiscorbutics." However, today this condition is usually treated as a separate disease. In the twentieth century, when the function of the thyroid came to be known, it was recognized that "bad blood" was often a symptom of hypothyroidism (Broda Barnes, 1976).

In Renaissance England, when the great herbalist Nicholas Culpeper wrote, this condition was called "humors in the blood." This phrase reflected the very ancient doctrines of Greek medicine. When the four "humors" were out of balance some of them were left over in the blood. This meant that the fire of life burning in the organism was not burning clean, but leaving waste products or "humors."

In nineteenth-century America, the traditional English terms "humors in the blood," "humor," or "canker" were replaced by a German term that translated as "impure blood." Another expression adopted at this time came from the Indians. The term "bad blood" is still widely used by Native Americans. (Indian languages usually don't have a word for "impure.")

In the twentieth century, as concepts about health evolved, the terms "toxins in the blood," "toxic blood," or "toxic liver" have come into use. Many modern herbalists feel embarrassed to use a folk medical term. However, the idea of "toxins" remains a popular explanation for disease down to the present, and folk medical terminology and concepts can be used in modern herbal practice—as long as they are identified as such.

Considering how often the names (and even the basic conception) for this condition has changed over the centuries, is there anything certain we can say about bad blood? Yes. The single symptom most commonly associated with this condition in the old literature is skin eruption or lesions of some kind. British herbalist Mary Thorne Quelch (1945, 17) writes, "Whenever any form of skin disease is present, be it an eruption of the slightest type, such as the appearance of blackheads or pimples, or a serious outbreak of boils or abscesses, it may be taken for granted that some impurity is poisoning the blood." The idea is that the toxins come to the surface for removal.

A good description of "bad blood" is given by Dr. John Scudder (1874, 311–13). His account is rich in detail, comprising one of the best descriptions of this folk medical diagnostic pattern I have been able to find in any of the old-time medical textbooks.

"You may say that 'bad blood' is a popular myth, and does well enough to base a nostrum advertisement upon, but it will hardly do for specific medication," writes Scudder. "There you are wrong, for 'bad blood' is a real, tangible entity, with definite expressions and a definite therapeutics." But "how will we recognize it?"

> The evidence of bad blood is best found in wrongs of excretion and of nutrition. There cannot be a wrong of this character without an effort upon the part of the skin, kidneys, and bowels to remove the unpleasant material, and we will usually find that all three of these emunctories show a lesion caused by the effort, though one may suffer more than another. In the case of the skin it manifests itself in cutaneous disease, taking the forms of the exanthemata in the simpler cases, and the graver forms of the pustulae, squamae, and tuberculae, when the lesion is more persistent and severe. This fact has long been recognized, in so far as the treatment of skin diseases has embraced means for removing effete and unpleasant materials from the blood.

Scudder emphasizes the "expressionless" aspect of the face and skin, and a pulse that is also lacking in full expression. It is, so to speak, "obscure" because there are humors or phlegm that hide and dull the sharpness of the pulse. I find this to be a very reliable indication.

"Bad blood" was originally known as "humor" or "canker" and associated with catarrh (heavy, thick mucus). Dr. Swinburne Clymer said that any coating on the tongue, other than clear, watery mucin, could be considered evidence of "canker." However, the other moist tissue state, relaxation, will produce moisture on the tongue or skin and yeasty overgrowths, including coatings of the tongue. The more these resemble "yeast," like the coating on Brie cheese, the more likely the condition is relaxation rather than stagnation. The latter will be associated with thickened, catarrhal discharges and coatings. Low thyroid function, one cause of "bad blood," actually produces mucopolysaccharides—that is, mucus-like material—in the interior cavities.

Bad blood responds to "blood purifiers" or "alteratives." These are mostly alkaloidal bitters, which stimulate the liver, though there are some exceptions. The most common alteratives used today are **burdock root, dandelion root** and **leaf, yellow dock root, scrophularia, red clover, nettles, sarsaparilla,** and **sassafras.** When there is bad blood it is often also necessary to keep the colon working, sometimes with laxatives—**yellow dock root, rhubarb root, butternut bark, buckthorn bark, senna,** and others. Refer to "Damp/Stagnation," under the tissue states (Chapter 1) for additional information.

LOCATION

High Blood. This term covers several overlapping conditions. First of all, it signifies that there could be too much red blood. This means that functions are overstimulated (as in the heat/excitation tissue state). High blood can describe hyperglycemia, from too much sugar in the blood. This would be called "high, sweet blood." Second, high blood indicates that the blood is high up in the body—superabundant in the head, especially, and toward the surface of the body. There are tendencies to headache, fullness of the head, an exploding feeling in the head on rising from a chair, the pulse beats toward the surface, and there is a pink-red or *carmine* complexion and fullness of the tissues, which are warm. Third, high blood can mean high blood pressure. Orthostatic hypertension (fullness in the head or exploding in the head on rising from a chair or lying down) is likely to occur in any of the above three conditions. All three can occur together.

Symptoms. A person suffering from "high blood" is prone to headaches, fainting, nausea, nosebleed, flushing of the face, fever, and high blood pressure (Cavender, 2003, 123). Symptoms are aggravated by heat in the summer and activity, and ameliorated by bleeding. The pulse beats against the top surface of the artery; it is elevated or "high." The tongue is likely to be elongated, red, and pointed, with a red tip.

Treatment. High blood was the state that was originally treated by bloodletting in European medicine. In German medicine it is still permissible to treat temporary bouts of high blood pressure with bleeding. However, herbal treatment is by diaphoretics, diuretics, and any other agent that lessens the oppression of the blood and the pulse. Typical remedies here are **yarrow, elder, peppermint, catnip, lemon balm, hawthorn, rose hips, peach leaf, blue vervain, boneset,** and **angelica.** Most of these herbs "release the surface," or promote sweating and reduce excessive circulation of blood to the skin or relax the kidneys.

Example. I often joke in class that bloodletting would be a good method to treat hyperactivity in children. One of my students in Maine then related the following story. She was keeping the most troublesome boy after school. He cut his finger on a piece of paper and looked up. "I feel better," he said.

Case History. A Welshman, long resident in the United States, came to see me for redness of the face, including spots of staph infection. He was much overweight, indicating "rich blood," and the pulse was rapid and elevated. I settled upon **elder,** a medicine he knew from his childhood. The redness was no longer an issue at his next visit.

Low Blood. This term also has three different definitions. First, the blood is low in one or more constituents. Hence, this kind of "low blood" often signifies iron deficiency anemia or malnutrition. Typical symptoms include pallor, exhaustion, pale inner eyelids, pale fingernails, a pale, dry tongue, pale, dry skin, and a hollow, easily compressed pulse. Second, the blood is positionally low. It tends to go down into the legs and not return up to the torso, head, and heart, creating varicose veins, sluggish, dark, clotted menses, and (especially in old people) dark patches and spots around the ankles. (This aspect of low blood is similar to "deficient heart blood" in Chinese herbalism.) Third, low blood can also refer to low blood pressure and orthostatic hypotension, so that the head feels empty, there is less blood to the head, with dizziness, memory loss, and fainting possible. Sometimes there can be high blood pressure, though one would not expect it, because the stagnation on the venous side of the circulation causes oppression against the heart.

Symptoms. The major symptoms of low blood are fatigue, pale, dry skin, weakness, dizziness, and listlessness (Cavender, 2003). Not enough blood is flowing to the brain, so thinking is diminished and memory can be poor. Low blood is the usual cause of senility, loss of concentration and focus, and poor memory in the aged. By the time dark blood has appeared around the ankles treatment for low blood is ten or twenty years late. The pulse is low. The tongue is pale and dry.

Treatment. Low blood can be treated by blood builders such as **blackberry, blueberry, elderberry, beet root, cooked rehmannia root,** and **yellow dock root;** stimulants to raise the blood, such as **sassafras, cayenne, safflower, yarrow,** and **elder;** and astringents to tone the veins, including **yarrow, witch hazel, collinsonia, horse chestnut,** and **white oak bark.** Low blood, as in low in the body, is harder to treat than blood deficiency. In my experience, important remedies for raising the blood are **rosemary** and **lavender**—not very Southern but effective. **Nettle** is a blood builder that is indicated when there is low blood pressure, according to Dorothy Hall.

VISCOSITY

Thin Blood. Blood is thinned out by the addition of water. Because water is cold, people with thin blood tend to be cool. The skin is less red and more pale, the blue veins more evident through the skin, and there may be a cool, clammy perspiration from excess water coming out through the skin. These people do better in summer and worse in winter.

Because it has an excess of water over solid constituents, thin blood is associated with anemia, but it is a different kind of anemia from low blood (or iron deficiency). When the blood is low the skin is dry, because the blood does not come up to the surface and because there is a lack of both fluid and solid constituents of the blood. However, thin blood has an excess of water so the skin is moist and cool. The anemia of low blood is due to nutritional deficiencies, including lack of iron, but the anemia of thin blood is due to low red blood cell production in the bone marrow. This in turn is due to low signaling from the kidneys or weakness of the bone marrow. The kidneys read the red blood cell level as the blood passes through and send a hormone—erythropoietin—to the stem cells in the bone marrow to get them to switch over to erythrocyte production.

When the blood is thin the urine is copious, clear, or thin, and frequent. So the kidneys are "damp." Indeed, water easily passes through the system with thin blood in the form of clear, copious expectoration, diarrhea, sweat, and urine. The kidneys have a hard time retaining the water, so they are "weak." A good remedy here is **sumach berry.**

When the kidneys are weak there is less stamina and staying power and the person is weakened by any loss of fluids. Therefore, exertion (producing sweat), diarrhea, and sex (fluid secretion) are weakening. There may be excessive menstrual bleeding with weakness after the period. Thin blood is the background for leucorrhea, or discharges from the vagina, especially those that are watery. A standard folk remedy for "watery blood" and leucorrhea is red oak bark, according to Dr. Ralph Russell (1911), of Birmingham, Alabama. If the discharge is white, the tongue has a white fur, or the mucus is white, like pastry starch, **white water lily** is indicated.

Blood that is both thin and low is called "tired blood." It wants to just sit around down in the feet and not rise up. If thin blood combines with high blood it rushes to the head, causing headaches, red cheeks, and menstrual cramps. These symptoms are more frequent just before the period.

Symptoms. Thin blood produces a relaxed, nonresistant pulse. Usually the skin feels cool and moist. There are often "streamers" running down the tongue on both sides. If the mucin condenses on the tongue the condition is turning more toward bad blood.

Treatment. Thin, watery blood responds to astringents, which tighten the pores and tissues to stop the loss of fluids. Good remedies for thin blood are **raspberry leaf, lady's mantle, red root, huckleberry** or **blueberry leaf, rose hips, sumach, white pond lily,** and **white oak bark.** Sometimes the blood gets congested, so warming, stimulating blood thinners such as **feverfew, chrysanthemum, angelica,** and **black cohosh** are needed.

Thick Blood. When the blood is thick there is a preponderance of solids over water. This can be due to a great number of causes. Almost unilaterally, thick blood is oily blood. However, it can also contain (1) an excess of nutritious substances or metabolites, (2) an excess of waste products, as in bad blood, (3) excess viscosity due to changes in essential fatty acids (this is the type of condition for which aspirin is given), and (4) clotting caused by the coagulation process in blood. Thick blood is oily, whereas thin blood is watery, so thick blood is a better insulator than thin blood.

Type (1). When thick blood is due to an excess of nutritional substances—sugar, lipids, and proteins—we can call this "rich" blood. It occurs due to a rich diet and a liver that is overactive on the anabolic side—building up useful metabolites in excess.

When thick blood is due to too much sugar, it will also taste sweet and is called "sweet blood." Blood sugar levels are higher, promoting hyperinsulinism, high cholesterol, high blood pressure, diabetes, vascular disease, stroke, and heart attacks. High cholesterol is usually due to excessive consumption of sugars, which are bound up as triglycerides and stored as LDL cholesterol—either in fat deposits or in the blood vessels. This results in tendencies to heart attacks and strokes. A person with thick, sweet blood tends to have more body fat and large, droopy, fatty tissues.

When thick blood is due to healthier dietary oils it is not necessarily a deleterious health condition. Good-quality dietary fats do not produce as much unhealthy cholesterol. Oily thick blood promotes sebaceous oil, which insulates and keeps the skin warm. The oil on the skin and in the blood keeps a person warm in the winter. The uptake of calcium will be higher and bone building will be increased, because vitamin D is made from oil on the skin in the presence of sunlight. So some people with thick blood have a large-boned build, whereas people with thin blood tend to have thin, long, narrow bones, less calcium, and (in the old days) more tendency to tuberculosis (which is controlled by calcium).

Thick blood due to high protein intake can create a healthy, muscular constitution. However, eventually there will tend to be problems. There are likely to be kidney problems because the kidneys are stressed by the exit of protein waste products through them. This is one of the serious problems with high protein diets. High protein can also stress the liver and cause bad blood. In addition, it can cause blood coagulation. Always consider **nettles** when there is stress from protein in the system.

Thick blood due to excess nutritional production requires sour, fruity remedies to cool off the constitution, such as **peach leaf, rose hips, strawberry leaf, blueberry, hawthorn, basswood bark** or **flower, honeysuckle, American viburnum, lemon, lemon balm, yellow dock root, sheep sorrel,** and **rhubarb root.** This cools the appetite, but to thin the thickness use **fenugreek, black walnut leaf,** or **sassafras root bark.**

Type (2). Bad blood due to a preponderance of waste material in the blood can be due to "toxins" or "humors" (phlegm). In the former case the thick blood tends to be more hot, because metabolic waste products burn off and create heat. When bad blood is due to phlegm the blood will be more mucilaginous (the urine more filmy), the kidneys colder, with more mucus discharge, and the system will tend to be cool. For this condition use the alteratives, **burdock root, dandelion root** or **leaf, scrophularia, poke root, red clover, chickweed, nettles;** the laxatives, **yellow dock root** and **rhubarb root;** and the thyroid stimulants, **black walnut hull, seaweed,** and **chickweed.**

Type (3). In medical terms, the viscosity of the blood is controlled by essential fatty acids. One set of EFAs thin the blood while the other thicken it. As we age, the ones that thicken the blood often start to predominate so the blood slowly becomes more viscous or thick. To remedy this, modern medicine puts people on low doses of salicylates (aspirin) to "thin the blood." Natural control of this mechanism is described by Dr. Barry Sears in *Enter the Zone.* In Southern folk medicine **tulip poplar** *(Liriodendron tulipifera)* is frequently given for this kind of thick blood—it contains small amounts of salicin.

My carpenter had a fully developed case of pneumonia. I told him to go to the veterans hospital and get antibiotics and take some support herbs. I recommended elecampane because it is such a strong antibacterial, and liriodendron because he was thin, wiry, and tense. As soon as he took the latter he looked up and asked, "Does this thin the blood?" "Hunh?" I replied. "Like aspirin," he continued. "It thins the blood and cuts down on pain." "Is that what you're feeling?" I asked. "Yeah." From this I learned that thinning the blood reduces pain (which is associated with heat).

Type (4). Finally, thick blood can be due to excess coagulation of the blood. This can arise from a number of factors but the symptoms tend to be the same: prominence of blue/red, blue/pale, blue/black, blue/green, blue/yellow, or blue/gray coloration around the veins of the wrists, or other places where the blood comes to the surface. (This is not the same thing as varicose veins—see "Low Blood"—though the two often occur together.) This is called "stagnant" or "congealed blood" in Chinese herbalism. It is called "bad blood" in American Indian medicine. It is said that it must be treated to prevent development of cancer. The tongue will be blue.

Congealed blood responds to sweet smelling aromatics, some warm, some cool. **Yarrow, safflower, angelica, cayenne, madder, tulip poplar, sassafras, feverfew, chrysanthemum, black cohosh,** and **rosemary.** When a stroke has occurred use **yarrow, sassafras,** or **tulip poplar.**

Thick blood due to nutritional excess causes a full pulse. Due to bad blood it causes an "obscure" pulse, as if the beat were hidden behind impurities, phlegm, or a curtain. Due to viscous and congealed blood it produces a "choppy" pulse (no two beats hit in the same place or have the exact same timing). Thick blood due to nutritional excess causes a full, thick tongue. Due to bad blood it causes a full, coated tongue. Due to viscous and congealed blood it causes a blue color on the tongue and complexion.

Case History. In September a nine-year-old boy came to see me; he had suffered from asthma since preschool. The condition starts in the fall, then continues from the end of September to mid-May. He also suffers from anxiety. The tissue is carmine red and puffy around the eyes, with dark underneath. The tongue is red and somewhat dry. Constitution full, plethoric, not overweight, but strong and large-boned. Although the symptoms indicated "high blood" (carmine red, anxiety, full build), I couldn't find a remedy that worked. Finally I gave more weight to the big-boned constitution and some blue complexion indicating "congealed blood." I told his mother I thought we needed to "thin the blood." "You talk just like my grandfather," she said. "He was full of all those old sayings." I gave the boy homeopathic honey bee (Apis mellifica) 30x, which is a specific for heat, fullness, and allergic swelling under the eyes, and an herbal tincture of safflower *(Carthamus tinctorius),* a good blood thinner and blood cleanser. From daily attacks of asthma he went to none at all. In January he was fiercely sick for four days with a head cold, but the asthma did not reoccur. I considered this to be a healing aggravation as the condition cleared his system. I saw him again next winter. He had been healthy for months.

SPEED

Fast Blood. When the pulse is rapid the blood is said to be "fast." This condition is associated with heat. Either there is too much heat, or the system is weak and cannot resist normal or slight elevations of heat. People with an abnormally rapid pulse who are not sick are often easily stressed and nervous. They need the simple sedatives like **melissa, skullcap, lycopus, motherwort,** and **poplar bark** *(Populus tremuloides).* There are tendencies to hyperthyroidism and hyperadrenalism, aggravated in hot weather.

If the pulse is rapid, full, and nonresistant, it means the "heat is having its way with the system"—that is, the body cannot resist the heat. A very good remedy here is **yarrow.**

If the pulse is rapid, nonresistant, and low it means the fever is chronic and is burning the person up. The heat has overwhelmed the body's defenses. This causes a "hectic fever," where there is redness on the cheeks, night sweats, and exhaustion. The sedatives mentioned above may be helpful but the old-fashioned specifics here were crawley root and cypripedium, two orchids we would no longer use due to environmental concerns. Chinese "yin tonics" would serve the condition.

If there is fever, and the pulse is rapid, strong, and hard, it means that heat has entered the system, but there is resistance and tension. A good remedy here is **barberry root bark.**

The pulse when fast also tends to be high or elevated, because fast, hot blood often goes up to the surface. The tissues are hot, red, full, and tender—the symptoms of inflammation in the acute stage. The high, fast pulse always means there is pressure on the surface, to open up, and treatment is by sedatives, diaphoretics, and diuretics.

When fast blood goes on for too long it lapses into sepsis. The tongue is dark red. Traditional remedies are stimulating antiseptics such as **baptisia** (small doses only), **woad** or **isatis** (small doses only), **scrofulawort** *(Helianthemum canadense)*, **echinacea**, **gravel root**, and **Virginia snake root** (small doses only). The doctors, and some folk practitioners, used acids (acetic, lactic, muriatic), in small doses.

Slow Blood. This condition occurs in chronic diseases, just as fast blood is associated with acute ones, even acute fevers that become chronic. Slow blood develops over a long time, due to chronic influences. Mr. John Lee said it could be caused by cold, thick, or low blood. When the blood is slowed down the person is slow and "feels slouchy" (Payne-Jackson, 1993, 23).

When the circulatory apparatus is burdened by excess or thick blood, especially when there is "bad blood" or metabolic waste products in the blood, it can slow down, according to Dr. John Scudder (1874, 309). He differentiates "full" excess blood (see "High Blood") from an "empty" excess blood, which he calls "asthenic plethora" (empty fullness). "There is another condition in which a large amount of blood is continuously made, but owing to exhaustion of the circulatory apparatus and nervous system by excesses, its circulation is sluggish." This "asthenic plethora will be recognized by fullness of blood vessels, oppression in the stroke of the pulse, and a turgid venous circulation, giving the surface the peculiar color of venous blood. The color is so characteristic, that when associated with the full animalized tissues, and the full blood vessels, there can be no mistake in the diagnosis."

If the blood is thick and coagulated it slows down. The tissues are full, as in thick blood, but increasingly there is stagnation and this produces a blue color around the veins. This kind of "slow blood" is similar to "stagnant blood" or "congealed blood," as described in Chinese medicine, or "thick blood" in the Southern system. The blood gets into a "pile up," as John Lee says, resulting in a clot or stroke.

TEMPERATURE

Hot Blood. This term refers to both psychological traits and physical symptoms. Hot-blooded individuals are likely to act before they think. They are impulsive because *they are driven by their blood.* They let the blood dictate their actions, rather than letting their mind rule over their impulses. They tend to get caught up in chauvinism involving racial, team, or local identity. They tend toward violent outbursts, worse from drinking alcohol, which is heating.

Hot blood can also refer to physical conditions. These are caused by overexposure to heat in different forms. Alcohol, as my great-grandfather explained to my dad, when he was a little boy, warms the blood. Phyllis Light adds that hot blood is also caused by diet, allergies, overexposure to the sun, excessive sexual desire or activity, acid blood, and fever. It causes sunburn, headaches, hives, rashes, and hot skin outbreaks. It also can cause the "hot-blooded" behavior mentioned above.

When the heat is in the surface or capillary blood there will be hives, allergic reactions, and sensitivity to the sun.

Treatment. If there is a fever where a rash is expected, like smallpox, but none comes, or the rash is slight and incomplete, this means there is hot blood bunched up in the interior that needs to be drawn to the surface. *It is not to be treated by cold (like immersion in cold water), which would drive it farther in,* but by agents that bring the blood out to the surface (make it high), move it faster, and make it thinner. The traditional herbs for this, in addition to the diaphoretics in general, were **black cohosh** and **safflower.** Treatment by cold and suppression would result in convulsions and fits.

Cold Blood. This term also refers to psychological traits. Cold blood lets a person think before they act. That is why a person who commits a premeditated murder is called a "cold-blooded killer." Of course, that kind of behavior is an extreme example, not the norm. A cold-blooded person is more likely to be a normal member of society, but from this group come the premeditated seducers, con men, and perpetrators of fraud.

In ancient law a crime of passion was considered less serious than a crime of seduction. This still shows up in Dante's *Inferno,* where rapists are found on a higher level of hell than seducers. Premeditated homicide is a more serious crime than unpremeditated.

Cold blood can also be a physical condition. It can be the result of chronic exposure to cold or an acute exposure to cold that does not get expelled from the system but becomes chronic. For instance, sitting out in a cold fishing boat, on a cold lake, would tend to cause a chill, if one didn't warm up with alcohol or something warming, and this could turn to "cold blood" if it became chronic. Cold blood can be the result of extended or chronic illness, exposure to a damp, cold environment, wind, sudden temperature change, not enough sex, or too many cold foods. It produces mucus in the lungs, bronchi, bladder, stomach, gallbladder, colon, small intestine, and vagina. People with cold blood have more colds, influenza, arthritis, fits, spasms, parasites, and strokes.

Cold blood is slow and the pulse is slow. When the pulse is slow and hard (it hurts the finger as you press on the artery), it means the person has been chilled by external wind and cold, or emotionally "cold" experiences. The muscles are tense, rigid, hard, and spasmodic. There are tendencies to fits and convulsions, but not as bad as when fast, hot blood is suppressed by application of cold. Treatment is by bitter warming remedies such as **wormwood, mugwort, elecampane,** and **wild lettuce.** If the pulse is slow, nonresistant, and low, it means the system has run out of heat and there is nothing left inside to warm it up. There may be hypothyroid; a good remedy here is the bitter warming **black walnut hull.**

CHAPTER THREE

Specific Medicine: Precision in Herbal Practice

In attempting to create an "American System of Herbal Energetics" we find much of the work has already been done. Rather than start over, we need to find, understand, and reclaim the knowledge of our elders and grandparents. Our future cannot ignore our past.

—DAVID WINSTON (1997, 199)

The capstone to the entire edifice of herbal medicine is the effective use of herbs, no matter what models we are using to understand the organism. Here we are served by a system of botanical practice known as "specific medicine," introduced by Dr. John M. Scudder (1829–94) in the mid-nineteenth century. Although specific medicine draws on well-established European roots, it is a production of American shores and was not adopted by British herbalists. Therefore, I have included it in the North American section of *The Earthwise Herbal*. An extensive discussion of the subject can be found in my book on the history and philosophy of homeopathy, herbalism, and the flower essences, *Vitalism* (1992). Eclectic Medical Publications, in Sandy, Oregon, has republished many of the important texts of specific medicine; others can be found online.

At the time Scudder began practice it was commonly asserted that "nothing is certain in medicine." Scudder rebelled against such uncertainty. He asserted that there must be specific solutions discovered by experience. Instead of looking for some principle or law upon which to found medicine, Scudder preferred direct, trained, personal experience. Careful observation of the organism and the effects of medicines should be the basis of medicine, not theories. "This is not a question of schools," wrote Scudder (1874, 27). "It is a question of sheer empiricism (call it quackery if you will)."

We learn to know the healthy man—know him by exercising all our senses upon him. We want to know how he feels, how he looks, how he smells, how he tastes, and what kinds of sound he makes. Then we want to learn the diseased man in the same way, and compare him with our healthy standard—certain expressions of life meaning health, and certain other expressions meaning disease....

Men live a lifetime, and know nothing of the manifestations of life. Students become conversant with books, attend their lectures, pass their examinations, and yet have no practical knowledge of human life. And physicians will practice medicine a lifetime, and yet fail to know what healthy life is (Scudder, 1874, 15).

In addition to careful observation, Scudder taught a return to proven remedies of the old practitioners. Old physicians, nurses, and lay practitioners, after years of experience at the bedside, must possess at least a few tried and true remedies, and if they have been kind enough to record these agents, then these will provide a platform upon which to construct a certain basis for the practice of medicine. Scudder therefore combed the old journals for descriptions of medicinal agents that acted reliably and the conditions or symptoms in which they were indicated. He would have agreed with Dr. Benjamin Rush, who wrote:

When you go abroad always take a memorandum book and whenever you hear an old woman say such and such herbs are good, or such a compound makes a good medicine or ointment, put it down, for, gentlemen, you may need it (Moss, 1999, 8).

In 1870 Scudder published the first fruits of his labor in *Specific Medication and Specific Medicines*. This was followed in 1874 by *Specific Diagnosis*. These were received with some controversy in the eclectic school, to which he belonged, but Scudder was an unusually magnanimous person. He pointed out that his work was not meant to replace anything that worked for anyone else, but simply to augment what was already effective. In time, his doctrine of specific medicine came to characterize the eclectic school.

Scudder defined a specific medicine as one that could be used time and again on certain grounds because it was suited to a well-defined symptom picture. If this had been the limit of his method, Scudder's specific indications would have been little different from leading, characteristic, or keynote symptoms used in homeopathy. However, the difference was that Scudder was looking for symptoms that were not only characteristic of a given remedy, but were common expressions of the diseases to which they were remedial.

It is a matter of interest to know the exact character of a lesion, but it is much more important to know the exact relationship of drug action to disease expression (Scudder, 1874, 14).

The reason Scudder's *Specific Medication and Specific Medicines* was followed by *Specific Diagnosis* was that he needed to teach his followers how to understand the diagnostic meaning of symptoms. Scudder, like Samuel Hahnemann, the founder of homeopathy, and Samuel Thomson, the herbalist, knew that diseases were basically just arbitrary names and not practically significant. It was not disease names he was treating, but pathological patterns. These presented characteristic symptoms as they came and went in the organism and at such times could be treated by specific medicines suited to those specific indications.

There are, of course, degrees of specificity. The degree is fairly low in a general, undifferentiated symptom such as "red, irritated eyes," and higher in a precise one such as "generalized redness and irritation of the eyes, as if one had just stepped out of a chlorinated swimming pool." The former could refer to many different conditions and remedies, though it has enough specificity to bring a few to mind quickly (eyebright, strawberry leaf, ragweed leaf, spikenard, and goldenrod, for instance). The latter, however, eliminates the red eyes of eyebright (which are usually also filled with mucoid gunk), the bloodshot eyes of ragweed leaf (with their engorged single swollen capillaries or rivulets in the conjunctiva), the redness of strawberry leaf (reddish eyelids and extensive, congested, irritated capillaries in the conjunctiva), and the red, terribly itching, irritated eyes of spikenard *(Aralia racemosa)*. It precisely describes the eyes normally treatable with goldenrod *(Solidago virga-aurea, S. canadensis)*.

The advantages of the specific system of medicine include the following, as tabulated by herbalist David Winston (1997, 199):

1. *It eliminates guesswork, giving the clinician more precise tools for therapeutic success.*
2. *It improves our understanding of materia medica by clarifying the fine distinctions between a list of herbs within one therapeutic category (e.g., diaphoretics).*
3. *We discover "niche" herbs that do not have a large scope of activity, but are very effective in a specific area (e.g.,* Euphrasia, Agrimonia, Nymphaea*).*
4. *In researching these "American systems of medicine" we rediscover forgotten or neglected herbs (e.g.,* Dicentra, Lycopus, Collinsonia, Lilium tigrinum*).*

5. *In gaining a "clear picture" of each herb's activity we have a better chance to substitute appropriately and find less toxic or more easily available [or less environmentally endangered] alternatives when necessary.*

I would take the environmental concern inferred by Winston in point five in a different direction. Specificity teaches us that sometimes there is no substitute for a given medicine. What then are we to do if it is environmentally challenged? We can use it in small or even homeopathic doses.

This brings up an additional point:

6. *Specificity reduces the amount of medicine required for treatment.*

Specific medicines can be used in much smaller doses than broad spectrum remedies. The less specific a prescription the more substance it takes to move the organism, the less efficient the herb or formula, and the more likely we are to force the organism to change, rather than gently stimulating it to renewed self-governance. The more specific the prescription, on the other hand, the less substance is required. Scudder himself usually recommended 1–20 drops of his special preparations, which he called "specific medicines." These agents, though carefully designed to remove unimportant materials from the preparation, are not that different from simple tinctures or fluid extracts—*especially those made from the fresh plant.* The dosage used by the eclectics continually demonstrates that specific medicines can be used in very small doses. This is environmentally preferable for many plants.

We also see that specific medicine is similar to homeopathy, especially in those departments where it uses herbs: organotherapy, drainage, and gemmotherapy. In the latter, remedies are made from the fresh growing buds of plants, reduced to 1 part in 10 and given in 50-drop doses.

It is sometimes thought that specific medicine is identical to homeopathy. I originally thought it was an adaptation of homeopathic ideas by Scudder, but subsequent study convinced me that there are important differences and that most borrowing actually went in the opposite direction. William Boericke's classic *Pocket Manual of Homoeopathic Materia Medica* (1927) clearly borrows extensively from Scudder and John William Fyfe (1909).

The major difference between specific medicine and homeopathy is that the former uses symptoms that are specific both to a remedy and to an important pathological expression. A specific indication for *Lycopus* is a rapid, tumultuous pulse. This indicates a fever that is pushing the blood around the body at will, wearing down resistance very quickly, leading to hemorrhaging and severe exhaustion. This indication is first mentioned, to my knowledge, by Constantine Rafinesque (1828–30) and illustrates Scudder's contention that he got specific indications from older practitioners and literature. It has been said that *Lycopus* is a specific for hyperthyroidism. That is relatively true—*Lycopus* is probably the single best remedy for this condition. However, it is specific for *hyperthyroidism when the pulse is rapid and tumultuous.*

In homeopathy a leading, characteristic, or keynote symptom is simply unique. It is not characteristic of some distinctive physiological imbalance, or at least that relationship is not developed. For instance, *Bryonia* is "worse from motion." This can be motion of the muscles, the bursa, the pleura, or the intestines (literally, a movement). In all cases, the *Bryonia* person usually winces with pain. This is a highly reliable indicator for *Bryonia,* but would it not also be valuable to know that the symptoms almost always arise from *inflammation and dryness?* That usually there is a lack of internal lubrication like synovial fluid in the joints or interstitial fluid in the muscles? When we understand the underlying physiology behind a symptom, we understand the context in which the remedy works and we are much more likely to use it correctly. A good specific indication for *Bryonia,* from my experience, is a *red, dry tongue.* Such a symptom not only is indicative of a whole state but differentiates the state and the remedy from one another. *Althaea* (marshmallow), for instance, is indicated by a *red, dry tongue with a glazed, shining surface.* This indicates a certain degree of hardening, to which *Althaea,* an emollient, is well indicated. *Amygdalus persica* (peach) is also indicated by an *elongated, red, dry tongue,* but it is usually more pink-red, compared to the dark red of *Bryonia,* indicating a more superficial level of inflammation. A *dark red tongue, with a dried, geographical coating,* indicates that the heat has gone deep and also is indicative of *Taraxacum* (dandelion root).

Because homeopathic symptoms are physiologically meaningless we get indications like the following (Phatak, 1977, 469):

> *Violent vomiting; with retching; desires death, to relieve vomiting; every few minutes. Hunger soon after eating. Easy vomiting, without nausea.*

Would anybody guess that these symptoms are specific to *Phytolacca?* Why yes, I suppose someone might say that, someone who had actually eaten uncooked poke root! However, anyone else would not particularly associate the above with this plant. These symptoms are associated with severe irritation of the mucosa from the actual impression of poke root and are not typical of the acute and chronic conditions for which this plant is usually used. By comparison, the following indications from John William Fyfe (1909, 657) describe a general physiological state:

> *Enlargement, inflammation or pain in glands; mucous surface of the fauces full and of dark color, the tonsils swollen, throat dry or covered with patches of tenacious secretions; fatty degeneration of the heart.*

Phatak's *Materia Medica,* cited above as an example of homeopathic literature, is not just any old book, but one of the most conspicuous used by modern homeopaths. Unlike the specific indications found in Fyfe, Phatak's symptoms are arranged with no relationship to internal pathology or recognizable physiological states. They defy intuition and experienced observation. They take homeopathy too far away from where it has been going in the last few decades: into abstractions and ivory towers far above the living organism. Specific indications, on the other hand, demand that the practitioner understand broad patterns of pathology in the organism—not the arbitrary names of diseases, but their natural history and symptomatic presentation.

CHAPTER FOUR

Holistic Pharmacology:
Integrating Energetic and Material Perspectives

Although pharmacy and herbal medicine used to be almost the same discipline, it is necessary today to deny this relationship.

—DOROTHY HALL (*CREATING YOUR HERBAL PROFILE*, 1988, 9)

In pharmacology, the action of a drug is understood in terms of its specific molecular structure and the function associated with that structure, in conjunction with the delivery system or other factors used to make the drug operative within the target organism or patient.

Reductionist science applies the same idea to the medicinal herb, even though a plant consists of a slurry of chemical components operating in combination together. Thus, the herb is reduced to its "active ingredient" and the other constituents are ignored. The herb product is then "standardized" to a certain level of the "active ingredient" to assure a basic level of strength.

The use of single constituents and "standardization" represents a rather wooden and materialist approach to herbalism in which medicinal plants are seen as analogs of drugs. A more sophisticated method values and interprets the entire complex of constituents, treating them as a complete entity with a specific influence of its own. This methodology has long been advocated by David Hoffmann. For instance, it was once thought that the active ingredient in *Hypericum* was hypericin. Later it was recognized that hyperforin was also active. As David Hoffmann (2003, 559) comments, "Based on currently available information, the whole extract must be considered the 'active ingredient.'"

Looking upon the whole plant as valuable provides a means through which pharmacology can become *holistic*. Ordinarily, pharmacology stops with the individual constituent, but when the synergistic influence of several major constituents working together is evaluated, we gain an understanding of the plant that treats it as a whole entity—and that is holistic in approach. As an example of this type of analysis I quote David Hoffmann's (2003, 560) treatment of *Inula helenium*:

This remedy provides a good illustration of the complex and integrated ways in which herbs work. The mucilage has a relaxing effect, while the essential oils bring about stimulation, so the herb both soothes irritation and promotes expectoration. These actions are combined with an overall antibacterial effect. Its bitter principles stimulate digestion and appetite.

In a lecture David Hoffmann gave more than twenty years ago he added that, as a consequence of this combination of constituents, elecampane is a remedy for children who swallow mucus and get an upset stomach—the bitters help digestion. This description of the properties of elecampane present a picture so clear that one can relate easily to it from personal or observed experience—many people remember swallowing mucus as children. Such a picture represents the holistic approach because it captures the "whole story," at least in one area in which the plant is used. From such a picture one can generalize, thinking about thick mucus, difficult to raise, all clotted up and stuck, or streaming out so rapidly that it creates new problems.

This sophisticated discussion of elecampane so impressed me that I commented to David, "I like the way you teach about the energetic properties of plants." To my surprise he responded, "I don't practice energetics." I was so shocked that I didn't say anything. His response flummoxed me for many years. Finally, I realized that the pharmacological properties of a plant could be used as the basis of an energetic system just as much as the four elements, the five elements, or yin and yang. This is particularly true when we speak of the pharmacological constituents in broad categories (flavonoids, tannins, bitters, volatile oils, fixed oils, mucilage, and so on) rather than specific chemicals. Years later I explained to David why I thought his approach was energetic. I guess he was flummoxed, because this time *he* didn't say anything.

A sound approach to herbal medicine would unite tradition and modern science. This would avoid some of the recent debacles in herbalism, where echinacea and black cohosh have been deemed ineffectual when tested *for uses that are not in line with their traditional uses,* but that were deduced from the theoretical action of constituents. Echinacea was introduced in the early 1980s as an "immune booster." The function of the immune system was not even well understood until the early twenty-first century. Black cohosh was hardly used, traditionally, for menopause; it was introduced for this purpose based on now-fallacious concepts of hormone replacement therapy.

Many attempts have been made to bridge Chinese or Ayurvedic medicine with Western herbalism, but I find these approaches are forced or superficial because *most Western herbalists don't know their own tradition* well enough to make a comparison. Herbs are not just stick figures; they are foci around which historical, cultural, and folk medical data have coalesced to produce complex icons. No one who has not mastered these traditions can represent them or attempt to analyze such a complex icon scientifically. It is not enough to know pharmacology. One must also use an herb. I find it preposterous that so-called "experts" who have never even tasted, much less used, an herb can pontificate about its "properties." Such a standard ought to make me an expert in any field I fantasize about.

One authority in the field of herbal medicine who has studied and mastered all these approaches is David Winston, a member of the American Herbalists Guild. My ability to understand pharmacology and reductionist science is very limited, so I have followed David's work in this field (Winston, 1999). The following notes, therefore, follow his path closely, with some additions from Rudolf Steiner and my own experience.

Energetics and Tastes in Traditional Herbalism

All traditional systems of herbalism in the Old World relied heavily on a system of energetics (yin/yang, the four elements, the five elements, the four qualities, the three doshas, etc.) to describe pathological and curative phenomena, and a system of tastes to analyze plant properties. Usually these are placed together. In Chinese herbalism there are five elements with five corresponding tastes (wood/sour, fire/bitter, earth/sweet, metal/pungent, water/salty). In Ayurveda there are six tastes: sweet (earth, water), sour (earth, fire), salty (water, fire), pungent (fire, air), bitter (air, ether), and astringent (earth, air). Samuel Thomson recognized three medicinal tastes: the hot, the rough (astringent), and the bitter.

When we place these systems side by side, they do not all agree. In Chinese medicine sour and astringent are placed together and associated with wood, which is on the tense/relax axis. In Ayurveda sour is warming, even though most of the sour fruits are considered cooling. In Greek medicine sour is cooling. In China the bitter flavor is warming; in Ayurveda, Greek, and modern Western herbalism it is cooling. Bitterness is pharmacologically complex since it includes cyanogens, terpenes, iridoids, anthraquinones, and other compounds, all of which have completely different uses. In most systems the pungent, aromatic, spicy herbs are warming. The effects and correlations of tastes are fairly complex; reducing them to elemental relationships and a specific number (four, five, six) is artificial. This is one of the important lessons in plant energetics I picked up from David Winston. Energetics are cultural; tastes and pharmacology are physical.

Tastes do reflect pharmacological properties. The cyanogens are bitter; they cool by slowing down the Krebs cycle. The flavonoids are associated with sour fruit acids. They cool by reducing immune response (quercetin) and improving capillary flow (rutin). Sometimes the effect depends on the part of the body affected. For instance, almost all the pungent, aromatic, spicy herbs are warming and stimulating—except those containing limonene, which are cooling. Yet, a few of the pungent herbs are cooling, primarily because they stimulate the capillaries and this removes local blood congestion and therefore reduces heat. Thus, lavender, yarrow, and echinacea are pungent, but cooling.

There are four actual flavors felt on the tongue: sour, bitter, salty, and sweet. The pungent or spicy flavor is actually a smell that produces the sensation of a flavor. Therefore, "aromatic" herbs are usually pungent or spicy. The Greeks called the pungent flavor "sharp" because they thought these plants had more fire particles in them, and fire particles are sharp, whereas air, water, and earth particles are dull-edged. Other "tastes" are actually sensations. This includes the astringent, mucilaginous (stickiness), resinous (tackiness), oily (nutty), meaty (proteinaceous), diffusive (tingling of nerve stimulation), and acrid.

Many traditions do not differentiate between the pungent, sharp, spicy, aromatic flavor and the acrid. Acridity, though burning and irritating, is very different from pungence or spiciness. It is correctly defined as the taste of bile in the back of the throat. In fact, the Greeks called this the "bilious" taste. Bile in the throat arises due to chaos in the autonomic nervous system, running the digestive tract, and was frequently associated with malarial chills and fever; bile in the throat is still found in digestive upset. Hence, acrid remedies are considered to be relaxing—switching from sympathetic to parasympathetic. They frequently open the pores of the skin, reduce fever congestion, and relax the nerves and muscles. Closely related, or perhaps identical, is the nauseant bitter flavor, which sends a shiver through the body. This is suited to conditions where chills and fevers are associated with shivering. It is also expectorant. Valerian, hops, cramp bark, catnip, and lobelia are all acrid; boneset, blessed thistle, wild lettuce, and blue vervain are nauseant bitters.

Pharmacology

Pharmacology is a division of modern reductionist science that classifies plants according to their constituents. Food plants are usually high in carbohydrates, dietary oils, and proteins. These are the essential substances necessary for the maintenance of life. Medicinal herbs are usually high in "secondary metabolites"—that is, substances that are not made by the plant for simple sustenance and reproduction, but are probably produced for survival. For instance, tannins are rich in the bark and probably help harden and protect the periphery from animal depredation and fluid loss, while cyanogens discourage predation through their toxicity. Some secondary metabolites may simply represent storage forms of substances created by stress that will revert to more digestible food forms when the stress passes.

Most secondary metabolites act on the "vegetative" level—that is, on cellular processes that are characteristic of plant life and organisms that lack a nervous system. However, some of them (mostly the alkaloids) act on the nervous system, and therefore on the higher animals and humans. Most of these are hallucinogens or poisons. Tamed, they become drugs.

Modern medicine, at least in the United States, largely ignores the secondary metabolites that act on vegetative processes, instead producing drugs from among substances like alkaloids that act on the nervous system and higher animal life. Thus, modern drugs very often have powerful side effects. In modern German medicine, on the other hand, important drugs are manufactured from the less active secondary metabolites. This is how standardized extracts of herbs, resembling purified drugs, have entered the modern marketplace and, to some extent, replaced traditional herbs.

Rudolf Steiner (1975) discussed the question of the difference between foods, herbs, and drugs. He differentiated between the effects of herbs, which act primarily on the vegetative level of the organism, and plants containing alkaloids, which act primarily on the "animal" level—that is, the nervous system. He suggested that when alkaloids are found in a plant it possesses animal-like qualities and these are often actually poisonous to the plant, stunting vegetative processes and growth. Hence, we get a plant like the hallucinogenic, alkaloid-rich *Mandragora*, which is vegetatively stunted but pharmacologically powerful (Pelikan, 1997).

Steiner also suggests that whereas stress causes disease in human beings, the plant adapts to stress by changes in structure and chemistry. Thus, long exposure to aridity or dampness will change or evolve the plant from an old form to a new one. The structure and chemistry of the plant therefore reflect the stresses it has survived. Thus, the appearance of the plant signifies its medicinal properties. In this way, Steiner defended the "doctrine of signatures" (the appearance of the plant is medicinally indicative) and promoted its study and use in medicine. These changes in the plant, it ought to be pointed out, are accompanied by the presence of secondary metabolites.

Pharmacology separates plants into three basic categories: foods, medicinal herbs, and drugs/poisons/hallucinogens. Of course, some possess qualities in two or more categories. However, we are able to see that there are important differences between herbs and foods and drugs. This difference has been observed in this materia medica. I have purposely eliminated from consideration the more forceful, toxic plants. Many of these are studied and used in homeopathy. I am not attempting to force some sort of classification scheme on herbal medicine; rather I am trying to uncover the lines that are already, to a large extent, used by herbalists, pharmacologists, and physicians themselves. "Herbs" are loved by herbalists, wildcrafters, growers, gardeners, cooks, aromatherapists, florists, artists, photographers, and many others. It is not artificial to define them as a distinctive group.

Energetics, Tastes, and Pharmacology

Now we can compare herbs in regard to their energetics, tastes, and pharmacology. Tastes are really the bridge or intermediary between energetics and pharmacology because they not only relate to hot and cold, damp and dry, tense and relaxed, but they also relate to secondary metabolites, and therefore to pharmacological constituents. For instance, mucopolysaccharides or mucilages are moist, soothing, and cooling. Sometimes they are sweet to the taste. Flavonoids are often known as "antioxidants." Oxidation is the fancy scientific word for burning (including weathering and rotting as well as burning). Thus, an antioxidant retards oxidation or, in a sense, fire. So, the flavonoids are "cooling," and indeed, they are found in the cooling sour fruits that satisfy animals and humans in the heat of midsummer. Most aromatic or volatile oils are pungent and warming, but limonene (in lemons, lemon balm) is cooling and promotes a sour taste. Some flavors do not easily fall into simple energetic or pharmacological categories. Despite exceptions, however, there are general relationships among these categories.

TISSUE STATE		TREATMENT		
Greek	Physiomedical	Taste	Action	Constituents
Heat	Excitation	Sour	Refrigerant	Flavonoids
			Sedative	Cyanogens
				Limonene
Cold	Depression	Pungent	Stimulant	Volatile Oils
			Antiseptic	
		Tingling	Diffusive	Terpenes
Dry	Atrophy	Bland	Mucilage	Polysaccharides
		Sweet	Nutritive	Carbohydrates
		Nutty		Fixed Oils
		Meaty		Proteins
		Salty	Emollient	Sodium
		Earthen		Minerals
		Bitter	Digestive	
Damp	Stagnation	Bitter	Bile	
	(Torpor)		Laxative	Anthroquinones
Lax	Relaxation	Puckering	Astringent	Tannins
(Damp)				
Tense	Tension	Acrid	Antispasmodic	
(Wind)		Nauseant	Antiperiodic	
		Bitter		

Most herbs follow this simple set of relationships. However, there are always exceptions. Whenever plant hormones are present we get extra effects not explained by the flavors because hormones are active in small amounts that need not change the taste. Also, when alkaloids and poisons are present in the plant there is a different kind of reaction in the body that is more complicated and moves us out of the successful use of the above classification scheme.

PART II

Materia Medica

Having fixed upon these general principles, as the only solid foundation upon which a correct and true understanding of the subject can be founded, my next business was to ascertain what kinds of medicine and treatment would best answer the purpose in conformity to this universal plan.

—SAMUEL THOMSON (1825, 1:44)

Using the Materia Medica

One of the most perplexing features of traditional—and regular—therapy is why so many seemingly diverse uses have been recorded for medicinal plants.

—JOHN CRELLIN AND JANE PHILPOTT (1990, 11)

*T*he Earthwise Herbal has been written to bring out the underlying unity behind the actions of a plant so that its application is not, as the above authors comment, "perplexing." The first volume (2008) covered the materia medica of Old World plants, or at least European plants, used in traditional Western herbalism. The present volume (2009) covers the herbs of the New World, especially North America. *The Earthwise Herbal* is less comprehensive in its coverage of plants introduced within the last twenty years. The emphasis has been placed upon traditional materials of medicine. As a formulary it is also less complete. No coverage of compounding has been undertaken, and the dosages given are suggestive.

The herbal is laid out in the following manner.

Latin Binomial (Genus and Species). Common Names.

I have sometimes used older Latin binomials when I felt that the original names are important. Botanists rename plants for their own convenience, not for herbalists, horticulturists, or pharmacists. I do not feel we need to follow botanists slavishly, but I also have tried to indicate the modern name, if it differs from the Latin binomial I have used.

Natural History, Plant Family, Historical and General Background, Pharmacology

Rather than crowding up the description of plant properties and uses with excess information, I have included a separate section, in italics, to provide the milieu of the plant.

The Essence, Nature, Logic, Properties, and Uses of the Plant

The main body of the text consists of a description of the plant uniting its diverse properties and uses into a whole profile that makes sense, empirically, intuitively, and pharmacologically. The greatest effort has been made to bring out the essential nature, personality, or logic of the plant. When this is understood the disparate traditional uses, modern uses, and physical properties usually form a unit that makes sense. Some case histories and anecdotes have been included to illustrate application and give the text some interest.

The reader has a right to know how many plants the author has actually used in practice, and how many he dares to write about without the basis of personal experience. I have not indicated this anywhere in the text, but most of the long accounts, commonly used herbs, and certainly all those in which I cite myself as a source have been used in my practice. There is another group of plants that I feel I know well because friends have filled me in on their experiences, and I trust and understand their methods. In a work of this magnitude there must be some herbs I have used but little or not at all. However, after more than twenty-five years of clinical experience and continuous study, always searching for the core essence of plants, my understanding of them has developed to such a degree that I write confidently even about plants I have yet to meet. I also have developed an eye for the literature, often quoting sources who clearly did understand their subject, while avoiding others who wrote without experience.

Young herbalists should know that the day will come when they will be able to look through the materia medica and it will simply make sense, because signatures, tastes, and constituents do correctly indicate uses, and the pieces integrate into whole pictures with definite properties.

Taste

The following template has been used: flavor • temperature and humidity • impression. As used here, the word taste includes the flavor, temperature (hot, cold), humidity (damp, dry), and impression made on the nervous system (diffusive, etc.). These properties often give us the best indications for the "energetics" or tissue state favored by the medicine.

I have done the best I could with plant tastes, working from experience. Out of habit and love of herbs, I taste virtually every formula or simple I give out and every plant I stop to seriously look at in the field or garden. On occasion I have quoted from some other author—this is always indicated. Yet, the sense of taste is subjective and I do not hold myself out to be especially keen in this area. I have been corrected in the past, and if the reader knows the taste more perfectly than the author, please correct me.

Tissue States

This follows the template: excitation (irritation, overstimulation), tension (constriction), atrophy, relaxation, stagnation, depression.

Each herb acts on a particular tissue state or combination of states.

Organ Affinities

Originally, this was a separate category, but I have worked organ affinities into the arrangement of specific indications. Thus, there are now headings lumping symptoms under location, organ, system, and sometimes constitution. Strong organ affinities are italicized.

Specific Indications

These are the collection of symptoms and indications that come down to us in the literature or from the personal experience of practicing herbalists. Symptoms that are "poorly developed" (like "diarrhea") are listed, but an effort has been made to collect and develop more detailed symptoms or "specific indications." For instance, sometimes we just have "gastritis." This is not a specific indication, but it is the best we have. With more experience we have more definition: "gastritis; gurgling, nausea, mucus in vomitus," or "gastritis; with liver involvement," and so forth. A fully developed specific indication is so detailed that it leads to the selection of a small number of remedies or even just a single medicine. At this level the specific indication not only contains detail, but it tends to indicate the specific affinities in tissue state and organ that characterize the plant. For instance, "gastritis; gurgling, nausea, mucus in vomitus" indicates an astringent.

Of least value are the names of illnesses: "diabetes." What kind of diabetes? Yet, we must include even these indications, nonspecific as they are, because the account would be incomplete without them.

When an indication is italicized it may be taken to be particularly characteristic and reliable, or often proven by experience.

David Winston, registered herbalist (AHG), makes it a point not to include new indications unless they have been tried out in practice more than twenty times. I set more liberal standards. If a newly discovered usage makes sense, in keeping with the general logic of the plant, and has been verified a half dozen times, it will be included. A few suggestive indications that have not been proved out in practice are included from time to time because they ought to be investigated more fully. The only symptoms taken over from traditional literature that I have thrown out are those where a mistake in the transmission of information is apparent and the symptoms clearly do not belong to the remedy.

Preparation and Dosage

It was not my intention to write a formulary, or workbook giving specific preparation methods, formulations, and standard dosages. I have instead merely handed on a collection of notes on preparation from my own or others' experience that should prove useful and may, in the future, provide material for a formulary. For a good contemporary formulary refer to Richo Cech, *Making Plant Medicine* (2000). I do not feel that it is a good idea to copy the United States Pharmacopeia or National Formulary slavishly. Herbs are like condiments; they can be prepared in subtle, beautiful, and almost countless ways.

The standard of dosages given in this book is highly variable. My favorite source of posology (dosage) is John William Fyfe (1909). This is because he gives advice on dosage like: "1 to 60 drops." I personally use small doses, but I do not advocate small or large dosages for other practitioners. I simply use what works for me. Some herbalists dismiss my work as homeopathic rather than herbal, because they mistakenly think the effect changes with small or large doses. This is only true for poisons, which are harmful in large doses and toxic in small ones. *The Earthwise Herbal* is limited to nontoxic herbs. People who are doctrinaire about posology miss the main point: the healing virtue is in the plant, not the preparation or amount. What works best is the dosage level a practitioner feels comfortable with, rather than a doctrinal position.

Contraindications, Cautions, Toxicity

This section has been included when necessary. The reader may want to consult more conservative texts on the subject. However, these are often written by nonpractitioners and may contain warnings of far-fetched potential reactions. As an example: It is often stated that chamomile can cause severe allergic reactions, and the admonition to be careful has spread to its Asteraceae cousins, such as yarrow. Herbalist Daniel Gagnon, of Santa Fe, counted the number of reports of allergic reaction found in modern literature. Over a period of some twenty years, during which more than sixty million doses of chamomile were consumed daily throughout the world, there were six reported severe allergic reactions. It is, of course, good to know about toxic and allergic reactions, but it is also wise to keep these facts in perspective. A good reference here is Gagnon's *Liquid Herbal Drops in Everyday Use* (2000) because it is written by a practitioner.

Literature

Throughout *The Earthwise Herbal* I have attempted to give credit for original work, quotations, and case histories. In the "monograph," or main body of the text under each herb, credit is indicated by the usual methods: quotation marks, sources, dates, and pages. In the section on "Specific Indications" the sources for symptoms are given at the end of the account of the herb, under "Literature." The numbers following the authors represent the symptoms they contributed to, counting down from the top under "Specific Indications." Dates and page numbers here have been ignored—one will have to turn to the reference section to find the original book or lecture, and then to the index of that book to find the plant and the symptom. Some undated references refer to conversations or class notes that I saved on bits of paper or by memory and could not include in the References section.

Confirmation of an important or unusual symptom is often noted in the text with the symptom number followed by "-confirmed."

Abies balsamea. Balsam Fir.

Balsam fir is indigenous to the Canadian shield and to cold acid soils a little to the south. It has long been used by the northern Indians and is still widely used by them, being a safe, simple first-aid medicine. The Anishinabe name for this tree, according to the late herbalist Keeway dinoquay, translates as "elder sister," meaning someone very helpful.

"Balsam is stimulating and relaxing, chiefly influencing the kidneys and mucous membranes, acting rather slowly," writes William Cook (1869, 203).

PREPARATION AND DOSAGE:

"The balsam contained in the blisters under the bark, is the portion of this tree most commonly employed in medicine" (William Cook, 1869, 203). "It is obtained by puncturing the blisters and pressing out their contents into a spoon or other shallow vessel." This is also the method taught by Keewaydinoquay, who commented that it did not hurt the tree to take sap from the blisters. "Its relaxing power is greater in the fresh exudation than in that which has been long standing."

Achillea millefolium. Yarrow.

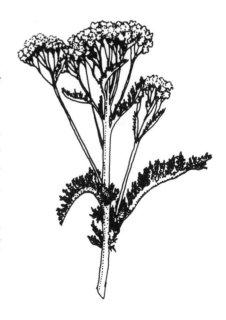

Yarrow (Achillea millefolium var. millefolium) *is a member of the aster family native to Europe and Asia. A clone of this species seems to be native to North America* (Achillea millefolium var. lanulosa). *It can only be differentiated under the microscope. The two are used interchangeably. Yarrow was used throughout the northern hemisphere as a medicinal agent.*

The constituents of Achillea are numerous and complex. The leaves and flowers contain flavonoids, vitamin C, bitters, tannins, alkaloids, sterols, phenolic acids (including salicylates), coumarins, sesquiterpene lactones (including achillein), volatile oils (including the toxic thujone, irritating borneol, stimulating camphor, antiseptic pinenes, etc.), and many other constituents.

Yarrow is one of the primal remedies of the Western herbal tradition. It can be called the "master of the blood." Through numerous devices—clotting, unclotting, neurovascular control, flavonoids, etc.—it regulates the flow of blood to and from the surface, in and out of the capillaries and venules, thickening and thinning. Through this it cures all manner of wounds, bruises, hemorrhaging, and clotting. The same property, combined with its diaphoretic capacity, makes it a "master of fever," moving blood to or from the surface to release or preserve heat and regulate fluids. Although pungent, bitter, and astringent in taste, it also contains high levels of flavonoids, which soothe the capillaries so the blood passes quicker. Thus, it is both cooling and warming, fluid generating and controlling. Remedies with contradictory but complementary properties are often of great utility since they are able to normalize opposing conditions. This is true for yarrow.

Through its action on the blood and vasculature, yarrow is suited to (1) lacerations, bruises, active hemorrhaging, and old, hardened bruises, (2) fevers, or fevers and chills, (3) heat and congestion in the digestive tract, portal vein, liver, and abdominal viscera, and (4) uterine congestion with excessive (or lack of) bleeding. Yarrow can be useful in almost any kind of acute inflammation with congestion of blood. It is specific for hemorrhages with bright, red bleeding and is contraindicated in passive, dark, coagulated flow (cf. shepherd's purse).

In addition to the evidence of heat there are usually signs of stagnant blood. Together, these give rise to characteristic pink/red and blue coloration. Yarrow is almost always indicated by an elongated, pointed, reddish tongue (the classic indication for heat), but with a blue undertone or middle, indicating venous stagnation. The tongue is usually dry in the center, indicating that heat is driving off fluids. There may be a crack down the midline; in severe cases it opens up to reveal a deeper layer of tissue, which is dark and crisscrossed by lines (chained or feathered). This is an indication that heat is burning deep into the tissues, especially of the digestive tract, or that the spine is inflamed. The pulse is usually rapid, full, and nonresistant, showing that heat is having its way with the tissues. The complexion is often reddish with blue veins (tongue and pulse indications from William LeSassier and Matthew Wood).

There are other cases, however, where yarrow is suited to a pale and dry tongue. As a bitter it increases secretion in the digestion tract and, with its ability to decongest the internal organs when blood is collecting in the interior, it brings blood to the surface and improves digestion and assimilation. It can provoke menses by bringing the blood to the surface just as it can curtail them when excessive. Likewise, it can provoke diaphoresis when the skin is in an atonic, weak condition.

In addition to its action as a hemostatic or normalizer of the blood and circulation, yarrow also acts on the skin as a diaphoretic and on the kidneys as a diuretic. Thus, it normalizes the distribution, secretion, and elimination of water in the body. A hot or warm cup of yarrow tea will open the skin, while a cold cup tends to stimulate the stomach, digestion, and kidneys. The influence of yarrow can also be changed and directed according to whether it is used fresh or dry or how long it is decocted or infused, since certain constituents come out at different temperatures and periods of extraction. Not all of these preparation differentials are understood.

TASTE:

bitter, pungent, acrid • diffusive • astringent, aromatic

TISSUE STATES:

excitation, depression, relaxation

SPECIFIC INDICATIONS:

CONSTITUTION, COMPLEXION, CHARACTERISTIC SYMPTOMS

- *Robust, sanguine persons, with red, full-blooded complexion; and sensitive persons, easily hurt.*
- *Complexion of skin red with blue veins showing through on the arms and legs; bruises are red and blue.*
- *Tongue elongated, pointed, red, blue in the center;* dry toward the center, not heavily coated, wet toward the edges.
- Tongue cracked down the middle and opening up to reveal criss-crossed, red tissues ("chaining" or "feathering"—looks like a feather or a yarrow leaf); this indicates "heat attacking the blood level."

- Tongue; purple line anywhere.

MIND, SENSES, NERVES, EMOTIONS, PERSONALITY
- The "wounded warrior, wounded healer" remedy; "people that jump in, put out the fires, get cut to the bone, emotionally and physically"; sensitive, delicate persons, easily hurt (Barbara St. Dennis).

HEAD
- Congestion of blood to the head; headache, vertigo, nosebleed, high blood pressure; in red, robust, sanguine persons, or during fever.
- *Nosebleed.*
- Earache, toothache, gingivitis.

RESPIRATION
- Stuffed sinuses (vapor, warm tea, tincture).
- Bronchitis, pleurisy, pneumonia; inflammation and pain in the chest; bleeding from the lungs with night sweats.
- Palliative in the bleeding and night sweats of tuberculosis (cold infusion).

DIGESTION
- Lack of appetite, bloating, digestive cramps, colic.
- Dyspepsia, colitis, diverticulitis, bleeding hemorrhoids; tongue red and cracked down the middle; with rapid, full, nonresistant pulse.
- Diarrhea in infants.
- Bleeding from the stomach or intestines.
- *Bleeding hemorrhoids (cf. Bidens, Rumex crispus).*

LIVER
- Liver inflammation, acute hepatitis (external, warm compress, once a day).

FEMALE
- *Lack of menstrual flow, difficult to start (drink 1 cup/day or 2 warm cups before); or heavy, hemorrhagic flow, hard to stop, excessive bleeding.*

- *Clumsy feeling just before the onset of the period.*
- Menstrual cramping.
- Endometriosis (cf. *Trillium*).
- *Uterine fibroids; with bright red hemorrhage* (cf. *Capsella,* fibroids, clotted, dark flow) (bath).
- Inflammation of the ovaries.
- Vaginal discharge.
- Uterine prolapse.
- Menopause: restlessness; night sweats.
- Pregnancy: morning sickness, restlessness, heat (but caution during pregnancy).
- Parturition: clumsiness twelve hours before delivery due to hormonal changes loosening the tendons; to prevent excessive bleeding and pain.
- Parturition: pain after delivery, suppression of the lochia.
- Lactation: sore nipples.

KIDNEYS AND BLADDER
- Nephritis; acute inflammation and bleeding from the kidneys.
- Acute cystitis; with or without bleeding; with mucoid discharges; scanty urine, also incontinence; *irritative conditions of the urinary apparatus, strangury, and suppression of urine* (infusion).

MUSCULAR AND SKELETAL
- Arthritis, gout, rheumatism.

CIRCULATION AND BLOOD
- Varicose veins (bath).
- High blood pressure where there is blood congestion.

FEVER
- In acute fever, pulse rapid, full, nonresistant.
- Fever; sudden onset, in robust persons, with or without chills.
- Fever; chicken pox, measles; brings out rash.
- Acute fever, early stages; skin cool, pulse weak, brings circulation to the surface and brings out the rash (hot infusion).

WOUNDS
- *Lacerations;* injuries to the arteries, of violent origin; hemor-

rhage, of bright red arterial blood; tenderness and oversensitivity in wounds.

- *Bruises* of violent origin; with cuts (cf. *Arnica*, bruises without cuts or bleeding); blood blisters.
- Old bruises that have become hard; especially on the head.
- Stroke, head injury, hematoma (external).
- Cerebral thrombosis.
- Psoriasis (bath).
- Pale, thin skin with poor circulation to the periphery and closed pores (infusion of the flower/herb).
- Bee sting (external).
- Wrinkles (external).

OTHER
- Fistulae.
- Reported antidote to radiation (cf. *Larrea*).
- Environmental allergies; cools heat and reduces sensitivity.

PREPARATION AND DOSAGE:

"The whole plant is used fresh gathered, but the best part is the tops," comments the eminent John Hill (1740, 392). The flower tops are harvested at their peak and dried for use as a tea or tinctured fresh in alcohol. The young leaves and roots may also be used. The situation, soil, and exposure to the sun change the properties somewhat. Infusion: 1 teaspoon to a cup of boiling water, cover to preserve oils, steep for 13 minutes (Harald Tietze, 1996, 47). Letting it stand longer can change the properties (Eva Graf). Dosage: 1–3x/day in chronic conditions; hourly in fevers. Tincture: 5–20 drops is a usual dose (Fyfe), 15–30 drops (Gagnon), 20–40 drops (Hoffmann). I use yarrow in 1–3 drops, 1–3x/day. A cup of the hot tea works better for pale skin with blood stuck in the interior.

CAUTIONS:

Allergies to yarrow are possible. It should not be taken in large doses during pregnancy, but it is sometimes appropriate in small doses at that time.

LITERATURE:

Traditional (8, 12, 14, 16, 22, 24, 25, 26, 36–42), Linnaeus (7), Maria Treben (19, 21, 23, 27, 35), Barbara St. Dennis (1, 6), William LeSassier (3–5), Matthew Wood (1, 2–5, 7, 20, 28, 33, 35, 43, 44), E. B. Nash (12), Jack Ritchason (15), Nicholas Culpeper (17), Richard Hool (17), Otto Wolff (18), Flower Essence Society (1, 6, 51), Christopher Menzies-Trull (44–46), Margi Flint (47), Julia Graves (13), Wendy Fogg (29), Robert Dale Rogers (9, 10, 22, 24, 25, 30, 31, 32, 48, 49), David Hoffmann, John Christopher (7, 13, 14, 17, 19, 31, 32, 33, 34, 50), John William Fyfe (11, 17, 19, 25, 30, 32, 33). An extensive account of yarrow is given in my earlier work, *The Book of Herbal Wisdom*.

Acorus calamus. Sweet Flag, Bitter Root.

Calamus is considered native to Eastern Asia, Siberia, India, and North America. It is one of the most highly esteemed medicines in the world. Those happy wanderers, the Mongols, brought it to eastern Europe in the Middle Ages. It was imported to England by John Gerard before 1595. Although it is prized in Old World cultures, I include it in the North American section of The Earthwise Herbal; *it is still widely esteemed by Indian people throughout North America.*

Calamus is widely known in traditional American Indian medicine as "muskrat root," named for the creature that builds his house among the reeds, cattails, and calamus stands. It probably was brought to North America from Siberia by Indian people. I asked herbalist Michael Moore about this and he relayed an interesting fact. The "native" American species is a single clone identical to one among dozens of Siberian clones. The fat rhizome of the American specimen, which is excellent for medicine, is incapable of sexual reproduction, so it seems to have been specially chosen as a medicine and spread across the continent by human activity. Today, however, there are also colonies of other strains imported from Europe by horticulturalists.

The rhizome is used; it contains a bitter volatile oil, terpenes (including sweet-scented eugenol), amines, tannins, resin, mucilage, gum, starch, acorin, and asarone. There is a great deal of pharmacological variation among wild populations and plant parts.

The Sanskrit name for calamus is *vacha*, related to the English "voice," meaning invocation, or the power of the voice. It acts prominently on the trachea (which the rhizome strongly resembles) to restore the voice and is used in American Indian culture as a remedy for singers. In China the allied species *Acorus gramineus* is used to reestablish the "bright yang of consciousness" (Bensky and Gamble), removing fine phlegmatous material from the cerebrum, increasing thinking ability and comprehension. The voice, in Greek and East Indian philosophy, is associated with intelligence and consciousness.

The rhizome of calamus is aromatic ("sweet flag"), bitter ("bitter root"), warm, and drying or astringent. This makes it useful as (1) a carminative to reduce gas and bloating and increase digestion, secretion, and neuromuscular strength in the GI, (2) a warming, drying joint remedy, (3) an anticatarrhal, warming and drying to the lungs, and (4) a mind and voice restorer. I have known cases where it appeared to be palliative in Alzheimer's. It is a smooth muscle relaxant used in constrictive or atonic conditions of the gastrointestinal tract and uterus. Also, (5) "the juice of the fresh root of acorus is excellent to promote the menses" (Hill, 1740, 177).

R. Swinburne Clymer (1973, 139) called *Acorus* "the water–brash (watery eruction) remedy. When every known remedy has failed to stop the eruction of the awful burning water from the stomach into the throat, a small piece of calamus slowly chewed and juice swallowed, nearly always will bring prompt relief."

A woman in her fifties fell down a mountainside and sustained a head injury. She was extremely debilitated, to the point where she would get lost for hours two blocks from home. We tried peony root without success, then calamus. She said the effect was immediate, profound, and highly beneficial. Each time she took the tincture (rhizome cold extracted in water and preserved with brandy), the plant seemed to say to her, "Concentrate." It taught her a new and different way of thinking and rescued her from an almost helpless state.

TASTE:

bitter, pungent, acrid • warm, dry • aromatic, astringent, resinous

TISSUE STATES:

depression, stagnation, constriction

SPECIFIC INDICATIONS:

MIND, SENSES, NERVES, EMOTIONS, PERSONALITY
- *Lack of comprehension, mental and verbal obtuseness, inability to grasp words.*
- Nervousness.

HEAD
- Headache.
- Head injury (cf. *Paeonia, Betonica*).
- Senility.

RESPIRATION
- Rhinitis, with reduced thinking, catarrh in head, loss of voice.
- Congested sinuses.
- *Laryngitis; hoarse voice; worse from overuse, singing in atmosphere with tobacco smoke.*
- *Tracheitis.*
- Bronchitis, asthma, chronic catarrh.

HEART
- Angina.

DIGESTION
- Bad breath, lack of saliva, lack of appetite.
- *Gastrointestinal indigestion, gas, bloating.*
- "Purely atonic dyspepsia"; gastritis, gastric ulcer, nausea.
- Colicky pains (mix with mallow, *Malva*) (Neil).
- Constipation.
- Typhoid.

MUSCULAR AND SKELETAL
- Joints cold, achy.

SKIN
- Burns, scalds, ulcers (external).

FEVER
- Chills and fever; influenza, malaria, epidemic disease.

OTHER
- Tobacco addiction (can cause aversion).

PREPARATION AND DOSAGE:

Cherokee author J. T. Garrett (2003) relates an elder emphasizing that it is important to know how to gather and prepare this plant. Herbalist Jim McDonald, of Michigan, has noted on his website many of the different properties based on variations in picking and preparation. The action of the rhizome differs somewhat from that of the rootlets. The properties also differ depending on whether it is found in water, submerged deeply, or growing in mud, or exposed to the sun, producing green on the rhizome. Almost all sources agree that the rhizome is traditionally extracted cold at room temperature by infusion overnight, about 1 ounce to 1 pint; 3 teacups a day. Tincture (cold infusion preserved in alcohol), 1–60 drops.

CAUTIONS:

Certain genotypes (not the original American clone) contain carcinogens, and calamus has been banned for internal use in the United States. European genotypes have now spread in North America, making the wild population unsafe. However, calamus is widely used in Europe and Asia as a carminative. It is often combined with gentian, orange peel, angelica, and other such agents.

LITERATURE:

Traditional (1–3, 5–13, 16–21), Lise Wolff (5), Matthew Wood (4), William Cook (14), James Neil (15), R. Swinburne Clymer (13, 14), Jim McDonald.

Aletris farinosa. True Unicorn Root.

Aletris is a member of the lily family native to central North America, similar in appearance and properties to its cousin Helonias (false unicorn root). Both were used as female remedies by the North American Indians and adopted into pioneer medicine. For a long time they were confused, but eventually independent indications for Aletris were determined (Fyfe, 1909, 357). Both are endangered, though cultivation of Helonias is now

*under way. In an effort to save the dwindling population of Aletris, prac-
titioners should limit themselves to small doses, in cases where the symptoms are well marked and the prescription is reliable and exact; to the
low homeopathic potencies; or to the use of plant populations for which
they take personal responsibility. Aletris is not generally available today
in commerce. It was used in homeopathy on the same indications as in
botanical medicine. It contains volatile oils, saponins, and resin.*

True unicorn root is one of the great female medicines of American Indian
provenance, widely adopted and used in the nineteenth century by lay
and professional doctors. "It is employed by many country practitioners, physicians, and Indian Doctors, and highly valued by them as well
as the Indians" (Rafinesque, 1828, 1:40). It is an important remedy in
infertility, exhaustion, and weakness, with well-developed, specific indications. It is a bitter suited to dry, anemic, malnourished cases, probably
increasing hormonal function along with appetite and weight gain. Dr.
John Christopher (1996) warns that *Aletris* should not be given if pregnancy is not desired.

William Boericke (1927) writes that *Aletris* is indicated in "an anemic,
relaxed condition, especially of the female organism. The patient is tired
all the time, and suffers from prolapsus, leucorrhea, rectal distress, etc.,"
with "marked anemia." Much the same indications are given by Fyfe
(1909).

TISSUE STATES:

relaxation, atrophy

SPECIFIC INDICATIONS:

CONSTITUTION, COMPLEXION, CHARACTERISTIC SYMPTOMS
- Thin, dry, atrophic, infertile, premature menopause.

MIND, SENSES, NERVES, EMOTIONS, PERSONALITY
- Mental energy weak; confused feelings; cannot concentrate the
  mind.

HEAD
- Fainting, with vertigo.

DIGESTION
- Much frothy saliva.
- Repugnance for food; least food causes discomfort; nervous dyspepsia; flatulent colic.
- Dyspepsia, colic, and flatulence.
- Paretic condition of the rectum; loads up with feces; stool large, hard, difficult to move, with pain.

KIDNEYS AND BLADDER
- Edema.

FEMALE
- *Too frequent menstruation, with labor-like pain and sense of debility in pelvis; complains of pelvic articulation, or inability to support the body on the feet.*
- Premature and profuse menses, with labor-like pains.
- Chronic uterine weakness; retarded and scanty flow.
- Increases the possibility of conception.
- Uterus seems heavy; prolapse, with pain in the right inguinal region.
- Leucorrhea due to weakness and anemia.
- Habitual miscarriages due to weakness.
- Muscular pains during pregnancy; morning sickness.

MALE
- Impotence and sterility.

MUSCULAR AND SKELETAL
- Chronic rheumatism.

PREPARATION AND DOSAGE:

Native to the Eastern Woodland environment of North America; the rhizomes and rootlets are picked in the spring and dried (the fresh agent is emetic and cathartic). "But small doses only must be used" (Rafinesque, 1828, 1:40). Since it is largely unavailable today, use the low homeopathic potencies (3x, 6x).

CAUTIONS:

Ecologically endangered. Traditionally considered safe during the entire period of pregnancy. It probably supports progesterone. However, Rafinesque (1828, 1:262) records that the Indians considered *Aletris* to be an abortifacient. The difference may depend on the dosage.

LITERATURE:

Traditional, John William Fyfe, William Boericke, John Christopher, Rolla Thomas (9).

Alnus serrulata. Tag Alder.

Tag alder grows in thickets along the edges of swamps and streams in eastern North America. There is a wide range of alder species that may be interchangeable, but this is the one most commonly used by the Indians, pioneers, and botanic physicians of the nineteenth century. At that time it was a central remedy in North American folk medicine, but today is largely forgotten in Western herbalism.

"Probably no indigenous remedy has such an extensive popular reputation as an alterative," wrote Dr. Edwin Hale (1867, 59). "It is resorted to by the country people in nearly all obstinate chronic diseases of the skin or glandular system, and often effects surprising cures after all other remedies used in regular practice have failed." Yet today it is almost unknown.

Tag alder is a bitter and astringent tonic that stimulates digestive secretion, hence assimilation and nutrition. Biloxi herbalist Darrell Martin says that it combines well with wild cherry and blue flag because the former increases digestive secretion, the latter promotes biliary flow, while alder increases uptake or assimilation. Internally, alder clears lymphatic congestion and enlarged glands. Coming out to the surface it enlivens the skin. As an astringent that improves peripheral circulation, alder can stop bleeding. This is an old Cherokee use (Garrett, 2003).

TASTE:

bitter • astringent

TISSUE STATES:

atrophy, relaxation, stagnation

SPECIFIC INDICATIONS:

CONSTITUTION

- Debilitated and elderly people with lack of secretion, digestion, assimilation, nutrition, and waste removal; with skin conditions.

DIGESTION

- Dyspepsia; especially in old persons, with a heavy, sleepy feeling after meals, flatulence, diarrhea alternating with constipation.
- Hemorrhoids (external, with *Cornus florida,* equal parts).

LYMPH/IMMUNE

- Lymphatic stagnation; swelling and suppuration; poor nutrition and waste removal; marasmus.

KIDNEYS AND BLADDER

- Cystitis, gravel.

FEMALE

- Leucorrhea, with erosion of the cervix, which bleeds easily.
- Amenorrhea with burning pains.

MUSCULAR AND SKELETAL

- Arthritis.

SKIN

- Chronic skin diseases; conditions resulting in boils; breakdown of surfaces, resulting in ulcerations of the skin, mouth, and throat; erysipelas; eczematous and pustular skin conditions.

PREPARATION AND DOSAGE:

Being an old folk remedy, methods of preparation are not fixed. "The tags, bark, boughs, or leaves may be taken freely in strong tea" (Horton Howard, 1836, 2:214). The bark is "easily acted on by water" (William Cook, 1869). A decoction or tincture can be made from the fresh or dried bark. The tincture, if it can be obtained, is used in doses of 1–60 drops (John William Fyfe). Dose: 5 drops (Yadubir Sinha). Directions for making a decoction, according to Dr. Ralph Russell (1911), of Birmingham, Alabama: pour 1 pint of boiling water over a handful of fresh roots, set 2 hours, strain, add 1/2 pint whiskey and take a teaspoonful before each meal. "Alnus is slow in its action, and should, therefore, be continued for a considerable length of time" (Fyfe).

LITERATURE:

Traditional, William Cook, Darrell Martin, William Boericke (6–7), John Scudder (3, 9), John William Fyfe (1, 3, 9), Edwin Hale, Eli Jones (1, 2), Yadubir Sinha, J. T. Garrett.

Aloe vera.

The aloes are natives of the Old World, now cultivated and naturalized in the New. Widely used in North America today, I accidentally included it in this volume. The outer skin contains a yellow latex that is highly purgative—from the presence of anthraquinones—while the inner gel is mucilaginous, cooling, and refreshing. Formerly Aloe socotrina *was the officinal species cited in medical textbooks and available in pharmacies as a purgative. Today* Aloe vera *is popularly grown as a houseplant and used as a domestic remedy, more often for the gel. This contains sugars and polysaccharides that are nutritious and immune building.*

Aloe vera is one of the time honored medicinal plants still widely used in modern folk medicine. It provides two completely different medicines: (1) the gel from the interior of the succulent leaf is moist and nutritive, while (2) the yellow bitter latex from the exterior of the leaf is a stimulating purgative. Today the nutritive, moisturizing, soothing, mucilaginous gel is much used in cosmetics and folk medicine for treatment of dried-out skin, bowels, and tissues.

TASTE:

(gel) sweet, salty • cool, moist
(yellow latex) bitter, pungent • stimulating

TISSUE STATES:

(gel) atrophy
(yellow latex) torpor

SPECIFIC INDICATIONS:

(gel)
- Persons who do not drink enough water.
- Premature wrinkling; from heat and dry weather.
- Worse in damp and heat.
- Tinnitus.
- Conjunctivitis.
- Canker sores.
- Asthma.
- Bloating.
- Peptic ulcer; ulcerative colitis; diverticulitis.
- Inflamed colon, dry bowels, stool dried out; constipation, hemorrhoids (the bitter aloe is contraindicated here).
- Anemia.
- Amenorrhea.
- *Skin;* acne, athlete's foot, bedsores, denture sores, fever blisters, wrinkles, bleeding, bruises, inflammation of the skin, ulcers, herpes, burns, sunburn, burns from atomic radiation, abrasions, eczema, psoriasis, shingles, ringworm, scar tissue, chicken pox itch, insect bites and stings (external).
- Sunburn; oversensitive to the sun; bad effects of exposure; burns (spray or mist, keep dressing continuously saturated).
- Bursitis, arthritic inflammation (internal and external).

(yellow bitter rind)
- "Persons of phlegmatic habits, weak stomachs, and sedentary life," but "it is injurious to bilious habits, and the piles, on account of its tendency to inflame the bowels" (Child).
- *Constipation;* full feeling in the upper right side, with discontent.
- Diarrhea from damp heat, monsoon diarrhea (small doses).
- Jaundice, hepatitis, enlarged liver, spleen, inactive gallbladder.
- Intestinal worms; pinworms, tapeworms.

PREPARATION, CONTRAINDICATIONS, AND DOSAGE:

The fresh gel is obtained from the inside leaf of a plant that is more than four years old. Commercial preparations of the gel or juice are easier to work with. The purgative property can be obtained by taking a cross section of the leaf or a commercial preparation of the powder (100–200 mg.). Aloe and most other yellow bitter purgatives containing anthraquinones should only be used in constipation from torpor and depression, not from inflammation or dryness. However, the gel can be used for intestinal dryness. The purgative is also contraindicated in pregnancy.

LITERATURE:

Traditional, homeopathic (17–18), Lydia Child (16), Dorothy Hall (1–2), Julia Graves (3).

Ambrosia artemisiifolia, A. trifida. Ragweed.

Two species of ragweed are native to North America. They have the same properties, for better or worse. They are the most common cause of hay fever in the late summer, not goldenrod, which is often blamed for this condition because it produces a beautiful golden flower during "allergy season." The ragweeds and goldenrods bloom at the same time and are members of the same family (Asteraceae) but the former are wind pollinated while the latter are insect pollinated. Thus, ragweed pollen travels on the wind and is the true source of the allergy, whereas goldenrod pollen travels only with the bees. Not despite this fact, goldenrod is also a good remedy for allergies, but more generally for cat and animal dander than for pollen allergy.

Ragweed pollen causes an allergic reaction by virtue of its size and shape, which lodges in the nasal turbinates and causes irritation. The characteristic symptoms are sneezing, runny nose, bloodshot eyes (goldenrod has a generalized glazed redness of the conjunctiva), swollen capillaries in the eyes, itching of nose and eyes, and in long-term reactions a bronchial congestion. A nip of the leaf, taken at the time of the allergy, will almost always abort such an attack. A homeopathic dilution or the herbal mother tincture in small doses is also useful.

Ragweed leaf has a mildly bitter, pungent, and slightly astringent taste that resembles so many of the Asteraceae and immediately suggests medicine. It is seldom used in medicine, but a good account is rendered by William Cook (1869, 240). "The leaves are stimulating and astringing, bitter, and permanent [not nerve stimulating] in action. An infusion is useful in diarrhea and dysentery of a passive character; in uterine, gastric, and pulmonic hemorrhages; and in degenerate leucorrhea as an injection and drink. It is also a valuable local styptic; and may be applied to bleeding surfaces, as in piles, epistaxis, wounds, etc., either in powder or infusion. A use of a strong decoction influences the kidneys considerably, sustains the tone of the stomach, and slowly elevates the circulation; and these actions render it useful in the treatment of chronic dropsies, especially when combined with hepatics and stimulating diaphoretics." It is also used as a poultice on purulent ulcers.

TASTE:

bitter, pungent

SPECIFIC INDICATIONS:

- Hay fever with congestion at the root of the nose, bloodshot eyes, itching eyes and nose.
- Fevers characterized by a tendency to putrescence.
- Diarrhea and dysentery.
- Hemorrhoids.
- Mucus flux.
- Passive hemorrhage.

PREPARATION AND DOSAGE:

Gather the leaves before the pollen appears, tincture fresh at 1:2 in 95% alcohol, water down to 70%. Give 1 drop initially, since a very few people are sensitive to the leaves. If they are better, give 15–20 drops (herbalist 7Song). Dose: 5–10 drops every 2–3 hours (Fyfe).

CAUTIONS:

The pollen is a sinus irritant.

LITERATURE:

William Cook, John William Fyfe (2–6), William Boericke (1), 7Song.

Anemopsis californica. Yerba Mansa.

Yerba mansa ("herb of the manse" or "household herb") is a member of the aster family native to wet ground in deserts of the Southwest and California. It is an important Spanish and Anglo-American folk medicine. It contains volatile oils and is bitter, astringent, and pungent.

This is an extremely important and effective remedy for head colds when the mucosa are boggy, relaxed, and full, with mucus discharge. "Chronic forms of inflammation of the Schneiderian membrane with considerable relaxation and profuse discharge. Chief value in catarrhal states, with full, stuffy sensation in head and throat. Useful in cuts, bruises, and sprains; and as a diuretic and in malaria." Also "found useful in profuse mucous or serous discharges; in nasal and pharyngeal catarrh, diarrhea, and urethritis. Recommended in heart distunes, as a quieting agent when unduly excited. Flatulence; promotes digestion" (William Boericke, 1927, 52). It kills amoebas and giardia.

Yerba mansa is a stimulating antiseptic similar to elecampane and other members of the aster family. San Francisco herbalist Tony Seiffert used it successfully in a case of suppuration in a badly infected foot. The active infection subsided fairly rapidly.

Ampelopsis quinquefolia.

See *Parthenocissus quinquefolia.*

Aralia nudicaulis. Wild Sarsaparilla.

Wild sarsaparilla is very common in the woodlands of North America, north into the boreal forests. It resembles its cousin, wild American ginseng, in appearance and taste, but not in properties. Like other members of the ginseng family, it has hormonal influences. The root contains sugars, essential oils, and minerals (calcium, phosphorus, potassium, magnesium, copper, zinc, iron, manganese, chloride). It is cooling, moist, and nourishing. The Cree consider wild sarsaparilla to be a rabbit medicine—a nutritive tonic.

Wild sarsaparilla was accurately defined by the old folk tradition, which saw in it an analog of sarsaparilla (*Smilax* spp.). Both of these remedies, though botanically unrelated, are "blood cleansers" used for acne. William LeSassier considered wild sarsaparilla the best remedy for acne in young people and teenagers. It is clear that both kinds of sarsaparilla act on acne by normalizing androgen levels—high levels being a common cause of acne in young people.

Wild sarsaparilla is little used in modern Western herbalism but it ought to be valued more highly. It was officinal in the U.S. Pharmacopoeia from 1820 to 1882. It is not only dependable in the acne of youth but has been suggested as a tonic for older men (Prairie Deva flower essences). Because it is high in minerals, especially calcium and phosphorus, it ought to have a powerful effect on bone growth and healing, which is also stimulated by the androgens. It has been used for arthritic joints and venereal disease—the latter, in the nineteenth century, usually meant diseases of the bones and cartilage. Androgens activate the thyroid receptors and immune tissues, so it may have a regulating effect on the thyroid. (Low thyroid is a common cause of "bad blood," for which both the wild and commercial sarsaparillas are used.) It has been used for diabetes, which often has an imbalanced hormonal background. Arthritis may be due to excessive immune activity in the cartilage of the joints.

In folk medicine wild sarsaparilla has been used to open the kidneys and the skin, soothe the lungs, and expectorate mucus. "Knowledgeable midwives encourage sips of the root infusion to help relax a hard cervix before delivery," writes Canadian herbalist Robert Dale Rogers (2000, 177). The decocted root is used to make a douche for irritation of the vaginal mucosa.

The Cree name for *Aralia nudicaulis* translates as "rabbit root," according to Rogers. This indicates their conception of the therapeutic direction of the medicine. In the Far North, on the Canadian shield where the Cree live, the rabbit is associated with starvation and emaciation. When the snow is high, only the rabbits can get out on top of the snow, so the deer population dies out and the people have to rely on the rabbit. However, the latter does not provide a complete diet because it lacks good-quality oils. Thus, rabbit medicines are used to antidote the ill-effects of emaciation and atrophy. They are largely nutritive and support the bones and muscles. Compare with other rabbit medicines like *Dioscorea, Urtica, Gnaphalium,* and *Celastrus.*

PREPARATION AND DOSAGE:

Decoction: 1 tablespoon of the dried root to 1 pint of boiling water. Cover, steep overnight. Gently warm in the morning. Dose: 4 ounces up to 4x/day (Rogers). Tincture: macerate the fresh roots in a sweet alcohol (brandy). Dose: 5–30 drops, up to 4x/day (Rogers).

LITERATURE:

Traditional, Robert Dale Rogers, William LeSassier.

Aralia racemosa. Spikenard.

Spikenard is a member of the ginseng or Aralia family that is highly respected as a medicine by the Indian people of North America. "All of the Spikenards or Aralias are popular medical plants throughout the United States," wrote Constantine Rafinesque (1828, 1:55). "They make part of the Materia Medica of the native tribes, and are extensively used by country practitioners." It was adopted as an "alterative" or blood purifier by the pioneers and early professional doctors of America, but specific indications are lacking in the old literature. It can be understood as a warm analog of eleuthero—in other words, it is an adaptogen that is warming and oily. It is not related to the biblical spikenard.

Spikenard is pungent, sweet, warm, stimulating, and oily. The oily brown root has a furry tuft where the stem arises from the ground—the signature of a "bear medicine." Cherokee herbalist J. T. Garrett (2003) notes it under the names bearberry bush and Indian root. Bear medicines stimulate the adrenal cortex, either directly through some hormonal connection, or nutritionally by improving metabolism of fats and oils.

David Milgrom, DC, of Flagstaff, Arizona, says spikenard "cleans out clogged ducts." It is especially beneficial for mastitis or clogged milk ducts in the breast. He also notices the influence on the adrenocortical side. It regulates the appetite and reduces blood sugar swings. "It's a good medicine to take before a fast." In other words, it pumps up the cortisone so that the body can pull lipids and proteins out of storage.

When cortisone is down hyperimmunity is up. Spikenard has a very powerful influence on autoimmune sensitivity in the mucosa. It is an excellent remedy for upper respiratory allergies, irritable membranes with sneezing, coughing, and free secretion of clear mucus. These are the few symptoms for which it is valued in homeopathy. It goes deeper and "has long been used with much success in chronic pulmonary diseases" (Fyfe, 1909). The cough reflexes are exhausted and the mucus is thick and heavy. It thins the mucus and strengthens the cough reflexes. "In asthmatic breathing and in the early stage of bronchitis it is a useful remedy. In chronic catarrh, some forms of rheumatism, and enlargement of glands, its action is also satisfactory."

Adirondack herbalist Kate Gilday has used spikenard in female problems. It warms and stimulates the uterus, breaking up stagnant blood and promoting a healthy menstruation. "It is especially beneficial for women who are somewhat weak and fearful. They tend to assume a fetal position, as if in self protection. The pulse is usually weak and low." A somewhat similar account was given by J. I. Lighthall and W. O. Davis (1882). They wrote that "spikenard is a tonic to a weak, debilitated condition of the nervous system, where the patient is easily startled and has night sweats and a nervous cough."

Lighthall and Davis's comment is the only specific information I could find in nineteenth-century literature. However, here is an interesting old formula in which spikenard plays the major role, showing its usefulness as a stimulant in sepsis. When "debility of the system has been the predisposing cause" for sepsis, "Dr. Ferris has recommended a poultice in cases of mortification, which has been very successful. It is composed of scraped carrots and bruised spikenard, which are boiled together till they are soft, in a small quantity of water, with Indian [corn] or oat meal [added], and applied warm" (Taylor, 1860, 232). Although carrots have long been used for poultices, clearly the spikenard is the major ingredient here.

TASTE:

pungent • warm • stimulating, diffusive

TISSUE STATE:

depression

SPECIFIC INDICATIONS:

CONSTITUTION, COMPLEXION, CHARACTERISTIC SYMPTOMS

- *Enfeebled state of the nervous system, anemia, general debility.*
- Thin, weak, dry.
- Enlarged glands.

MIND, SENSES, NERVES, EMOTIONS, PERSONALITY

- *Fatigue, weakness, timidity, fear of stressful situations.*
- *Easily startled;* hunches over in self-protection.

THROAT

- Chronic laryngitis with excessive, abundant mucus.
- Chronic pharyngitis with thick, tenacious mucus.

RESPIRATION

- *Itching of the mucosa of the upper respiratory tract, eyes, ears, nose.*
- *Hay fever, colds.*
- Itching of the lungs, with irritable coughing; palliative in tuberculosis.
- *Chronic catarrh and cough;* stringy, tough mucus.
- Dry, wheezing, irritative cough, with difficult inspiration; weak lungs.
- Respiratory problems in persons with weak voice and lungs.
- *Cough at night, on lying down.*

DIGESTION

- Blood sugar swings.
- Lack of appetite.

KIDNEYS AND BLADDER

- Accumulation of uric acid in the system.
- Irritation of the bladder, with scanty urine; mucus in the urine, no odor.

FEMALE

- Menstrual problems in weak, timid women; cramping, vaginitis, leucorrhea.
- Menstruation: suppression of menses from weakness and cold.
- Menstruation: dysmenorrhea.
- Acrid leucorrhea with offensive odor.

- Postpartum: suppression of the lochia, with pain in the uterine region.
- Mastitis; stimulates the ducts (American Indian usage).

EXTREMITIES
- Rheumatism.

GENERAL
- Tongue dry, narrow, and red.
- Pulse weak and low.

FEVER
- Night sweats, weakness, hectic fever.

PREPARATION AND DOSAGE:

Fluid extract, tincture, 5–40 drops (Fyfe).

CAUTIONS:

Not recommended during pregnancy. Environmental concerns.

LITERATURE:

Traditional, William Cook, John Scudder (8, 10, 11, 25), J. I. Lighthall (5), John William Fyfe (3, 10, 12, 17–23, 26), William Boericke (8, 9, 14), David Milgrom (16, 24), Kate Gilday (5, 18, 26, 27), Corey Pines (13), Matthew Becker (24), Michael Moore (6, 7, 11, 18).

Arctostaphylos uva-ursi. Bearberry, Kinnikinnick, Uva Ursi.

Bearberry has a circumpolar distribution and is used in the herbal traditions of Europe, Asia, and North America as a urinary antiseptic. It is highly esteemed in Indian medicine, as the name "bearberry" indicates. The name "kinnikinnick" demonstrates that it is an Indian smoking herb. Uva ursi contains arbutin and methylarbutin (which turn into antiseptics in the presence of water), tannins (15–20%), flavonoids, volatile oils, iridoids, and resin. It is a typical antiseptic astringent of the heath family.

As a fragrant astringent and antiseptic uva ursi acts principally upon relaxed mucosa to give better tone and restrain excessive discharges from bacterial infection. It is useful in swollen mucous membranes as far up as the throat and as far down as the intestine, bladder, and uterus. An American Indian name for the uvula is "bearberry," so the plant is credited with a relationship to the throat (Yagho Tahnahgah).

Uva ursi is especially famous for bladder infections with green, phlegmy discharges. These symptoms were more common in the old days, when gonorrhea was difficult to treat. It is used today for bladder infection and yeast infection. Contemporary herbalists consider it best indicated when there is highly acid urine. I do not use it much, as one does not see mucoid discharges like in the old days.

"In cases of dysury [painful urination] from a variety of causes, I have given the decoction of this plant with very satisfactory success," writes Dr. Jacob Bigelow (1817–20, 72), of Boston. "In Dr. Mitchell's experiments on the pulse with this medicine, it appears that the pulsations were sometimes, not always, slightly increased after taking it, but that in every case they soon sank below the normal standard and remained so for some time."

TASTE:

slightly pungent • astringent

TISSUE STATES:

relaxation, depression

SPECIFIC INDICATIONS:

- Relaxation of mucous membranes with chronic mucus discharges; sometimes ulcerative, mixed with blood.
- Sore gums, canker sores.
- Bronchitis; discharge from the lungs.
- Supposed to strengthen the heart muscle.
- Indigestion; nausea, phlegm in the stomach; slow emptying of the stomach and sluggish discharge of pancreatic enzymes and bile; chronic diarrhea and dysentery; an ulcerated condition of the bowels.

- Diabetes mellitus with profuse urination and weak digestion (cf. *Vaccinium*).
- Kidney and bladder problems where the urine is acid; mucus discharges, relaxed mucosa of the bladder; aching and congestion.
- Ulceration of the bladder with prostate involvement, involuntary seminal emissions, incontinence of urine.
- Chronic urethritis.
- Incontinence; loss of control over the bladder.
- Passive menstrual bleeding.
- Gonorrheal discharges, lingering, in females, due to poor tone of mucosa.
- Leucorrhea, especially when connected with a flaccid condition of the womb and vagina; uterine prolapse; ulceration, discharge.
- Parturition; when the parts are moist and flaccid, expulsive power weak, labor pains trifling.
- Postpartum; resolves tendency to flooding, increases tissue tone (cf. *Capsella*) and discourages infection.
- Arthritis, lower back pain.
- Fever: hectic.
- Rapid pulse.

PREPARATION AND DOSAGE:

The dried leaves are the part used in commerce. As a urinary antiseptic it is often given by infusion, 1–2 teaspoonfuls per cup of boiling water. It is also used as a tincture or extract.

CAUTIONS:

Can turn the urine green—not a dangerous symptom. Tannins can cause constipation. Contraindicated during pregnancy according to some authors. Large doses can be toxic, causing liver impairment in young children.

LITERATURE:

Traditional, William Cook, Finley Ellingwood, Jacob Bigelow (17, 18).

Arum triphyllum. Jack-in-the-Pulpit.

This common woodland plant has a tuber that is intensely irritating when fresh, but was prepared for consumption by the Indian people. It is hardly used in herbal medicine, but Constantine Rafinesque (1828, 1:68) provides us with the early traditions and uses. "It has been found beneficial in lingering atrophy, debilitated habit, great prostration in typhoid fevers, deep seated rheumatic pains, or pains in the breast, chronic catarrh, &c.," flatulence, stomach cramps, and asthma. It "quickens circulation."

Asarum canadense. Wild Ginger, Canada Snake Root.

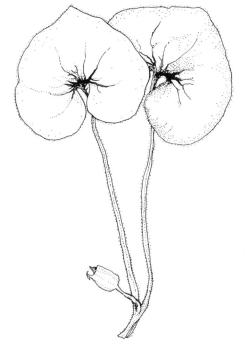

Wild ginger is a member of the Aristolochia family native to woodlands in eastern North America. The rhizome is an old Indian remedy adopted and used by the pioneers and their doctors; it is still well known to the northern Indians. The little heads coming up in the spring in a group look like a den of snakes, hence the name "snake root."

Wild ginger is similar to cultivated ginger; both are warm, pungent, and sweet, but wild ginger is somewhat more acrid and less mucilaginous. It possesses many of the same uses, warming the stomach, relaxing tense, cold muscles and spasmodic uterus, and expelling phlegm. Both can be used as a warm tea. Constantine Rafinesque (1828, 1:72) gives an early and valuable description of its properties. "It is useful in cachexia, melancholy, palpitations, low fevers, convalescence, obstructions, hooping cough, &c." These indications resemble those he gives for *Aristolochia serpentaria,* a more active cousin, and may be derived from those uses by analogy. The latter plant has not been included in *The Earthwise Herbal* because of its potency and toxicity.

William Cook (1869), much experienced with the native flora of the United States, describes the general properties and contraindications of *Asarum*. This aromatic is "stimulating and relaxing, rather prompt in diffusiveness, and somewhat tonic." In other words, it is suited to cold and constriction, and is somewhat nutritive and moistening. "Its influence is expended largely through the circulation and nerves, both of which it arouses and sustains. Through these channels it warms and invigorates the surface, and secures a favorable perspiration in languid constitutions; but this soon subsides, and is followed by an increased warmth of the skin and a little dryness. These facts make it objectionable to use in all cases where the skin is already dry and hot; and it should not be used indiscriminately as a diaphoretic. It is best for recent colds and such functional suppressions as follow colds." It is used in mouthwash; stimulates gums.

Asarum is well suited to back spasms in long-standing back problems—that is, spasms associated with cold (Lise Wolff, registered herbalist, AHG).

TASTE:

pungent, acrid, slightly sweet • aromatic • mucilaginous

TISSUE STATES:

depression, constriction

SPECIFIC INDICATIONS:

RESPIRATION

- Acute nasal catarrh; where the discharge has not appeared, or has been suppressed, with headache and general oppression, muscular aching and general discomfort.
- Conjunctivitis, from taking cold, with profuse and constant lacrimation.
- Recent colds; suppression of colds, followed by amenorrhea and gastroenteritis.
- Pneumonia; with considerable exhaustion.
- Painful or long-standing spasmodic coughs; whooping cough, bronchitis, sometimes concomitant with nausea and diarrhea.

HEART
- Heart palpitations; angina.

DIGESTION
- Stomach tense, better from warm drinks and food.
- Intestinal spasm, colic, flatulent colic, cholera.

FEMALE
- Uterus congested, spasmodic, weak expulsive power (cf. *Angelica sinensis*).
- Early menstruation in young girls.
- Metrorrhagia and menorrhagia; hemorrhages of a passive character with sluggish uterus, cold surface; flow steady but not free; with cutting pains in the abdomen and groin, extending down the thighs, with aching in the back, the patient nervous and irritable.
- Menstruation: amenorrhea following a chill.
- Menstruation: premenstrual backache; cramping with cutting pain in the lower abdomen, groin, and thighs; violent back pain, interferes with the breathing.
- Pregnancy, early part: melancholy and nervous disturbance, miscarriage threatened.
- Parturition: pain and weak expulsive power (cf. ginger, *Zingiberis*).
- Postpartum: depression.

MUSCULAR AND SKELETAL
- *An incredible specific for back spasm, especially chronic lower back trouble.*

FEVER
- Scarlet fever, smallpox, typhoid fever.
- Snake bite with low, tedious fever and exhaustion (cf. *Aristolochia serpentaria*).

PREPARATION AND DOSAGE:

Tincture: 1–3 drops, 1–3x/day. Externally, as a spray (Lise Wolff). "Many times added in small portions to tonic-expectorant and tonic-emmenagogue preparations" (Cook, 1869). One of the original ingredients in Thomson's Composition Powder.

CONTRAINDICATIONS:

Asarum is toxic in large doses and has been banned for internal consumption by the FDA. It was considered to be a reliable abortifacient (Finley Ellingwood). Considered to be contraindicated in active inflammatory states with excitement; sensitive stomach, bowels, uterus, warm, dry skin (William Cook). It is a common woodland wildflower but should not be overpicked.

LITERATURE:

Traditional, Finley Ellingwood (1, 2, 4, 8, 11, 12, 13, 14), Lise Wolff (16), William Cook (3–5, 7, 9–13, 15, 17), Matthew Wood (7, 16-confirmed), William Boericke (3).

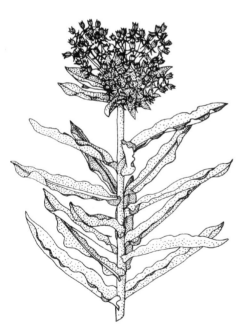

Asclepias tuberosa. Pleurisy Root, Butterfly Weed.

Pleurisy root is a cousin of milkweed native to North America. It was known to Native Americans. "While it is unknown how it was used," relates Cherokee author J. T. Garrett, an elder said "it was known in earlier days as wind root for its ability to carry a message to the Great One." It is an "East Medicine" because the flower is bright orange red and it acts on the heart. Pleurisy root was used by the earliest colonial root doctors of whom we have record. It was popular in the nineteenth century as a moistening diaphoretic. It was widely appreciated in the days when a reliable diaphoretic was an essential for the treatment of acute fever. Although it was one of the most important agents in the nineteenth-century materia medica of professional and lay medicine, pleurisy root is less often called for or used at the present time. It contains flavonoids, sugars, steroids, and cardiac glycosides.

Asclepias was almost universally classified in nineteenth-century literature as a sedative or relaxing diaphoretic that opens the pores of the pleura
and the skin to decongest water and heat. It was considered the prime
example of a "relaxant" by Alvah Curtis, William Cook, and Joseph
Thurston. Diaphoretics relax the autonomic nervous system, which is
responsible for regulating the pores of the skin. However, the taste of
pleurisy root indicates that it does not relax and open the pores according to the normal pathways. Because it is mildly bitter and sweet I would
guess that it also generates fluids at the same time that it relaxes the surface. I asked William LeSassier about this before he died, and he was of
the same opinion as myself: the mild relaxant effect is intensified by the
fluid generating side.

Michael Moore (2003, 202) also has an interesting take on this plant.
"Pleurisy root, as a gestalt, tends to stimulate skin and mucosal circulation, sebaceous secretions, and sweat; therefore it can be used with great
success in tonic formulas for both dry skin and hair, frequent nighttime
urination, and generally poor adaptability to changes in heat and humidity." He goes on to explain that pleurisy root shifts the balance of fluids
in the body away from the kidneys, toward the lungs and skin, and is
therefore beneficial for the sympathetic excess type, who often has dry
skin and compromised respiratory function with excessive urination.

Asclepias moistens internal membranes, brings moisture to the surface, opens pores, and decongests internal fluids that have become stuck
or stagnant. When the skin is hot and dry, *Asclepias* produces a mild perspiration that feels cooling and relaxing. In other instances stuck fluids
in the interior cause a continuous flux of moisture to the surface, with
profuse sweating, or diarrhea. In these cases pleurisy root reduces internal oppression and fullness, relaxes and sedates, drying the too active
skin or mucosa. The cough becomes fuller, easier, and more successful as
the oppression abates. Pleurisy root is indicated by a full, stuffy, oppressed
feeling in the chest and a full pulse oppressed, as it were, by some obstacle in the way of the bloodstream.

"In any disease in which we may have a hot skin, either dry or with
a tendency to moisture, a flushed face, a full, or even bounding pulse,
with sharp pain that may be worse upon movement, *Asclepias* becomes
an efficient remedy. It can be used alone or in combination with other
indicated remedies. These symptoms frequently present in the early state
of catarrhal affections generally, in pneumonia, in pleurisy, in pleurody-
nia [pleuritic pain]—in short, in chest affections particularly. *Asclepias*

may be given with great reliance in pneumonia in the early stages, and especially in children. It may be given alone or in combination, or in alternation with other indicated remedies. It will act under these conditions as a synergist to any other indicated remedy. It is par excellence the child's remedy in chest affections. It deserves as much praise in the delayed appearance of exanthematous diseases, like rubella, measles, etc. *Asclepias* is also a remedy in bronchitis and consumption. It will lessen the cough, and free the secretions, and act as a sedative. In coughs generally, that are tight and dry and constricted, if the direct cause cannot be located, *Asclepias* should have due consideration as a possible remedy.

"In rheumatism, especially of the costal variety [affecting the ribs], and in neuralgia with suppressed secretions and symptoms as above, *Asclepias* is the remedy. The same may be said of it in asthma with dryness, difficult breathing and a sense of constriction.

"Besides in these chest troubles, *Asclepias* is an excellent remedy in digestive disturbances. With the symptoms above named predominating, it is very efficient in dyspepsia; in headache due to gastric troubles; in diarrhea, from cold, catarrhal, especially in children; in dysentery; enteritis, etc. It has received the highest praise as a remedy in the distressing flatulent colic of babies. It has also been highly recommended in cases of "nervous irritability" of children presenting the above symptoms. For many cases of syphilis [dryness of fluids] and of scrofula [swollen glands], for gout, *Asclepias* should have a fair trial. The same may be said of it in certain forms of dropsy, and in some skin diseases when the skin is dry and scaly" (Bloyer, quoted by Fyfe, 1909, 396).

Here is a case history from Dr. J. V. Cerney (1976, 72). A man gets cold chills after sitting in a duck blind on a "wet miserable fall day." Afterward "he had stabbing pains in his left lung. It became worse when he tried to breathe deeply or when he coughed. His fever went up to 103°F. His face was pale. He had a perplexed or anxious look about him and when I walked into the examining room he was lying on the side that hurt him most." The pain shot down into the belly. The condition was aggravated by hiccoughs. Dr. Cerney recommended pleurisy root, at which the patient laughed. However, a prescription drug had already failed. For a "few cents" his pain and fever were cured in twenty-four hours.

I have a note from a student (name lost) giving a case history where pleurisy root helped the irritable cough caused by radiation therapy (cf. *Althaea*).

TASTE:

slightly sweet, slightly bitter, slightly salty and earthen

TISSUE STATES:

atrophy, constriction, excitation

SPECIFIC INDICATIONS:

CONSTITUTION, COMPLEXION, CHARACTERISTIC SYMPTOMS

- Conditions where the skin is dry, full, hot, or with profuse perspiration; pulse full, oppressed, or bounding; fever with closed, oppressed skin.

MIND, SENSES, NERVES, EMOTIONS, PERSONALITY

- Nervous irritability of children with dry skin; full, hot, or profuse sweat.

HEAD

- Headache due to gastric troubles.

RESPIRATION

- "Snuffles, or acute nasal catarrh of infants; flatulent colic in young children."
- *Dry skin; full, stuffy feeling in the chest.*
- *Cough, dry in the upper lungs, wet in the lower lungs.*
- Early state of catarrhal affections generally, pneumonia, pleurisy, pleuritic pain.
- *Pneumonia in the early stages,* especially in children.
- The child's remedy in chest affections par excellence.
- Bronchitis and consumption, lessens the cough, frees secretions.
- *Coughs that are tight, dry, and constricted.*
- *Chronic pleuritic stitches following old cases of bronchitis and pneumonia; sharp, stitching pains in the chest; pain in the chest from coughing.*
- *Pneumonia with water in the bottom of the lungs.*
- Asthma with oppressed breathing and pulse, dryness, difficult breathing and a sense of constriction.

- "In the convalescing stages of pneumonia, bronchitis, influenza, and in phthisis when the cough is dry and expectoration difficult."
- Whooping cough.
- Weak, debilitated, asthenic stages of croup.

CARDIOVASCULAR
- Oppression of the chest and heart area; pulse strong, oppressed, tense.

DIGESTION
- Digestive disturbances, dyspepsia.
- Diarrhea, from cold, catarrhal, especially in children; in dysentery, enteritis, etc.
- Flatulent colic of babies.

KIDNEYS AND BLADDER
- Dropsy.

MUSCULAR AND SKELETAL
- *Acute bursitis and arthritis* with redness, swelling, tenderness, pain, and lack of perspiration.
- Rheumatism, especially of the ribs, neuralgia with suppressed secretions and symptoms.
- Old cases of bursitis and arthritis with *adhesions in the joints* that crackle on movement (will sometimes lubricate the joint instantaneously).
- *Frozen shoulder;* with atrophy, weakness, crackling, and limitation of movement.

SKIN
- *Dry skin; inflamed, full, hot; also profuse sweat.*
- *Hot skin, either dry or with a tendency to moisture,* a flushed face, a full or even bounding pulse, with sharp pain, worse upon movement, in fevers.
- Delayed appearance of exanthematous diseases, like rubella, measles, etc.
- Skin diseases when the skin is dry and scaly.

PREPARATION AND DOSAGE:

Decoction: infuse a small handful of roots 20 minutes and drink while hot (Ralph Russell). Tincture or fluid extract. Acute pleurisy, 10–20 drops every 15–20 minutes until the pain stops (Dorothy Hall). Chronic pleurisy, 3–10 drops, 1–3x/day (Matthew Wood).

CAUTIONS:

Nontoxic, but probably should not be taken by people on digitalis or other cardiac glycosides.

LITERATURE:

Traditional (10–13, 27), William Bloyer (1, 2, 3, 7–9, 14, 19–22, 24, 27–30), Frederick Petersen (28), John William Fyfe (4), Grover Coe (15, 16, 17), John Scudder (23), Matthew Wood (5, 6, 18, 25), Jennifer Tucker (26).

Berberis aquifolium, Mahonia spp.
Oregon Grape Root.

Oregon grape is a member of the barberry clan native to the Rocky Mountains. Consequently, it does not enter into the Western herbal tradition until the late nineteenth century, when that region was colonized. Today it is one of the indispensable articles of herbal materia medica. It was first used as a bitter tonic to promote internal and external secretion in dry and atrophic diseases. Today it is sometimes used (or abused, really) as a "natural antibiotic" because of the presence of germ-killing berberine. This is a materialistic way of viewing a plant by its "active ingredient" rather than by the overall influence of its numerous constituents working together.

Mahonia is a powerful bitter that increases secretion from the gastrointestinal tract, improving digestion, assimilation, and metabolism. It also acts on the liver and gallbladder. Scudder (1870) wrote that *Berberis aquifolium* "rights the wrongs and cleans the Augean stables, sharpens the appetite, gives new tone and new blood to the body, and comes as near to curing consumption as any remedy known to us at the time. It is both a blood maker and a blood cleanser, and as there is no known remedy so virulent to microorganisms of nearly all varieties, as healthy blood serum, berberis becomes, indirectly if not directly, a microbicide." This interesting comment directs us to the fact that the "antibiotic" properties are supported by other actions of the plant. Herbal remedies kill microorganisms, not only through proven antibiotic effects, but by cleansing and changing their environment.

I thought of the "Augean stables" remark when confronted with a forty-two-year-old woman who felt "toxic." She had been through a lot of alternative therapy and felt like it was all working, but the "toxins" were all stuck and she felt bad. The skin was slightly dry, the abdomen bloated, with constipation. *Mahonia* made a huge difference. She felt like she was detoxifying, the stool was "furry" though no longer constipated, and the abdomen was no longer bloated. In three months she felt like a new person. She said, "I can feel my body more now and that I can appreciate it more."

Closer to our era than Scudder, Dr. Christopher (1996) noted that *Mahonia* creates appetite, improving digestion and absorption, heals the lymphatic system, purifies the blood, and stimulates the liver to promote strength and vitality. However, it was Michael Moore (2003) who has really taught the modern herbal audience to appreciate this important plant. He says that it is much like its cousin, *Berberis vulgaris*, but acts on *dry cases*. When the body is dried out it cannot move metabolites. Therefore, as he notes, *Mahonia* is suited to situations where there is both faulty anabolism and catabolism—that is, tissue building and cleansing. Typical symptoms are lack of appetite, constipation, thinness, and dry, scaly, irritated skin. Catabolic waste products can build up in this environment, causing irritation and mucus production. The mucus is typically thick, and tenacious, due to the systemic dryness. Since not a lot of blood is being made, and the liver is generally underactive, there is a tendency to a lack of bile, hence constipation.

By improving metabolism and elimination, *Mahonia* proves to be a very important remedy in the therapeutics of the skin. It is indicated when muscles, joints, and bones are inflamed and sore. This is largely due to poor cleansing and removal of waste from connective tissue.

TASTE:

bitter

TISSUE STATES:

atrophy, stagnation

SPECIFIC INDICATIONS:

CONSTITUTION AND COMPLEXION

- *Poor anabolism, with withering, wasting, dry skin, scalp, or mucosa, constipation from lack of secretion; at the same time a buildup of catabolic waste products with lack of secretion from skin and mucosa.*
- "A general preference for 'yinny' foods [carbs], and adrenaline, food, drug, or lifestyle 'rushes'" (Michael Moore).
- Anemia and malnutrition in children.

MIND, SENSES, NERVES, EMOTIONS, PERSONALITY

- Paranoia, the whole world is hostile (flower essence).

RESPIRATION

- *Allergies.*
- Chronic catarrhal conditions of the upper respiratory tract, nose and throat; thick, gummy, tenacious mucus; with wasting; with soreness in the muscles, cartilage, bones.

DIGESTION

- Incipient or chronic indigestion, loss of appetite, wasting, constipation.
- Catarrh of the mucosa of the gastrointestinal canal.
- Constipation, dry intestine.
- Ulceration of the intestines, Crohn's disease.
- Car sickness, nausea.

LYMPH/IMMUNE
- Lymphatic congestion; chronic swelling and induration of glands, with dry, atrophic condition; mononucleosis.

LIVER AND GALLBLADDER
- Hepatitis, jaundice, cirrhosis.

FEMALE
- Amenorrhea, vaginitis, leucorrhea, uterine weakness.

SKIN
- *Dry, scaly, itching patches;* facial eruptions; psoriasis, eczema, dandruff, acne.
- Waxy, yellow, dry, parchment-like appearance of the skin, similar to what is sometimes seen in the beginning of jaundice or diseases of the spleen, where there is poor assimilation and wasting of flesh.
- *Inability to sweat, especially when active or feverish.*
- Eruptions on the face, at puberty.

MUSCULAR AND SKELETAL
- Arthritis; pain as from a blow, with lameness and stiffness; rheumatoid arthritis.
- Muscular, bone, and periosteal pains, worse at night.

FEVER
- Intermittent chills and fever.

OTHER
- Diabetes.
- Blood sugar lability, sugar cravings.

PREPARATION AND DOSAGE:

The yellow root is used per decoction, tincture, fluid extract, powder, or capsules. Usual dose of fluid extract, 5–30 drops (Fyfe); of the tincture, 30–60 drops (Christopher). "When effective, we like the small dose; when necessary we give the large one with equal delight" (Scudder). I use it in small doses (1–3 drops).

LITERATURE:

Traditional, Michael Moore (1, 2, 5, 15, 17, 23), John Scudder (13, 14), John William Fyfe (6, 7, 8, 13, 15, 16, 19–22), Flower Essence Society (4), Julia Graves (11), William Mitchell.

Bignonia capreolata. Crossvine, Trumpet Flower.

Crossvine is a valuable remedy, but little known outside the South, where it grows over trees and thickets. It was used by the Indians and taken up by the pioneers, who applied it as a rejuvenative to tired work animals. Tommie Bass observed this use in his youth; in later years crossvine was one of his favorite tonics for humans. He often combined it with American ginseng, sarsaparilla, sassafras, and green briar *(Smilax)*. This combination shows his understanding of its properties. He is thinking of it as an "adrenal tonic." His favorite combination was crossvine and pipsissewa, used as a renal rejuvenative.

Crossvine would be what a modern herbalist would call an adaptogen, but unlike American ginseng it works quickly and the effects are felt in three or four days (Darryl Patton, 2004, 119).

TASTE:

sweet

TISSUE STATE:

atrophy

PREPARATION AND DOSAGE:

Dried leaves, 1 cup to a quart of water, boiled on low heat for 10 minutes. Strain and take 1/2–1 cup of tea 2x/day.

CAUTIONS:

None known.

LITERATURE:

Tommie Bass, Darryl Patton.

Cactus grandiflorus, Selenicereus grandiflorus. Night Blooming Cereus.

Cactus was introduced by Dr. Rubini, a homeopath, and later adopted by eclectics and botanical physicians. It still occupies a niche in homeopathy, herbal medicine, and European phytotherapy today. The modern botanical name is Selenicereus grandiflorus. *It contains flavonoids (including the vascular stabilizer rutin), isoquinoline alkaloids, and amines.*

Cactus is particularly called for in cases where there is heart trouble against a background of sympathetic excess, nervous weakness, neurasthenia, or asthenia (Frederick Petersen, 1905; Finley Ellingwood, 1918). The people are often thin, nervous, and exhausted. These are the kinds of people, according to the old authors, in which valvular changes of the heart are most likely to occur, and cactus is suited to such cases.

Ellingwood called cactus "the heart tonic par excellence." John William Fyfe (1909) gives one of the richest accounts in eclectic literature. "The range of usefulness of cactus is extensive, and the more fully one becomes acquainted with its valuable properties the more successful will one become in the treatment of a class of wrongs of life which is numerous. In impaired action of the heart, whether functional or organic, cactus is a most efficient remedy. Of course, it cannot be expected to cure structural diseases of the heart, but in such diseases when the action of the heart is irregular or intermittent, or when there is regurgitation due to valvular insufficiency, it will strengthen the impaired muscle. Cactus will not close dilated openings, or overcome valvular deficiency, but it will do much toward sustaining and bringing about a better action of the permanently diseased heart. In fatty degeneration of the heart, it acts equally well, but in mitral it is said to be contra-indicated.

"In endocarditis, pericarditis and myocarditis much benefit is derived from the use of cactus, and in angina pectoris it may well constitute a part of the treatment. It is an absolutely needed remedy in cardiac weakness and threatened heart failure due to exhaustion from overexertion. In neurasthenia of old age, and in nervous exhaustion, the judicious administration of cactus will produce results pleasing alike to patient and doctor. It also constitutes a medicament well adapted to the treatment of the 'tobacco heart' of cigarette fiends and the inveterate smoker. In these cases the patient will complain of precordial oppression, or the sensation of a band tightly bound about the body or the organ or part affected. With this latter symptom—it matters not where it is located—we have call for cactus which should never be neglected."

Among the modern authors Christopher Menzies-Trull (2003, 825) has a detailed account. He recommends it in cases where the person sighs from air hunger, or where there is a sense of weight on the chest (note the "band-like" sensation mentioned above), oppression of breathing, with feeble heart action, anemia, nervousness, and even panic or apprehension of some danger or death. The pulse is rapid and feeble. In my experience the pulse "tumbles," like water tumbling down rocks without much regularity, but without skipping beats. I do think of it when *vata* or asthenics present with heart trouble; also, it is for "broken-heartedness."

TISSUE STATE:

atrophy

SPECIFIC INDICATIONS:

CONSTITUTION, COMPLEXION, CHARACTERISTIC SYMPTOMS
- *Thin, nervous, neurasthenic* [vata] *persons, with heart palpitations and irregularities.*
- *Band-like sensations around the throat, heart, uterus, and other body parts.*

MIND, SENSES, NERVES, EMOTIONS, PERSONALITY
- Depression with foreboding; panic, apprehension of danger.

HEAD
- Congestive headaches; vertigo, temporal arteries swollen, pulsations felt in the brain and all over.

CARDIOVASCULAR
- Irregular, feeble action of the heart; uneasy sensations, weight, oppression, band-like sensation, in the region of the heart.
- Sensation as if a band were tightly bound around the chest, head, or other part.

- Palpitation, fibrillation, mitral valve irregularities, progressive valvular inefficiency, regurgitation.
- Shortness of breath on slight exertion; sighing, air hunger.
- Cardiac weakness and irregularity accompanied by coldness of extremities, numbness of the left arm.
- Periodic attacks of suffocation, fainting, cold sweats.

FEMALE
- Nervous women afflicted with cerebral congestion, heavy pain and weight in the head, numbness of the arms and legs, inability to lie on the left side, and menstrual troubles, menopausal hot flashes.
- Menses heavy and clotted, too early, too abundant.

OTHER
- Persistent and almost excruciating pain in the deep muscles of the back, over the region of the kidneys.
- Pulse irregular, uneven, "tumbling"; rapid and feeble.
- Electric shock.
- Worse at night.
- Hyperthyroidism, heart palpitations.

PREPARATION AND DOSAGE:

Cactus is usually used in the tincture, 1–10 drops (John William Fyfe), or 10 drops to 1 dram diluted in 4 ounces of water (Rolla Thomas).

CONTRAINDICATIONS:

With cactus, "the action of the heart is always impaired, never increased" (Rolla Thomas).

CAUTIONS:

Generally regarded as safe.

LITERATURE:

Homeopathic provings (2, 4–11, 13, 15, 16), John Scudder (13), John

William Fyfe, Finley Ellingwood (3, 12), Wade Boyle (1, 2), Christopher Menzies-Trull (3, 8), Matthew Wood (1, 14), Julia Graves (16).

Capsicum annuum.
Cayenne Pepper.

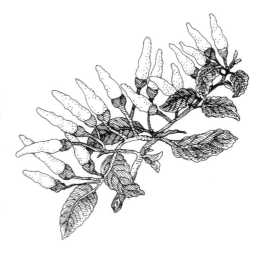

Hot pepper is native to the New World but spread around the world after the voyage of Columbus almost as rapidly as syphilis. It was widely adopted in hot, tropical climates, where its inclusion in the food kills worms and opens the sweat pores. The hottest peppers are grown in West Africa, even though it is a native of Central America. It is used throughout the world as a condiment and medicine. Cayenne contains albumin, pectin, gum, starch, a volatile oil (capsaicin), and minerals (including calcium carbonate, iron sesquioxide, potassium phosphate, alum, and magnesium).

Samuel Thomson introduced red pepper into American herbalism about 1806. Coming down out of the mountains he had on his mind the need for some agent to move the blood. He first saw some peppers tied up on the wall at a coastal house, and one taste told him he had found the remedy. Cayenne pepper came to be looked upon as a "diffusive" (John Thacher) to "equalize the circulation" (Wooster Beach). In other words, the distribution of the blood in the vasculature can become unequal. Due to weaknesses in the system, there could also be disparities between different circuits of the vasculature. For example, overeating might cause an excess blood supply to the digestive organs, smoking to the lungs, drug abuse or drinking to the liver, constipation to the large intestine, or there might be stagnation around the heart itself, or in the surface, the capillaries. When this inequality occurs a burden is placed upon the heart. In treating cardiovascular conditions, one had first to equalize the circulation to remove this burden. An orderly approach to cardiovascular disease, according to Beach, was to first relieve the inequality in the circulation, so that the burden is removed from the heart. After this has been accomplished, it is possible to see the real condition of the heart, and to treat it with heart-specific remedies, if necessary.

The highly stimulating and heating properties of cayenne pepper rouse the circulation, move the blood to the surface, and clear the capillaries of stagnant engorgement. It is therefore used as an assistant remedy to move stagnation in the mucosa, in either sudden checking of secretion from acute disease, often bacterial, or in chronic sequelae. Thus it is frequently used with bayberry and horseradish in head colds, and with black walnut in diarrhea. Derby herbalist George Slack (1919, 106) writes, "The author on one occasion being from home was seized with a severe pain in his stomach and bowels, also with sickness and purging. He had a pint of milk boiled, and a teaspoonful of Cayenne pepper put into it. This was stirred up and drunk in tablespoonful doses every few minutes. In one hour he was in good perspiration and quite free from pain, etc."

The great champion of cayenne in modern times was Dr. Christopher, who called it "one of the great herbs of all time." He used it as a specific for hemorrhaging, high and low blood pressure, heart troubles, heart attacks, varicose veins, and hypoglycemia. "It equalizes the blood stream from the top of the head to the bottom of the feet." By spreading out the blood, he explains, there is less of it in the area of the hemorrhage, which very quickly—"by the time you count to ten"—stops.

A good portrait of the cayenne constitution can be derived from homeopathic literature. *Capsicum* was given a homeopathic proving. It is called for in patients of lax fiber and flabby muscles, who don't exercise and who eat the wrong foods. They have a red face, yet the face feels cold to the touch and is generally chilly. At times they gasp for breath, or can't catch the breath. Worse from slight drafts, cold air, cold water, uncovering, dampness, bathing, drinking, and eating; better from continued motion and exercise. These symptoms describe a patient with poor circulation.

One of the most characteristic symptoms, in my experience, is what I call the "unequal pulse." This can appear in several different ways. The artery is flaccid in some positions, but sharp as a knife blade in others. Sometimes the beat is not synchronized from one arm to the other. Another characteristic symptom is the facial and skin color, which is not just "red," as the homeopathic literature explains, but a reddish-purple—like the hot pepper itself. One quickly gets the picture of stagnation in the capillaries. This is especially evident on the cheeks.

Capsicum also has an application in more precipitous cardiovascular problems. Thomson reasoned that during a heart attack the blood pooled in the interior and congested around the heart, while it was absent in the extremities—which were cold and blue. As a consequence, cayenne was his remedy of choice in the treatment of acute heart attack. The late Dr. Christopher said that cayenne never failed him in more than thirty years of use as a remedy for heart attack. Here the crude substance should be used, rather than the potencies.

TASTE:

pungent • hot • diffusive

TISSUE STATE:

depression

SPECIFIC INDICATIONS:

CONSTITUTION, COMPLEXION, CHARACTERISTIC SYMPTOMS

- Middle-aged persons, poorly exercised, flabby, with reddish-purplish complexion, congestion and stagnation in the capillaries.
- Reddish, dusky hue to meaty tissues; pulse "unequal," sharp and taut under some fingers, languid and relaxed under others, or pulse on one arm not synchronized with pulse on the other arm.

MIND, SENSES, NERVES, EMOTIONS, PERSONALITY

- Nostalgia, homesickness; life was better in the past.

HEAD

- Cluster headaches.
- Fatigue, senility.
- Hangover.
- Shock, profuse sweat, stagnation of blood, red/blue complexion.

RESPIRATION

- As a preventative in the beginning of a cold or fever (combine with horseradish).
- Tonsillitis, sore throat, gum disease (gargle).
- Respiratory catarrh, colds, asthma, pneumonia.

CARDIOVASCULAR AND BLOOD

- Weak peripheral circulation, pooling of blood in the extremities, skin red and dusky blue, but cool to the touch.
- Stress on the heart from pooling of blood in the center and lack of circulation to the periphery and weak, senile heart.
- Acute remedy in heart attack (on tongue or extremities).

DIGESTION

- Lack of appetite, lack of digestive juices and digestion, stomach ulcer.
- Diarrhea from bad water and food (combine with *Juglans nigra*).
- Severe bleeding from viscera.

MUSCULAR AND SKELETAL, EXTREMITIES

- Weak circulation to legs, varicose veins, ulcerated veins, phlebitis.
- Arthritis, paralysis, Parkinson's disease, convulsions.

FEVER

- Fever with weak peripheral circulation, skin cold and inactive, or with collapse, profuse sweating, fever and chills.

WOUNDS

- First aid: sprinkled on viscera when torn open in severe injuries requiring surgery (antiseptic and antihemorrhagic).
- Severe hemorrhage.

PREPARATION AND DOSAGE:

The dried or fresh fruit, soluble in vinegar, 98% alcohol, vodka (folk remedy), or boiling water (Hutchins, 1991, 68). Fluid extract, 1–3 drops; tincture, 15–30 drops (John William Fyfe). "It is best given in cream or milk as it is less irritating to the mucous membranes in this form" (Petersen, 1905, 63). "Remember that it is an agent that is seldom used alone, as by itself the power is soon extinguished." Hence, combine with burdock, ginger, goldenseal, slippery elm, etc. (Alma Hutchins, 1991, 68).

CAUTIONS:

May cause dermic, gastric, or intestinal irritation (Daniel Gagnon). Can be addictive when used as a food long term.

LITERATURE:

Traditional, Samuel Thomson (8–12), Wooster Beach, John Christopher (13, 20, 21), homeopathic literature (1, 3), Matthew Wood (1, 2, 3), Jack Ritchason (4).

Cascara Sagrada.

This small tree, native to the Pacific Northwest and a member of the Rhamnaceae or buckthorn family, was introduced into medicine in the nineteenth century by Dr. J. H. Bundy. It shares the purgative to cathartic properties of the buckthorns and was the laxative of choice for many physicians in the late nineteenth century. It is still officinal in the U.S. Pharmacopoeia.

Cascara sagrada, like its buckthorn cousins, contains purgative anthraquinones. It was introduced into medicine in 1878, by Dr. J. H. Bundy. It is still used today as a moderate purgative, occupying a position somewhere between senna and yellow dock root. Although purgatives are often used in a general sort of way, Bundy's account shows that cascara has a specific application. "It acts upon the sympathetic [i.e., autonomic] nervous system," writes Bundy. "Especially upon the solar plexus, stimulating the nutritive and assimilative forces, increasing the digestive processes generally. It acts upon the secretory system in a marvelous manner, especially where the secretions are deficient and perverted, and this seems to be one of its special indications."

Ellingwood (1918) elaborates on this description. Cascara sagrada is "especially indicated in torpidity or atonicity." It restores functional activity of the intestine and stomach, increasing peristaltic action and secretion. It also acts in catarrhal conditions to rectify excess secretion. Cascara sagrada "is not a cathartic in the common acceptation of the term, but by restoring normal function ... bowel movement of a natural character follows. It does not mechanically liquify and empty the intestinal canal, but it restores normal elasticity and tone to the relaxed structures, and natural vermicular motion and peristaltic action, exercising a direct influence upon muscular structure of the intestinal walls. It materially influences the venous and capillary circulation of the entire intestinal tract, thus proving of much value in hemorrhoids."

Ellingwood explains that smaller doses are preferable to larger ones, because they tonify the intestines to cure the constipative condition, whereas the large dose causes catharsis and weakens the bowel. "If a single dose, so large as to produce a cathartic effect be administered, subsequent small doses will prove insufficient to restore tone, and the constipation will remain unless the large dose is constantly repeated. If a dose of from two to ten drops in a proper vehicle be given, three, four or five times daily for many days, even if the constipation does not at first yield, the effects after a few days are usually salutary. There is a normal movement in the morning and the habit of regular evacuation can be soon fixed." As improvement continues, decrease the dose until it is just a drop at a time. Medium doses are efficient in gastric or intestinal catarrh. "It is a useful remedy in many cases of chronic indigestion and in chronic disease of the liver. It has been used in cirrhosis with the best of results. It is useful in jaundice with deficient excretion of bile, and corrects catarrh of the bile duct. It is useful in diarrhea, subacute or chronic, depending on deficient liver action, and upon catarrhal and atonic conditions of the intestinal tract." The anthraquinone-containing purgatives stimulate the peristalsis of the colon.

By toning intestinal peristalsis, the gallbladder function is improved by *Cascara sagrada*. Hence, it is an old remedy for "biliousness" (Mary Thorne Quelch, 1945, 45).

PREPARATION AND DOSAGE:

Fluid extract or tincture, 1–10 drops per dose, 1–4x/day. Not recommended for pregnancy; causes griping and constipation in large doses. Fluid extract, 1/2 teaspoonful in water night and morning (adult), 5 drops (children) (Ralph M. Russell).

LITERATURE:

Finley Ellingwood.

Caulophyllum thalictroides. Blue Cohosh.

Blue cohosh, a member of the Berberidaceae family, is a native of hardwood forests in eastern North America. Its presence is always an indicator that the woods in which it appears has never been subjected to grazing and has never lost its basic integrity, although it may have been subject to heavy or light logging. Blue cohosh grows in combination with other native wildflowers like bloodroot, wild ginger, and wild sarsaparilla.

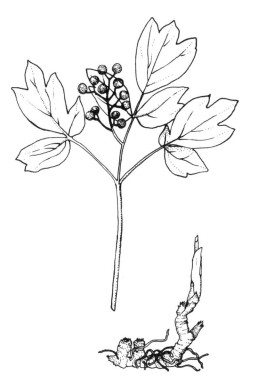

Blue cohosh is an old American Indian female remedy, as the name "cohosh" indicates. It has a threefold leaf shape, which often is found in plants used by the Indians for female problems (see *Trillium* for a discussion of this signature). Samuel Henry (1814) records it under the name "come-pappose."

The nineteenth-century physicians used blue cohosh in small doses as a tonic during the last few weeks of pregnancy. John William Fyfe (1909, 457) writes, "As a measure preparatory to confinement [delivery], this agent, when used for two or three weeks previous to labor, is of much service to the childbearing woman. It so acts upon that part of the nervous system which control the uterus and pelvic region that there is perfect coordination of muscular powers or contractions. Through this kindly action caulophyllum becomes an efficient remedy for atonic or irritable false pains, and relieves or cures many manifestations of uterine irritation."

In modern practice blue cohosh came to be used to initiate labor, when it was delayed. The old use as a tonic, to improve the quality of the labor, has been forgotten. Unfortunately, when blue cohosh is used at the end of pregnancy, in large doses, to initiate partus, the labor is often forceful. The "baby always comes out crying," says Native herbalist Karyn Sanders. Thus, when given in large doses to initiate labor it does not have the tonic effect it would have if given in small doses over time. "If you have to use blue cohosh to induce labor you did not do your job earlier in the pregnancy"—that is, preparing for a healthy labor. Furthermore, because it is a mild heart stimulant, blue cohosh can be damaging to the heart of the baby. It is therefore not used as much for this purpose today.

Here is an old case history showing the interface of American Indian and white herbal medicine in the nineteenth century. "Mrs. V., an Indian woman, the wife of a white man, in labor with her fourth child. Had always had a very quick time. Indian doctors had been with her over twelve hours, and after exhausting their skill I was summoned in haste. Labor was not advancing, though the pains were frequent and strong. Gave caulophyllin [concentrate triturated in sugar] every half hour. Delivery was completed after taking the second powder," but the child was born dead. This was submitted by Dr. S. L. Grow (*Eclectic Medical Journal*, 1864; reprinted by Brinker, 1995). The same doctor gives two more cases. "After taking the third powder, the pains were so much stronger that I anticipated a speedy delivery," which occurred successfully about two hours later. In another case, Mrs. S. had "been unwell for a week or ten days. To use her own words, her hips had given out, and she was obliged to keep her bed. After twelve hours of labor she was fainting and vomiting regularly. As I entered the room she remarked that if I could not soon help her she must die." Two doses of the *Caulophyllum* brought out a "healthy child" and a "rapid convalescence followed." So there were cases in which blue cohosh proved appropriate in parturition.

Finley Ellingwood (1918) was one of the best obstetric writers among the eclectics. He describes the use of blue cohosh as a tonic. "The effect of caulophyllum is to prolong gestation till the fetus is fully developed, labor being a physiological process at full term, and not pathological, therefore less protracted, less painful, and less liable to accidents. . . . It prevents premature delivery by a superior tonicity, which it induces in all the reproductive organs. It has caused many cases to overrun their time a few days, and yet easy labors and excellent recoveries have followed." In exhausted labor, it revives good contractions. As a menstrual remedy blue cohosh is used to remove congestion of the uterus from muscular and vascular constriction and tension. This is often accompanied by malposition of the uterus.

Anishinabe herbalist Keewaydinoquay used blue cohosh to increase or restore fertility in older women. It appears to be a remedy for low estrogen. This conclusion is supported by a side effect noted by herbalist Daniel Gagnon (2000, 58): it can cause spotting in sensitive women at ovulation. Pain and bleeding at ovulation is usually due to high estrogen or intolerance to the hormone.

In homeopathy *Caulophyllum* is used on the same indications as in herbalism. An interesting symptom that was added is: arthritis in the fingers and sometimes the toes, or in the small joints, during pregnancy. I have found this to be a good indicator for blue cohosh in a few nonpregnant women as well. There is pain and stiffness and sometimes swelling in the digits. When the blue cohosh is given, the entire frame relaxes, including muscles and tendons in the hands.

Caulophyllum is an acrid remedy, and thus we should find it to be a relaxing remedy for contracted and tense conditions. Traditional Appalachian herbalist Phyllis Light remarks that blue cohosh really has a more general use as a muscle relaxant, outside of its reputation as a menstrual remedy. She notes that it probably will turn out to have a cardiovascular application.

TASTE:

acrid

TISSUE STATES:

constriction, atrophy

SPECIFIC INDICATIONS:

CONSTITUTION, COMPLEXION, CHARACTERISTIC SYMPTOMS
- General debility in women who are worn out, especially sexually, who complain of pain, heaviness, and weakness in the lower extremities.
- Fullness of the tissues with exhaustion.
- General tension in the tendons and muscles, with arthritis in fingers.
- Women, with low estrogen conditions; delayed menses, cramping, infertility.
- "Uterine pains and tenderness in persons of full but lax habit; rheumatic pains in asthenic plethora" (weak fullness).

MIND, SENSES, NERVES, EMOTIONS, PERSONALITY
- Weariness, depression, hysteria, nervousness, neurasthenia.

RESPIRATION
- Whooping cough.

HEART AND CIRCULATION
- Heart palpitations with weakness, high blood pressure.

KIDNEYS
- Edema.
- Bladder infection.

FEMALE
- Amenorrhea of young women (give at the commencement of the period).
- Painful menstruation, or pain and soreness of the uterus, connected with rheumatism; ovarian irritation, pain in the breasts, accompanied by general irritation and chorea.
- Chronic uterine disorders, in broken-down constitutions; subinvolution of the uterus; uterine pain, with fullness, weight and pain in the legs.
- Insomnia in nervous women, with disturbing bladder troubles, urethritis, and even albuminuria.
- Debilitated conditions where there are spasmodic muscular pains, articular pain, rheumatic pains, impaired muscular power, spasmodic affections of the respiratory tract, bronchitis, asthma, and whooping cough, rheumatism of the small joints of the hands and feet, shifting pains in the limbs, cramp-like pains in the stomach and bowels, worse after eating.
- Sexual debility, with excitability and weakness.
- Spasmodic uterine contractions, dysmenorrhea, irregular menstruation, metritis, endometritis, ovaritis, urethritis, vaginitis, thrush, menopausal pains and discomforts.
- Drawing pains in the joints, shifting and erratic; stiffness in small joints; articular rheumatism; especially during pregnancy.
- Partus preparator: used in small doses to prevent abortion and improve the eventual delivery; especially beneficial in older pregnant women.
- Labor: softens rigid os and uterine spasm, improves contractions, and reduces prolonged labor.
- Severe afterpains, false labor pains, hourglass or spasmodic uterine contractions.

MALE
- Orchitis, with rheumatic symptoms.

MUSCULAR AND SKELETAL
- *Arthritis; especially in the small joints, fingers, toes; with tendino-muscular tension.*
- *Cramps, fits, epilepsy.*

FEVER
- Intermittent fever.

PREPARATION AND DOSAGE:

The root is dried for use by decoction or tinctured fresh in alcohol. Only small doses (1–7 drops) should be used for a gentle, tonic effect.

CAUTIONS:

"May cause mid-cycle spotting and cramping in sensitive women" (Daniel Gagnon). Not used during the first seven months of pregnancy, and only to be used in the last two months with great care. Can stress the baby's heart.

LITERATURE:

Traditional, William Cook (2), John Scudder (1, 15), Matthew Wood (3, 4), Rolla Thomas (5), John William Fyfe, Finley Ellingwood, homeopathic provings and literature, including E. B. Nash (14, 22), Louise Tenney (9–10, 24–25).

Ceanothus americanus. Red Root, New Jersey Tea.

Red root is native to dry, unshaded soil in eastern North America. Numerous species native to the West have been used instead of the single eastern species. It was probably used by Native Americans, but documentation is slim. This is one of the few native American medicinal plants whose place in our herbal materia medica was assured by an English homeopath, J. Compton Burnett. Red root contains tannins, coumarin-like substances, and many other constituents.

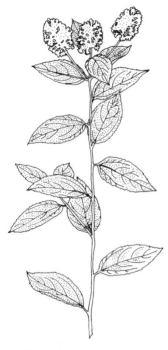

Huron Smith interviewed a Meskwaki medicine man who valued *Ceanothus* highly in intestinal problems because, he explained, the S-shaped root looked like an intestine. It is, indeed, a tonic astringent for failure to thrive due to diarrhea and lack of absorption in the gut. Tommie Bass recorded several such case histories. Furthermore, the S-shaped root is surround by nodules that fix nitrogen; they look like lymphatic glands surrounding the intestine. Shortly after picking they shrivel up and disappear. It is an important remedy for swollen glands and water-filled cysts.

As early as 1835 *Ceanothus* was used by surgeons in Boston to stop internal hemorrhaging during operations. It became popular during the Civil War as a remedy for "ague cake," the swollen spleen associated with malaria and intermittent fever. However, it was an English homeopath, Dr. J. Compton Burnett, who introduced this American herb into medicine as a remedy for swollen spleen in the late nineteenth century. Although he was a homeopath, he used it in drop doses of the tincture—as an herb.

In 1900, Dr. J. C. Fahnestock gave *Ceanothus* a homeopathic proving that verified the enormous swelling of the spleen described by Compton Burnett. "To my surprise the first symptom noticed was a sticking pain in the spleen, and after the continued use of the remedy, there was quite an enlargement of that organ, worse by motion, but at the same time unable to lie on the left side; following this there was pain in the liver, a congestion and enlargement, with sticking pains worse by motion and touch." An East Indian practitioner, Yadubir Sinha (1962), comments, "The more enormously large is the spleen, the more *Ceanothus* is beneficial."

Today in the West we do not as often see swelling of the spleen, since it is usually associated with malaria. However, it sometimes occurs in mononucleosis or glandular fever. I have often used red root for spleen complications. *Ceanothus* (4 parts) and *Berberis vulgaris* (1 part) for swollen spleen (William Mitchell).

"*Ceanothus* is considered to be the spleen remedy," wrote R. Swinburne Clymer (1973, 89), "though it is probably second to *Chionanthus* in general practice." He gives the specific indication: "Whenever there is a tendency during any ailment to despondency and melancholy and a tenderness to the touch of the skin over the region of the spleen, *Ceanothus*" is indicated. The spleen was anciently associated with melancholy. I have verified this symptom many times. Red root is specific for "artistic funk," which is a more modern way to say "melancholy."

Herbalist Michael Moore (2003) deserves credit for reintroducing this herb into modern herbalism and for bringing our understanding to a higher level. He determined that *Ceanothus* improves the electrical charge on cell walls. The outside walls of cells are positively charged, the insides negatively, so in health they repel one another. The better charge on membrane walls helps keep water and blood flowing through vessels, preventing internal hemorrhage and lymphatic congestion. Thus, red root is an important remedy for increasing lymphatic and vascular uptake of fluids and decongesting cysts and congestions of fluid and blood.

I saw a case of congestive heart failure in which there was a continuous discharge of albuminous sputum, like partially congealed egg white. This type of discharge is a classic indicator in this condition. It seemed to me most likely that the discharge was caused by blood proteins seeping out of the vessels around the heart and lungs with the serum they are supposed to be keeping in the vessels. Within three days the discharge was largely stopped, though we also had to contend with other complications from a damaged aorta and vascular spasm. When the symptoms reoccurred eight months later they were promptly checked by red root.

In his proving, Fahnestock noted swelling and coating of the tongue. The characteristic tongue in my experience is enlarged, with a dirty, slick yellow, gray, white coating.

TASTE:

sweet ● astringent

TISSUE STATE:

relaxation

SPECIFIC INDICATIONS:

CONSTITUTION, COMPLEXION, CHARACTERISTIC SYMPTOMS
- Enlarged spleen, sallow skin, and expressionless face.

MIND, SENSES, NERVES, EMOTIONS, PERSONALITY
- Melancholy, artistic funk, unable to think one's way out of a problem.

HEAD
- Thickheaded, oppressive frontal headache after fatty meals.
- Profuse, thin discharge from the sinuses.
- Watery earlobe cysts.

MOUTH AND THROAT
- Acute pharyngitis (gargle).
- *Tongue swollen, dirty coating.*
- Tooth and periosteal abscesses.
- Swollen sore throat; acute tonsillitis.

RESPIRATION
- Bronchorrhea; clear, profuse discharge, with violent shortness of breath.

CARDIOVASCULAR
- Blood, slow coagulation.
- Blood; thick, viscous, red blood cell clumping.
- Pulmonary edema of congestive heart failure (cf. *Taraxacum, Rosmarinus*).

LYMPHATICS
- *Weak, water-logged lymph nodes and tissue* (Michael Moore).
- *Swollen glands, lymphatic stagnation, edema, watery cysts, pelvic congestion, swollen prostate.*
- *Spleen; enlargement and inflammation, subacute, chronic, or secondary to hepatitis or malaria.*
- *Mononucleosis,* with widespread lymphatic involvement.
- *Mononucleosis* (with *Baptisia, Helianthemum*).
- Lymph glands; chronic swelling under jaw, in groin; with chronic debility.

DIGESTION
- Loss of appetite, loss of flesh, general weakness, pain and weakness in the umbilical region, anemia, pallor.
- Diarrhea, weakness, unable to assimilate food; especially in children.

LIVER
- Sluggish portal circulation, inactive liver.

KIDNEYS
- Pain in the liver or back, from congestion or fluid retention.

FEMALE
- Mastitis, acute (internally with *Gossypium* and externally with *Phytolacca*).
- Fibrocystic breast disease, water-filled cysts.
- Edema, diarrhea, bearing down pains in the abdomen and rectum, constant urging to urinate, profuse menstruation, extravasation of blood, and leucorrhea; worse in damp, cold weather.
- Watery ovarian cysts; swollen cervical lymph nodes in some instances.

MALE
- *Swollen prostate*; constant urging to urinate.
- Hydrocele.

OTHER
- High blood pressure.
- Swelling from injuries; from histamine overreaction.
- "Doughy, sallow skin, expressionless face, pain in region of the liver or spleen" (Petersen, 1905, 65).

PREPARATION AND DOSAGE:

This remedy is commonly used in material doses. Michael Moore recommends the cold infusion of the root and the tincture of the fresh or dried root. Dosage of the cold infusion: 1 ounce steeped overnight in a quart of water, 2–4 ounces per dose. Dosage of the tincture: 30–90 drops, up to 4x/day. I use small doses, 1–3 drops, 1–3x/day.

CAUTIONS:

J. Compton Burnett found that material doses can cause aggravations. I have seen this myself. For instance, I gave a patient *Ceanothus* tincture, 3 drops, 3x/day. The next day he complained that his tongue was massively swollen and the taste buds were visibly swollen and elevated. I ran into another person who had the same reaction from red root given by another practitioner.

LITERATURE:

Traditional, Rolla Thomas (1), Howie Brounstein (5, 8, 16, 25), James Compton Burnett (16), R. Swinburne Clymer (2), J. C. Fahnestock homeopathic provings (7), Matthew Wood (2, 4, 7, 9, 10, 13), John MacIntosh, informant to anthropologist Huron Smith (12), Michael Moore (3, 6, 11, 12, 14, 15, 16, 17, 18, 19, 24, 25, 29), Tommie Bass (20, 21, 28), William Boericke (10, 15), Daniel Gagnon (23, 26, 30), Frederick Petersen (1, 22, 32).

Celastrus scandens. Bittersweet Vine, False Bittersweet.

Celastrus scandens *(bittersweet vine, false bittersweet) should not be confused with* Solanum dulcamara *(bittersweet, woody nightshade), a toxic nightshade native to Europe and widely naturalized in North America. This confusion is often seen in nineteenth-century medical literature.*

Bittersweet vine was greatly valued by the Indians as an emergency food and was adopted by the early explorers. The French explorer Radisson, caught on the Mackenzie River without provisions in the winter, survived with his men on *Celastrus* bark. It grows in thickets along the margins of woods and roads. It was considered wise to place a winter village near such a thicket.

Like many emergency foods bittersweet vine is associated with the rabbit in northern Indian medicine stories. This is the only animal available in a hard winter, since it can walk on deep snow that kills the deer. However, it does not provide a complete diet, like venison, and the brain needs to be stewed with the rest of the meat to prevent neurological complications (Clara NiiSka). The southern Indians will not eat rabbit, since they do not want to adopt its traits. On the Seminole reservation, where I spent the first two years of my life, it was considered bad luck for a woman to see a rabbit before conception—she might have twins.

There is an old story that Nanabozho, the Trickster (who is a rabbit in the Great Lakes region), was walking across the ice on a lake in northern Minnesota when he noticed something clunking around on the ice behind him. Oops! His intestines had fallen out and were already frozen. He grabbed a piece and threw it to the shore, where it snagged on a tree branch. He said, "This will be a medicine for my relatives." That's why it is called *Nanabozho onagic*, intestine of Nanabozho.

The early frontier root doctors picked up the use of bittersweet vine from the Indian people. Dr. William Cook (1869) devotes three pages to a discussion of the properties. However, it eventually dropped out of popularity and is little known today.

Celastrus acts on the small intestine to improve absorption and nutrition. It is indicated in wasting or withering, but also in congestion and edema due to weakness of the lymphatic vessels surrounding the intestines and the kidneys. It is even beneficial in diabetes insipidus and bedwetting, not as an astringent, but by nourishing the parts to retain fluids. Cook used it in combination with agrimony for enuresis in delicate, nervous children. "It is very good, combined with mild tonics, for young women about the age of puberty, when they get blue bands under their eyes, with general paleness, precarious appetite, nervousness, feebleness, and vaginal weakness," he writes.

Bittersweet vine was also used for swollen, indurated glands, "caked breasts," mastitis, and "breast cancer" (diagnosis uncertain). It definitely has an influence on the endocrine system, the adrenocortical situation, and sex hormones. It probably has an effect on the hypothalamus.

TASTE:

sweet, bitter

TISSUE STATE:

atrophy

SPECIFIC INDICATIONS:

CONSTITUTION, COMPLEXION, CHARACTERISTIC SYMPTOMS
- Thin, withered, dry, but with swollen glands and lymphatic disease.
- Dry, thin, delicate persons with poor nutrition, low anabolism, adrenocortical deficiency, nervousness and debility; easily exhausted by fluid loss from the sexual-urinary tract.
- Girls in puberty; blue bands under the eyes, general pallor; precarious appetite, nervousness, feebleness, adrenocortical deficiency, vaginal prolapse.

MIND, SENSES, NERVES, EMOTIONS, PERSONALITY
- Psychologically, it helps people with weak boundaries, who get wrapped up in other people's problems.

LYMPHATICS
- Swollen, indurated breasts, mastitis; lymphatic enlargements in scrofulous constitutions.

KIDNEYS
- Diabetes insipidus; loss of fluids from the sexual-urinary tract; debility, nervousness, dryness, thirst.

FEVER
- Fever; hot, dry inflammatory conditions with nervousness, weakness, loss of fluids.

SKIN AND EXTERNAL
- Dry, chafed, inflamed, irritated skin.
- External application on swollen, indurated glands; inflamed and threatened abscess of breasts in nursing women; hemorrhoids; light burns, sores, chafed skin, irritable surfaces.

PREPARATION AND DOSAGE:

Decoction of the root bark (preferable) or branch bark is made by boiling 2 ounces in a quart of water. Tincture, dosage 1–3 drops per dose.

CAUTIONS:

Nauseous and emetic in large doses. Fruit toxic. Do not confuse with the other bittersweet.

LITERATURE:

Traditional (1, 2), Jonas Richel, Constantine Rafinesque, Beal P. Downing, William Cook (3), Leonard Thresher, Matthew Wood (1, 4).

Chimaphila umbellata. Pipsissewa.

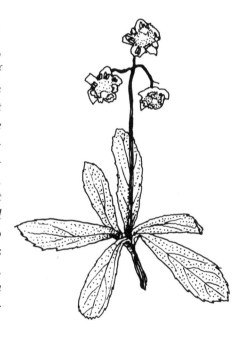

This is a small evergreen plant native to boreal forests in the northern parts of Europe, Asia, and North America. (This is called a circumpolar distribution.) It is a member of the heath or Ericaceae family, the source of so many renal antiseptics (uva ursi, cranberry, trailing arbutus, etc.). Chimaphila *contains tannins, like many members of this clan, but unlike many of them it is a powerful stimulant. It is even irritant enough to raise blisters on the skin. It contains quinones (hydroquinone or arbutin), napthaquinones (chimaphilin), gum resins, flavonoids (quercetin), triterpenes, methyl salicylate, and tannins.*

Pipsissewa is an old Indian remedy, as the name indicates, adopted at an early date by white settlers as a remedy for scrofula (lymphatic stagnation and inflammation). It was used in the Revolutionary War as a tonic in typhus fever (Eberle, 1834, 2:369), where a stimulant would often be desirable. It is especially adapted to chronic, lingering affections that give rise to mucus or mucopurulent discharges (John William Fyfe, 1909). About 1810 its efficiency in scrofula was documented by James Craig, Governor-General of the Canadas, leading to its adoption by allopaths as a specific for scrofula. They liked the fact that it raised a blister—hence was a "counter-irritant" and had a rational explanation for use. Thomson

(1825, 1:140, 2:76) used "pipsisway" for "cancers" (diagnosis uncertain), "all scrofulous humours," and called it "rheumatic weed." The eclectics, in their search for specifics, were attracted to *Chimaphila*. Dr. Edwin Hale introduced it into homeopathy on empirical grounds and it subsequently received a homeopathic proving that justified its traditional uses. Thus, *Chimaphila* is indicated in homeopathy for the same sorts of conditions for which it is remedial in herbal literature. Today it is little used in Western herbalism.

Pipsissewa is a great "eliminator of *kapha*," if I may coin a phrase. It warms and activates the lymphatics and kidneys, the carriers and dispersers of water in the body. It is indicated when the tongue is swollen and coated white in the middle. This might be an indication of "spleen yang deficiency" in traditional Chinese medicine, a category similar to "scrofula" in old-time Western medicine. There is usually congestion and stagnation of fluids, compromised lymphatic and renal function, with thickened, catarrhal fluids and buildup of waste products. It warms and dissolves these congealed fluids and moves the wastes. Thus it is useful in cold, swollen, sluggish conditions and patients. In addition, it contains tannins that astringe the tissues and return them to good tone. It is indicated in the sluggishness, water retention, and weight gain of middle age.

Dr. R. Swinburne Clymer termed pipsissewa "the dropsy remedy." In domestic medicine it is the standby "in diseases of the kidneys, especially dropsy." Dr. Hale wrote, "It is chiefly in chronic rheumatism that its curative powers have been most observed" and notes that it is called "rheumatism root" in folk medicine. I use *Chimaphila* when arthritic pain is better from the use of diuretics to remove water pressure from the joints, or when arthritis accompanies edema. There can be pitting on the leg from the edema.

TASTE:

bitter • hot • astringent

TISSUE STATES:

relaxation, torpor, depression

SPECIFIC INDICATIONS:

LYMPHATICS AND GLANDS
- Middle-aged person with weight gain and water retention.
- Tongue swollen and coated white in the middle.
- Lymphatic and renal stagnation; swollen, indurated glands, with dirtiness of the internal fluids shown in discharges of heavy, viscid, catarrhal substances; *arthritis worse from buildup of internal dampness; worse in cold and damp.*
- Enlarged glands in the neck associated with skin diseases.
- Swollen parotids (cf. *Trifolium pratense*).
- Loss of appetite, wasting and debility.
- Enlargement of glands, breasts, prostate.
- Breasts; congested, indurated, wasting, tumors.
- Breast cancer; "in women with quite large breasts with considerable of the gland affected by the cancer, yet not ulcerated, chimaphila is the needed remedy. Dose, tincture chimaphila twenty drops three times a day" (Eli Jones).
- Swollen mesenteric glands in the abdomen.
- Inflammation of the liver with abdominal and renal edema; enlargement of the mesenteric glands; obstinate constipation and hemorrhoids.

KIDNEYS AND BLADDER
- Prostate swollen and inflamed; prostatic discharge.
- Chronic bladder and renal affections; mucopurulent discharges; smarting pain and frequent urination; sensation of swelling in the perineum (prostate) and bladder.
- Urine thick, ropy, bloody sediment; itching and smarting pain in the urethra and bladder, strangury.
- Bladder infections where the urine is scanty, containing offensive and nonoffensive pus, mucus, or pus and blood mixed.
- Urine scalding or burning, in chronic urethral and prostatic irritations, chronic relaxation of the bladder, and chronic prostatitis with catarrh of the bladder.
- Renal and bladder problems, especially when the urine is scanty and loaded with a mucopurulent sediment.

- Dribbling of urine or incontinence of urine in any form.
- Chronic diseases characterized by discharge of mucus, pus, or blood from the bladder.
- Edema, with debility, loss of appetite, swollen glands; after scarlatina and measles.

FEMALE
- Leucorrhea.
- Swelling and inflammation in the labia of the vagina.

EXTREMITIES
- *Arthritis; swollen and painful joints* (fomentations applied externally until perspiration sets in; internal preparations as well); pitting edema.

FEVER
- Hectic fever, with night sweats.

PREPARATION AND DOSAGE:

The leaves are the part used in medicine. They are prepared by decoction, rather than infusion, as is usual with leaves. Boil a tablespoonful of the leaves in a cup of water. Dose of the tincture, 2–15 drops in water, 3–4x/day (R. Swinburne Clymer).

CAUTIONS:

Because it is a powerful stimulant it is contraindicated in acute inflammatory conditions (cf. *Juniperus*). The fresh plant can burn the skin and mucosa. Environmental concerns.

LITERATURE:

Traditional, John William Fyfe, Finley Ellingwood, Eli Jones, R. Swinburne Clymer, Matthew Wood (1, 2).

Chionanthus virginica. Fringe Tree.

This beautiful tree is native to the southern United States. Southern folk doctors used the bark of the root to purge bile from the liver and gall ducts, and to cleanse the urinary tract and the lymphatics. These usages probably come over from the Indians. The bitter taste and the doctrine of signatures—the inside of the root bark is yellow—suggest the liver/gallbladder use. Physiomedical and eclectic doctors adopted the use of Chionanthus *as a specific for jaundice, and it has long been used to dissolve and expel gallstones. It is the great remedy for expelling gallstones. It works so well it's "like God himself came down and recommended it," said Mississippi herbalist Darrell Martin. It was William LeSassier's favorite remedy for gallstone colic. Fringe tree contains bitters and saponins.*

In the nineteenth century, *Chionanthus* was considered nearly a specific for jaundice not dependent on serious organic disease. "It has been much used as a remedy among the Negroes in agues, and lingering intermittents," writes Dr. William Cook (1869). "Its merits probably depending upon its tonic and slow hepatic properties, rather than upon any antiperiodic action." (Remember that the older Western doctors saw a relationship between periodic or intermittent chills and fever and the hepatic system.) It is associated with "periodic sick headache"—that is, migraines associated with periodic or relapsing chills.

The eclectics learned to use fringe tree with diabetes mellitus. "Dr. Fearn claimed to have early made the discovery of the use of *Chionanthus* in reducing the quantity of sugar in the urine. Patients with no appetite, losing flesh, listless, increasingly anemic with a little sugar in the urine were those to whom he first gave it, ten drops four times a day. Later he used it in severe cases of diabetes mellitus" (Ellingwood, 1918). Other doctors confirmed these observations.

The use of fringe tree as a digestive and nutritive tonic is mentioned by Appalachian herbalist Tommie Bass. He noted that it was fed to horses and mules to make their coats shine when he was a boy. He used it to increase the appetite, digestion, and nutrition. Herbalist Phyllis Light, of Arab, Alabama, has long used it on the traditional indications carried down in her area and family—scrofula (lymphatic congestion) and torpor of the urinary tract. "It is especially used where there is no active inflammation of the bladder but the urine is cloudy."

Overdoses show that *Chionanthus* produces the same symptoms it cures, hence it entered into the homeopathic pharmacopoeia as a remedy for jaundice with pancreatic complications. However, these "provings" or poisonings did not produce a well-developed profile and most of the indications for its use remain empirical.

TASTE:

bitter

TISSUE STATES:

atrophy, depression, stagnation

SPECIFIC INDICATIONS:

- *Dirty, sallow skin, expressionless eyes, lusterless hair, associated with hepatic tenderness, light grayish stool, constipation, and scanty urine.*
- Headache in association with digestive congestion; irregular or periodical.
- Migraine following a conflict with people, weather changes, or digestive upsets.
- Yellowish or greenish discoloration of the eyes.
- Gastric and duodenal troubles dependent upon deficient action of the liver; defective appetite, acute dyspepsia, chronic gastritis, chronic duodenitis, chronic intestinal inflammation; irritation of stomach and bowels associated with chronic dietary indiscretions (Felter).
- Acute congestion of the liver, with imperfect discharge of bile or catarrh of the common bile duct; indicated by acute jaundice, yellowness of the conjunctiva first, subsequently of the skin, with distress in the right hypochondrium and cramp-like pains in the abdomen (Ellingwood).
- Hepatic engorgement and portal congestion; with jaundice, pain over the region of the gallbladder, stomach, or abdomen; nausea; occasional vomiting; constipation with dry feces; temperature slightly above normal; skin usually yellow (Ellingwood).
- Liver pain from slight uneasiness; feeling of weight, fullness, and soreness; becoming an intense pain; radiating from the gallbladder to the umbilicus, from the umbilicus to the abdomen; attended with nausea, vomiting, and prostration.

- Hypertrophic liver due to obstruction of the bile ducts; of a malarial origin; swollen spleen. Acute catarrhal jaundice of children and the jaundice of the newborn.
- Swollen spleen associated with hepatic problems (cf. *Ceanothus*).
- Pancreatic problems, diabetes mellitus, associated with hepatic problems; sugar in the urine.
- Urinary tract problems; cloudy urine without inflammation.
- Intermittent bilious fevers.
- External: wounds tending to heat, congestion, infection, and suppuration of pus.
- Skin resembling copper in color, but shading a little more on green.

PREPARATION AND DOSAGE:

The dried bark of the root is used to make a decoction or alcoholic extract. Dose of the tincture, 1–60 drops, usual dose 5–10 drops (John William Fyfe). In toxic doses Chionanthus produces a slow pulse and a yellowish-greenish tongue, fullness in the hepatic region, nausea, and the sort of full, dull frontal headache commonly associated with hepatic and digestive disturbances. These are general symptoms pointing to a torpid, congested liver. In large doses it is a cathartic cholagogue that stimulates the release of bile, but drains and exhausts the chylopoetic structures. In smaller doses (up to 20 drops of the tincture), it stimulates and builds up exhausted hepatic functions, removing mucus, thickened bile, and inflammatory swelling in the gallbladder and bile ducts.

Chionanthus, Chelidonium, Taraxacum (equal parts) for congested liver or gallbladder (William Mitchell, 2003, 14).

CAUTIONS:

Too bitter for large doses to be taken; generally regarded as safe.

LITERATURE:

Traditional, William Cook, John Scudder, John William Fyfe (14), Finley Ellingwood, Harvey Felter, Julia Graves (3), R. Swinburne Clymer (10), William Boericke (11), Phyllis Light (12), William Mitchell.

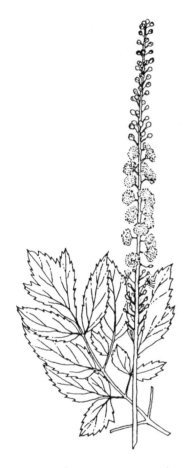

Cimicifuga racemosa.
Black Cohosh.

Black cohosh is a member of the butter-cup family native to rich forest floors in eastern North America. "It is an article of the materia medica of the Indians, much used by them in rheumatism, and also in facilitating parturition, whence its name of Squaw Root" (Rafinesque, 1828, 1:85). The word "cohosh" seems to indicate a female remedy in some Algonquin language. It was also used for snake bite and called "black snake root." The roots are black and interwoven, like a den of snakes, and the ripened stalk looks like a snake (or spine).

Black cohosh or black snake root is one of the great American Indian female remedies of the Eastern Woodland region, learned from them by the pioneers and their doctors. Modern research shows that it is "estrogenic," contains phytoestrogens, and is suited to estrogen deficiency conditions (dryness, amenorrhea, premature aging, menopause). However, black cohosh goes far beyond this superficial designation. It is a remedy that both generates fluids and unbinds them, so that there is better flow of fluids in the organism, especially the all-important cerebrospinal fluids surrounding the nerves. Hence it is indicated in nervousness, spasm, convulsions, menstrual cramps, back pain, and spinal injury. A peculiarity of black cohosh, or a specific symptom really, is *better from onset of menstrual flow.* Consequently, black cohosh women are worse from the cessation of menses at menopause. This tends to bring on fibromyalgic pains (rheumatism), more than hot flashes, for which black cohosh is somewhat overused (cf. *Salvia, Verbena*).

Black cohosh has a deep psychological vein; in fact, this remedy is suited to deeply psychological, brooding persons who are quite psychic and aware of psychological and sexual energy. They have often suffered from an abusive, possessive, manipulative relationship or business dealings. They become brooding, withdrawn, and melancholic, especially before the onset of the flow, which gives relief. The black cohosh woman (more often than a man) is sometimes dark and mysterious, whereas her cousin, the pulsatilla woman, is more often emotionally labile.

TASTE:

(fresh root) sweet, slightly acrid

TISSUE STATES:

atrophy, constriction

SPECIFIC INDICATIONS:

CONSTITUTION, COMPLEXION, CHARACTERISTIC SYMPTOMS
- *Magnetic women, brooding, pensive, with possessive, manipulative partners; businesspeople involved with money, manipulative business partners; after the end of strong sexual or financial relationships, depression, brooding.*

MIND, SENSES, NERVES, EMOTIONS, PERSONALITY
- *Depression like a black cloud; brooding, introspective, worse before the period.*
- "Children and adults who need to stand up to bullying and abuse; makes them sit up straight and take a stance."

HEAD, NECK, AND SPINE
- *Bunching-up of the cerebrospinal fluids, with muscular cramp, spasm, spinal pains, menstrual problems, depression, and brooding.*
- *Whiplash, congestion of the cerebrospinal fluid, tightness of the attachments of the trapezius muscles to the scapula; with brooding, dark state of mind, chronic pain and depression.*

RESPIRATION
- Bronchitis chronic, pneumonia, asthma, *stuffy feeling in the chest.*
- Whooping cough in children (5 drops in sweetened water).

CARDIOVASCULAR
- Angina, with back problems.

LIVER AND GALLBLADDER
- Liver and gallbladder problems; cramping and spasm in the gall ducts, retarded secretion of bile, biliousness, upset digestion, diarrhea, gallstone colic; diabetes.

KIDNEYS AND BLADDER
- Edema.

FEMALE
- *Premenstrual syndrome; brooding, introversion; cramping, pain; aggravation of back and muscular pains; better immediately with the onset of the period and the decongestion of fluids.*
- *"Rheumatic pains, uterine pain with tenderness; false pains, irregular pains; rheumatism of the uterus; dysmenorrhea"* (Rolla Thomas).
- *Menopause; drying, withering, premature cessation of menses, amenorrhea, rheumatism, achiness,* hot flashes.
- *Parturition; ripens the uterus, descends the cervix, prevents cramping.* Used in small doses in the last month; contraindicated in early pregnancy as an emmenagogue.

MUSCULAR AND SKELETAL
- *Rheumatism of the "belly of the muscle"; the underside of the upper arm, the thigh, or such structures as "hang" from the bones.*
- *Rheumatic symptoms worse after menopause, when the relief caused by menstruation ceases.*
- *Rheumatism; "when the pulse is open, the pain paroxysmal, the skin not dry and constricted"* (Rolla Thomas).

FEVER
- *Fever; chicken pox, skin rashes and nervous complications during fever; spinal meningitis. Helps bring out the rash in measles and eruptive disease.*
- *Anyone who has ever had measles or meningitis; it clears the debris of this sickness out of the system.*

OTHER

- Snake bite, insect bite, neurological symptoms, cramps, convulsions, paralysis.

PREPARATION AND DOSAGE:

The dried root (rhizome) is used in herb commerce, but there is no substitute for the fresh rhizome, which has a "living taste" reminding one of the floor of a rich forest. Fresh root in alcohol; dose of the tincture, 1–3 drops is easily sufficient (Matthew Wood), but most people use much more (10–25 drops). John Scudder recommended 1–2 teaspoonfuls of the tincture every 3 hours for rheumatism and neuralgia. "It must be given to the extent of producing cerebral symptoms—a feeling of weight and fullness in the head, with a headache. Sometimes a very disagreeable prostration and sickness of the stomach follows its administration in large doses, but this soon passes off when the remedy is suspended" (*Eclectic Medical Journal,* 1864, 2,1:31; reprinted by Francis Brinker, 1995; also see Dr. Brinker's own article on *Cimicifuga* in the same publication, 1996, 2,2:2).

CAUTIONS:

Moderate to large doses cause mild unpleasantness, cramping, etc. Phytoestrogens are mildly carcenogenic, but less so than the estrogens they replace. Contraindicated in early pregnancy as an emmenagogue.

LITERATURE:

Traditional, John Uri Lloyd, homeopathic provings, J. V. Cerney (7), Matthew Wood (1, 2, 4, 5, 11, 16), Julia Graves (3), Rolla Thomas (12, 17).

Collinsonia canadensis. Stone Root.

Collinsonia is a member of the mint family native to rich, shaded, moist soil in eastern North America—not a usual environment for a mint. It was used as an indicator for soil fertility, hence the name richweed. The dried roots are extremely hard, explaining the most common name, stone root. These are a signature for its use in removing gallstones. It was much used by the eclectics in the late nineteenth century. It contains glycosides,

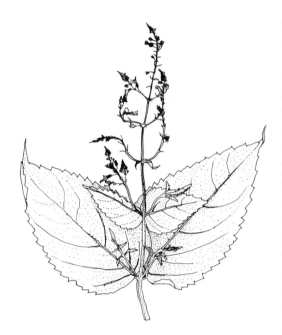

resins, mucilage, tannins, and volatile oils.

Collinsonia was one of the most important organ-specific remedies of the late-nineteenth-century physicians. They considered it to be a remedy for passive venous stagnation. It is a stimulating astringent with an affinity to the veins, so it is suited to conditions where there is passive venous congestion—that is, the blood lingers on the venous side of the circulation, causing blockage and tension. This gives rise to the specific indication often mentioned by the old authors, *passive congestion with dark discoloration of mucous membranes.* Even though it is an astringent, it settles tension due to this kind of blockage. It is most famous for hemorrhoids, for which it is one of the great specifics, but this is only the tip of the iceberg, indicating deeper venous stagnation, often extending throughout the portal vein, thus engorging the liver and gallbladder, resulting in gallstones. Dr. Royal Lee introduced it for gallbladder congestion backing up into the portal vein, resulting in venous and pelvic congestion. It also has a profound effect on the cardiovascular system, releasing venous stagnation causing high blood pressure and distending the right side of the heart. Like all such remedies (especially cf. *Aesculus hippocastanum*) it also has an effect on asthma.

"The tonic action of this drug upon the heart is direct, decided and permanent. It is one of our most efficient remedies when the heart is debilitated from long-continued disease, and especially in protracted rheumatic troubles. It relieves the irritation of the heart, and increases its power and regularity of contraction. In mitral regurgitation it may be administered with confidence in its modifying power. In all functional wrongs of the heart its tonic influence is promptly made apparent. In doses of from two to five drops of the specific medicine it almost invariably relieves the distressing cough which frequently accompanies diseases of the heart.

"Collinsonia has a specific action upon the vascular system, and the power of the capillaries is markedly increased under its influence. In passive hemorrhage, when the capillary circulation of the part is enfeebled, it exerts a speedily manifested controlling influence, and in all conditions showing a lack of tonicity of the walls of the blood-vessels it is specifically indicated. The power of increasing the tone of the circulatory system makes it an energetic remedial agent in many cases of dropsy. The dose employed in these conditions should be ten drops of the specific medicine every two or three hours" (Fyfe, 1909, 476).

TASTE:

pungent • astringent

TISSUE STATES:

relaxation, depression

SPECIFIC INDICATIONS:

CONSTITUTION, COMPLEXION, CHARACTERISTIC SYMPTOMS
- *Sensations of congestion, irritation, constriction; especially affecting the throat and rectum.*
- Blood pools in the center of the body and does not warm the surface; cool hands, feet, and forehead; *passive congestion with dark discoloration of mucosa.*

MIND, SENSES, NERVES, EMOTIONS, PERSONALITY
- Mental tension.

RESPIRATION
- Chronic laryngitis; *irritation and constriction in the larynx.*
- Cough arising from excessive use of the voice, or associated with heart disease (right side of the heart); asthma.
- Catarrh of the respiratory, digestive, or urinary tract.

HEART AND CIRCULATION
- Functional diseases of the heart; oppression of venous and capillary flow.
- Varicosities and *hemorrhoids.*

DIGESTION

- Stomach, weakness and atonicity of the walls, with poor secretion and digestion, *oppression, tightness,* defective circulation (cf. Hydrastis).
- Specific for *hemorrhoids;* sensation of *painful constriction of the rectal sphincter;* sense of a foreign body in the rectum; hemorrhoids of pregnancy; relaxed mucosa of the lower bowel.

LIVER AND GALLBLADDER

- Gallstones and congestion of the gallbladder; spasm of the gall ducts and sphincters.

KIDNEYS AND BLADDER

- Edema, catarrhal affections of kidneys and bladder; stimulates the kidneys and lymphatics to remove water (cf. *Chimaphila*).

MUSCULAR AND SKELETAL

- Spasms, chorea.

PREPARATION AND DOSAGE:

Dose of the fluid extract, 1–60 drops (Fyfe); 5 drops in water, 2–3x/day (Ralph M. Russell). "Dr. Scudder advised the use of this agent in small doses. I have been obliged to give it in doses from ten to twenty minims to secure the desired results. I am confident that the larger dosage will give more satisfaction" (Finley Ellingwood, 1918, 264).

LITERATURE:

Traditional, John M. Scudder, John William Fyfe (cardiac symptoms), Wade Boyle (2), Royal Lee (11).

Comptonia asplenifolia. Sweetfern, Spleenwort.

This is one of the most important tonic medicine plants of the Eastern Woodland Indian people. It was adopted and used by the pioneers, but not much by the professional doctors and is today largely forgotten— except by the Indians. It has properties somewhat similar to its cousin,

Myrica cerifera, *which did become a basic remedy in Western herbalism. However,* Comptonia *is more gently warming and astringent, and somewhat sweet. In my knowledge, it is the plant that comes closest to the idea of "warming the center" or "warming the spleen" in traditional Chinese herbalism. At least, this is how I use it, sometimes in combination with* Myrica *and* Hydrastis.

Sweetfern "warms the center," or mildly stimulates the assimilative and nutritive functions of the body. It is an immune tonic acting on the vital arc from the small intestine (digestion), through the lymphatics (absorption), to the bone marrow (immune development). Thus it is a remedy for poor digestion, lymphatic weakness, emaciation, low immunity, and poor bone development. The variant name "spleenwort" indicates its folk associations with the spleen—that is, the lymphatics, absorption, and nutrition.

Sweetfern was officinal in the U.S. Pharmacopoeia for some years as an astringent for diarrhea, but it is also sweet and oily (thus nutritive) and spicy/stimulating (it contains clove oil). Cook (1869) writes that the leaves "very gently promote digestion, especially in convalescence from acute forms of disease; and appear to exert an excellent influence upon the mesenteries and general assimilative apparatus, on which account they are good in scrofulous, rachitic, and mesenteric debility." It "is a popular family remedy in subacute diarrhea and laxity of the bowels."

I use sweetfern when the tongue is enlarged and pale. If there is a thick white coating in the center I would add *Myrica*.

John Monroe (1824), who studied with an Indian medicine man, cited sweetfern as a remedy for worms. Wood and Ruddock (1916) write that it is a "prompt and efficacious remedy for expelling the tapeworm. A pint of the decoction is to be taken in frequent doses during the day, for four or five days, when it is followed by a cathartic."

Sweetfern is a good remedy for poison ivy. Once I found myself blistering up. Though I caught it elsewhere, just then I was at Sunstone Herb Farm, in Ulster County, New York. There wasn't a lot around but white pine and comptonia. The poison ivy was gone in twelve hours.

TASTE:

sweet, spicy • warm • astringent, oily

TISSUE STATES:

relaxation, atrophy, depression

SPECIFIC INDICATIONS:

CONSTITUTION, COMPLEXION, CHARACTERISTIC SYMPTOMS
- Black rings under the eyes, sunken eyes.

RESPIRATION
- Chronic colds and bronchitis, low immunity.

DIGESTION
- Laxity of the bowels, diarrhea, dysentery, cholera.
- Convalescence after illnesses attended with fluid losses, sweating.
- Rickets, failure to thrive, poor nutrition and absorption.
- Tapeworm.

LYMPH/IMMUNE
- Poor absorption and nutrition, low immunity, poor bone development; strengthens the small intestines, lymphatics, marrow, and bone.

FEMALE
- Vaginal discharge.

FEVER
- Profuse sweating.

LITERATURE:

Traditional, John Monroe, William Cook, Matthew Wood, Julia Graves (1).

Cornus florida. Dogwood.

This small tree is native in the mild to medium climes of the Eastern Woodland region of North America. It was an important agent in the Native American pharmacopoeia and was handed on to the early pioneers and botanical doctors. William Byrd already mentions it as a substitute for quinine bark in the treatment of intermittent fever (malaria, influenza) in 1728 (Moss, 1999, 181). The three great antimalarial barks—

Cornus, Liriodendron, *and* Prunus serotina—*were recommended for use in the Confederate army by Dr. Francis Porcher (1863) during the Civil War, when quinine was blockaded. This formula is analogous to one of the main Chinese formulas for malaria—dogwood and magnolia (of which* Liriodendron *is a close cousin). Such patterns should be of interest to those who desire testimony from different parts of the globe to indicate a valuable property. Today dogwood is much less used due to the decline of malaria.*

"The bark is intensely bitter, and among the common people is used largely as a tonic, and as a substitute for quinine," wrote Dr. Edwin Hale (1875, 2:206). Such intense bitters, which literally shake the frame, are specific for the shivering intermittent chill and fever caused by malaria and influenza attacking the system and knocking out the equilibrium of the autonomic nervous system (which does the shaking). As the shivering continues unabated, the digestive tract, which is so dependent on the autonomic, is knocked out of tune, resulting in one of the most common symptoms of our malarious ancestors, biliousness. The bile doesn't come at the right time, the food sits in the wrong places, or for too long or too short a period of time, upset causes regurgitation, and the tissues lose their tone. In such cases an astringent would combine well with the acrid bitter to provide toning properties, and this is the combination that was often used to treat malaria and that we find in dogwood. Thus, writes Cook (1869, 384), "It may be used to advantage in such intermittent difficulties as are accompanied by general laxity of the fibers," though as an astringent it may be "disposed to confine the bowels, and should not be used without the strictest attention being paid to the hepatic and alvine function"—that is, to make sure they are flowing. It is not suitable for active inflammatory diseases—thus for typhoid, until the fever and cramping has died away—only in "nearly passive stools" from loss of tone.

Hale developed a somewhat different picture from Cook, which was adopted by homeopaths and eclectics. He looked for sharply marked intermissions of fever and chill, producing a great deal of exhaustion, debility, and the aforementioned atonicity. Dogwood was recommended in heartburn from gastric atonicity, in tendencies to fermentation, and in leucorrhea.

Chills and fever were also a consequence of deep wounds that became infected. Here is a case history given by Samuel Henry (1814, 299) from the War of 1812. "A young man was shot by an Indian, and received two bullets which entered below the shoulder blade and came out at the side of his breast, was perfectly cured in five weeks, by the use of slippery-elm bark as a poultice, and taking daily the extract of dogwood made into pills."

The branches of the dogwood look somewhat like antlers. This remedy is one of the "elk medicines" of the Indian pharmacopoeia (at least in my opinion) used to treat the kidneys and the sexual function. Some of the elk medicines are astringents that tone the sexual-urinary tract, while others act on what would have to be described, in modern terms, as androgen excess—that is, liver trouble indicated by acne, propensity of chills and fevers, stiffness and achiness in the joints, and sexual frustration (but not incapacity). Androgen, more than any other hormone, is hard on the liver and sometimes combines with other weaknesses (perhaps the chills of malaria or influenza) to depress hepatic function. Strong bitters and some elk medicines act on the liver, chill/fever, uncontrollable shivering or movements, acne, "bad blood," and the reproductive sphere. They are beneficial for men and women alike, more than half of the female population suffering from androgen excess at some time during their childbearing epoch. We do not have such symptoms recorded in the literature for Florida dogwood, but compare the Chinese dogwood *(Cornus officinalis)*, used for impotence.

"From a variety of experiments made by Dr. Walker upon the healthy system, it was found that this medicine uniformly increased the force and frequency of the pulse, and augmented the heat of the body" (Bigelow, 1817–20, 79).

TASTE:

bitter/acrid • astringent • slightly aromatic

TISSUE STATES:

constriction, relaxation

SPECIFIC INDICATIONS:

CONSTITUTION, COMPLEXION, CHARACTERISTIC SYMPTOMS

- *Chronic malaria* with digestive atonicity from repeated chills; indigestion, acidity, acid heartburn, nausea, diarrhea, relaxed tissues, and great exhaustion.

- Pulse weak, tissues relaxed, sodden, and feeble, temperature subnormal.

FEMALE
- Leucorrhea.

FEVER
- Night sweats and fluid losses with great debility.
- Feels cold, but is warm to the touch.
- Great exhaustion in intervals, followed by chills.
- *Intermittent fever;* the hot stage accompanied by violent headache with throbbing, stupor, confusion of intellect, vomiting, sharp pain in the bowels, diarrhea, hot, moist skin, quick pulse; cold stage preceded by days of drowsiness, sluggish flow of ideas, cold, clammy skin, and a dull, heavy headache.

EXTERNAL
- Ulcers and foul sores (powder of the bark, externally).

PREPARATION AND DOSAGE:

The bark is the part usually prepared in traditional nineteenth-century herbal medicine, but R. Swinburne Clymer notes that the flowers are even more effective than the bark for malaria. Dose: fluid extract, 5–60 drops (Fyfe); tincture, 5–10 drops every 2 hours (Hale). Large doses upset the stomach. A decoction of the small branches and twigs is less upsetting (John Eberle, 1833, 1:303).

LITERATURE:

Traditional, John Eberle (7), Rolla Thomas (1, 2), William Cook (1, 3), Edwin Hale (1, 2, 4, 5, 6, 7), John William Fyfe (1, 6, 7, 8), Frederick Petersen (2), Jacob Bigelow (2).

Dicentra canadensis. Turkey Corn, Corydalis.

This plant is included more for historical interest than practical application. It is native to old-growth forests and, because of overharvesting in the nineteenth century, is now rare. I have seen it only once. It is an early spring ephemeral. Later in the year the herbage dies back and the little roots sticking out of the ground look like kernels of corn. Turkey corn was an important remedy for the Indian people and the pioneers. The bulb contains alkaloids, resin, and fumaric acid.

Dicentra was traditionally used in sluggish digestion, where the food sits in the stomach, ferments, and is delivered in a rotten state to the intestines, where bloating and inflammation occur. Toxins are absorbed into the bloodstream and lymph, giving rise to "bad blood." It slowly increases the circulation to provide warmth and vitalization, and opens the skin and kidneys to promote elimination. Christopher Menzies-Trull (2003, 578) classifies it as a vasostimulant and vasotonic alterative. William Cook (1869, 401) remarks that the perspiration produced is mild and insensible, but the urine is perceptibly increased, including both the liquid and solid parts. It appears to have properties similar to its European cousin, fumitory.

TASTE:

pungent, bitter • diffusive

TISSUE STATES:

depression, stagnation

SPECIFIC INDICATIONS:

CONSTITUTION, COMPLEXION, CHARACTERISTIC SYMPTOMS
- General malaise and indisposition to exertion; after protracted disease; with sluggishness of the digestion, glands, skin, kidneys, and circulation; with "bad blood" (sometimes hypothyroidism).

DIGESTION
- Bad breath.
- Tongue persistently coated.
- Ulceration of mouth and tonsils; of glands (i.e., scrofula).
- Loss of appetite, indigestion.
- Full, bloated feeling, catarrh, in stomach and intestines.
- Swelling and enlargement of the abdominal structures.
- Irregular bowels, colic, diarrhea, constipation.

FEMALE

- Amenorrhea, dysmenorrhea, leucorrhea.

MUSCULAR AND SKELETAL

- Relaxed ligamentous supports of the uterus, prolapse, sometimes occurring from extreme debility following fevers.
- Rheumatism.

SKIN

- Chronic skin disorders, with marked cachexia; eczema with great relaxation of the tissues and general plethoric fullness.
- Persistent ulceration with breakdown of soft tissue (i.e., syphilis, scrofula).

FEVER

- Malaise, digestive torpor, glandular atonicity, impairment of nutrition; following a protracted intermittent fever, ague, or malaria.

PREPARATION AND DOSAGE:

Due to rarity, this should be used only in a homeopathic form or in small doses harvested from cultivated patches.

CAUTIONS:

Environmental concerns.

LITERATURE:

Traditional, Constantine Rafinesque, Edwin Hale (2, 3, 4, 5, 6, 8), Finley Ellingwood (1–14), Christopher Menzies-Trull.

Dioscorea villosa. Wild Yam.

Wild yam is an old North and Central American Indian remedy, adopted by the pioneers, and introduced into herbal medicine by Horton Howard, an early frontier doctor in the Midwest, where it grows most prolifically. Wild yam and its cousin, cultivated yam, contain steroidal saponins that make them a source for the manufacture of steroids used in the pharmaceutical industry. It is another of the old American Indian female medicines.

Wild yam is found on brushy land, where the timber has been cut, or in old pastures going back into brush. When well established, the white, bone-like rhizomes crisscross under the ground like a rabbit running through the briar patch. The common name "devil's bones" refers to the appearance of these "roots" as they are dug from the ground. *Dioscorea* is therefore a "rabbit medicine"—that is, a nutritive tonic that builds up calcium to support the bones and sedate spasm in the muscles. Rabbits are thin-boned and twitchy-muscled, so this root is perfectly suited to that category. Although I was not taught this designation from a traditional old American Indian mentor, I believe I have the right to generalize from what I have been taught, and I can say that *Dioscorea* is a rabbit medicine.

The properties of wild yam depend upon the method of preparation. Nineteenth-century botanical physicians and the educated public, mostly in the Northern cultural zone, made a fluid extract or tincture from the fresh or recently dried rhizomes for use in small doses as an antispasmodic. The fresh "root" contains acrid properties that made it unpalatable, but that possess relaxant properties in small doses. To make it palatable as a tea it is dried for more than a year. However, Southern folk medicine, according to Phyllis Light, knows of additional preparations and uses. If it is cooked for longer than 20 minutes it starts to extract saponins that have a cortisone-like effect as anti-inflammatories. The brew now looks soapy and starts to turn red. After another hour or longer it starts to extract saponins that have a hormonal effect and turns intensely red—a signature for the blood and menses.

As a Northerner, by culture and training, I will represent only the Northern tradition, which follows the published accounts of nineteenth-century physicians of the eclectic, physiomedical, and homeopathic schools. Dr. Charles Millspaugh (1892, 699) writes, "Dioscorea has held a place in domestic and general practice for a long period as almost specific in certain forms of bilious colic, in which it is promptly efficacious." Indeed, the late Dr. John Bastyr specified that if it does not correct the gallstone colic within 20 minutes it is not the remedy (Mitchell, 2003, 20). His dose was 20 drops repeated frequently. To continue with Millspaugh: "As a visceral antispasmodic, and remedy for intestinal irritations, it has proved itself a valuable remedy in cholera morbus, spasm of the diaphragm, asthma, dysmenorrhea, and kindred afflictions." It promotes diaphoresis, emesis, and expectoration.

Dr. John William Fyfe (1909, 503) gives similar testimony. "*Dioscorea* has valuable properties besides those found useful in the treatment of colic. In the nausea attending pregnancy it often affords much relief, and as a modifier of after-pains it acts in a very satisfactory manner. In dysmenorrhea it aids in rendering the painful condition bearable, and in hysteria it may well constitute a part of the treatment. Hepatic diseases [gallstone colic], especially when accompanied with irritability of the stomach, are among the wrongs in which indications for this agent are likely to be seen, and as a remedy for dysentery and all spasmodic affections of the stomach and bowels, it is of frequent usefulness."

In the 1940s pharmaceutical researchers in Central America discovered that the Mayan Indian women used their local variety of *Dioscorea* for birth control. It subsequently became the raw source material for the manufacture of many steroidal drugs, including birth control pills. Wild yam was recently reintroduced into the marketplace as a "natural source" of progesterone. However, it had to be pharmaceutically processed to yield this agent. Phyllis Light points out that the Mayan women originally made their own birth control medicine by cooking the wild yam.

The following profile represents the traditional "Northern" approach to *Dioscorea villosa*.

TASTE:

sweet, earthen, acrid • moist

TISSUE STATES:

atrophy, constriction

SPECIFIC INDICATIONS:

CONSTITUTION, COMPLEXION, CHARACTERISTIC SYMPTOMS
- *Thin, undernourished people with spasms in the intestines, poor assimilation through the small intestine, decalcification.*
- Tongue usually coated.
- Skin yellow and dry, conjunctiva more or less yellow.

RESPIRATION
- *Asthma,* whooping cough, and bronchitis.

DIGESTION, LIVER, AND GALLBLADDER
- Spasmodic hiccough.
- Abdominal distention, gas.
- Belly muscles tender and contracted.
- *Abdominal muscles contracted, constant pain; colic, sharp, cutting pains;* in the gallbladder, abdomen, or ovaries; relieved by pressure, by supporting the abdomen, by drinking, worse from eating.
- *Bowel spasm;* many times the pains extend throughout the body.
- Hepatic disorders, accompanied by irritability of the stomach.
- Typhoid fever when there is tenderness on pressure and tympanitic swelling.
- *Abdominal cramping, uterine cramping, gallstone colic.*
- Stool thin and yellow, preceded by violent, twisting, colicky pains.
- Lack of blood in the abdomen; anemia, poor nutrition, decalcification.
- Facial neuralgia, gastralgia, pain in the uterus, and in painful and spasmodic action of the bladder and rectum, and in sciatica.
- *Nausea of pregnancy.*

FEMALE
- *Dysmenorrhea due to ovarian neuralgia* (45 drops in water, 4x/day) (John Bastyr).
- *Severe menstrual colic.*
- *Menopausal women with hip joint disease.*

MUSCULAR AND SKELETAL
- *Hip joint deterioration;* cannot find a comfortable position to lie in, tossing and turning at night.

PREPARATION AND DOSAGE:

Roots are harvested during the summer and fall. They can be dried or used fresh to produce a tincture or fluid extract. Dose of the tincture:

1–10 drops, 1–3x/day (Wood), 20–40 drops, 3–4x/day (Gagnon). For use as a tea the rhizomes are dried a year, then decocted about 20 minutes.

CAUTIONS:

Large doses may cause vomiting. Excessive doses have caused psychological upset. Environmental concerns when picked in areas where it is not naturally abundant.

LITERATURE:

Traditional, homeopathic provings and clinical experience (6–19), Horton Howard, John Scudder (2, 3), John Bastyr (17), Matthew Wood (1, 19, 20), John William Fyfe, Julia Graves (19, 20), Louise Tenney (4, 5, 6, 15, 16, 18).

Echinacea angustifolia, E. pallida, E. purpurea. Purple Coneflower.

Echinacea, a member of the aster family, is native to open areas and prairies in the eastern and central part of North America. The western species, E. angustifolia, was one of the most important plants of the Indians of the Great Plains and is still held in esteem and used by them today. It was introduced into popular medicine by H. Meyer, who sold it as the original "snake oil." It was adopted by the eclectics and picked up by German pharmaceutical companies in the 1930s. That led to the use of the eastern species, E. purpurea, which is easy to grow. It shows many pharmacological properties, but it is not clear that it is as powerful as the western coneflower. There is little record of the eastern Indians using this species, which should lead us to be suspicious that it is not equivalent to the western representative.

Echinacea was introduced into the modern marketplace as an "immune stimulant" based on the presence of polysaccharides in it that have stimulating influences on the immune system. Unfortunately, no attention was paid to the traditional uses of echinacea, even by the eclectics from whom the German pharmaceutical chemists learned about the plant. Thus, it was introduced as an "immune stimulant" on entirely theoretical grounds. It became a fad herb, producing more than $165 million in

2005 sales. This led to serious testing, first in an American pediatric journal and then in the New England Journal of Medicine. *Both studies found no evidence that echinacea helped treat minor head colds and acute upper respiratory tract illnesses in children or adults. One study involved naturopathic physicians from Bastyr University in Seattle, so there was even an effort at "integrated scientific research." After the* NEJM *study an editorial was included by Dr. William Sampson, a longtime opponent of complementary and alternative medicine (CAM), in which he stated that not only were results of the study negative, but there was no evidence in historical records that echinacea had ever been used in folk medicine to treat head colds and upper respiratory tract infections. He concluded that no funds should be spent investigating CAM products and practices. This, however, is the wrong conclusion. The real flaw was that researchers did not study historical and folk medical uses, as Sampson points out. Echinacea was traditionally used for septicemia, not mild infections. The use of echinacea for acute disease, as an "immune stimulant," was therefore entirely theoretical and, as it turned out, inappropriate. According to traditional sources, echinacea is only rarely useful in acute conditions. It was not traditional herbalism that led the marketplace astray, but theorists and commercial interests. Unfortunately, armchair "Western herbal experts," also with no clinical experience, jumped on the bandwagon and soon everyone was preaching the virtues of echinacea as an "immune stimulant." I never joined this irresponsible and ignorant fad, as my account of echinacea in* The Book of Herbal Wisdom *(1997) shows. I advocated only traditional uses.*

Echinacea is now a debacle damaging the reputation of herbal medicine, or is a belief that faddists cannot let go. It is also a historical monument to the evolving and changing view of the immune system. In the 1980s, when echinacea was introduced into the marketplace, there was very little understanding of the immune system. It was not yet appreciated that the immune system contains many pathways. Just because an agent stimulates one element of the system does not mean it is appropriate to another pathway.

Echinacea contains sugars, including polysaccharides that have immune-stimulating properties, betaine, echinacin, echinacoside, caffeic acid derivatives, resins, essential oils, and fatty acids. The substance that causes tingling in the mouth, xanthoxylin, is also found in Xanthoxylum.

Western purple coneflower is one of the "snake medicines" used by the

Indians of the Great Plains to treat snake bites, insect bites, septicemia, and various kinds of poisonings. It has a wide range of applications to heat conditions, both those arising from tissue depression, and those associated with allergy and excitation. Echinacea is one of a small number of stimulants that have a cooling taste and effect (cf. *Lavendula, Xanthoxylum*). It is also sweet, so it is indicated as a nutritive.

The eclectics defined *Echinacea* rather broadly as a remedy for "bad blood." "Wherever disease results from lack of vital force, from a tendency to morbific changes, from a depraved state of the fluids, from blood-poisoning, or from a tendency toward disintegration of tissue, echinacea should always constitute at least a part of the treatment" (John William Fyfe, 1909, 506). (Does "disintegration of tissue" sound like "rhinitis"?) *Echinacea* "is the ideal remedy in the treatment of boils, carbuncles and bruises; not because of their name, but because we have [in echinacea an antidote to] the pathological condition which manifests itself in an edematous, doughy condition of the muscular tissue, and, [that] under palpation, gives to the touch a sensation ... like unto that where there is deeply burrowed pus" (Ross, quoted by Fyfe). (Does that sound like "head cold"?)

From a deeper, traditional, and holistic perspective, we would say that echinacea is suited to cases where white cell production is required in high amounts to combat putrefactive conditions, or where health has been compromised due to a long-term septic drain on the system. Not only in boils and abscesses, but in snake bites and poisonings, and in long-term stress and exhaustion.

Echinacea is suited to a high level of exhaustion. Overwork, long hours, and lack of vacation are sometimes a component. The immunity is down and the person gets sick when they get a chance to relax. There may be swollen glands. The veins are full and dark, showing that there is stagnation on the venous side of the circulation—so typical of a depressed tissue state. If there is an injury, the veins leading away from it are swollen (George Royal). There is a tendency to the formation of boils (William Boericke, 1927).

Echinacea belongs to the group of antiseptics including *Baptisia, Isatis, Helianthemum,* and *Scrophularia*.

TASTE:

sweet • cold • diffusive (tingling), stimulating

TISSUE STATES:

depression, irritation

SPECIFIC INDICATIONS:

- Dull eyes; dull feeling of mind and body; shattered in mind or body.
- Fatigue, exhaustion; from overwork, poor work habits; often accompanied by the production of boils; dirty, gray visage of the face.
- Ulcerative pharyngitis, tonsillitis, and stomatitis (canker sores).
- Tongue coated dirty brown or black.
- Gastric and duodenal ulcers.
- Enteritis.
- Swollen lymphatics.
- Swollen, blue veins.
- Septicemia, prostrating fever, chills.
- Septic infections; veins leading from the wound are swollen, purple; promotes suppuration (discharge of pus).
- Boils, abscesses, carbuncles; semi-active, low-grade character, with exhaustion and atrophy; chronic, constitutional tendency.
- Eczema from toxins in the blood.
- Bee stings, snake bites, venom; histaminic irritation; applied directly it has a cooling and detoxifying effect.
- Deepened, bluish or purplish coloration of the skin or mucosa, with a low form of inflammation.
- Putrescent odor from excess of broken-down material being eliminated from the system; as in scarlet fever, diphtheria, spinal meningitis, and typhoid fever (cf. *Baptisia*).
- Old sores, wounds, necrosis, gangrene.
- Chilly.

PREPARATION AND DOSAGE:

The traditional preparation is made by the Plains Indians from the roots of *Echinacea angustifolia*, four years or older. Dried for use by decoction or capsule; extracted fresh in alcohol. Dose for specific usage need not be great (1–10 drops, 1–3x/day). It works poorly in the homeopathic potencies (beyond 3x).

CAUTIONS:

Overuse can lead to an exaggerated white blood cell count. Not to be taken during leukemia. There are environmental concerns. *Echinacea angustifolia* is overharvested, and its environment and distribution have been reduced by chemical spraying of prairie pastures. *Echinacea purpurea* can be easily grown in the garden, but may not be as powerful.

LITERATURE:

Traditional, H. M. Meyer, John King, George Royal (homeopathic provings: 8, 10), William Boericke (11), A. W. Priest and L. R. Priest (3, 5, 6, 10, 12), Matthew Wood (1, 2), John William Fyfe (4, 7, 11, 14, 15), Flower Essence Society (1).

Epigea repens. Trailing Arbutus.

This is a widely admired plant medicine among the Indian people. It was adopted into folk medicine in Canada, at a very early date in European settlement, and recommended to the medical profession by Constantine Rafinesque. It is one of the more effective diuretic remedies in the heath family and should perhaps be more widely known and used, as it was in former times. The following two authors reflect eclectic literature, though it was also used in other nineteenth-century medical schools. Today it is little used.

"Trailing arbutus is successfully employed in cases where there is an excess of uric acid. In the nauseating backache met with in cases where the crystalline constituents of the urine are not well dissolved and washed out of the tubules it is also a potent remedy, and where there is renal sand or gravel in the bladder it has a corrective influence. In cases in which the urine is dark and heavy, with irritation, causing congestion of the kidneys, epigea is used with markedly beneficial effects, and when precipitated solids irritate the bladder and induce cystitis, with thickening of the walls and the formation of pus, it constitutes a most valuable remedial agent. In diseases of the kidneys and bladder the dose should be administered in about an ounce of hot water—not warm water" (Fyfe).

"Epigea is generally classified as a tonic and astringent diuretic, and there are to be found in any general practice of any size a great number of cases in which epigea may be used with advantage to both patient and physician. They are of a chronic nature. The acute symptoms of irritation have given way to atony and relaxation. There is debility and backache. The urine is usually heavily loaded with mucus, or in some cases it is bloody, and in others more or less purulent" (Bloyer, quoted by John William Fyfe, 1909).

Epilobium angustifolium, E. parvifolium.
Fireweed, Willow Herb.

The Epilobiums are members of the evening primrose or Onagraceae family, native to temperate regions of the New and Old Worlds. The usual common names are willow herb (some of them are like an annual willow) and fireweed (the E. angustifolium grows best on ground that has been burnt). They occupied a modest niche in Western herbalism until Maria Treben introduced willow herb as a specific for the prostate. Fireweed leaf contains flavonoids, quercetin, mucilage, sugars, starches, pectin, tannins, vitamin C, and calcium salts. There has been considerable modern pharmaceutical work on fireweed and it has been shown to suppress inflammation more effectively than cortisone and to enhance the action of some drugs.

Scudder used willow herb during the Civil War for "camp fever" and taught its use to the eclectic profession. "It is especially valuable . . . in chronic diarrhea and dysentery; sometimes effecting cures where all other means had failed. Thus, I employed it extensively in the treatment of the chronic diarrhea during the civil war, and with a success not to be obtained from other remedies." It is an astringent and nutritive tonic.

"This agent exerts a specific influence upon the intestinal mucous membrane, relieving irritation, and promoting normal function. It is, therefore, a good remedy in acute diarrhea, dysentery and colic. In chronic diarrhea with large passages of half-digested food it has given excellent results, and in cholera infantum it constitutes an efficient medicament. In the diarrhea of typhoid fever it exerts a controlling influence over the discharges and quiets gastrointestinal irritation" (John William Fyfe, 1909).

In the twentieth century Maria Treben introduced the use of willow herb *(Epilobium parvifolium* and other *Epilobiums)* for swollen prostate.

She considered it to be nearly a specific. The success and specificity of *E. parvifolium* as a specific in prostate problems is given further testimony by herbalist Hilde Hemmes, of Australia. "I am not a laboratory scientist, but the simple fact that I have thousands of responses from men (and their wives thanking me for giving them back their husbands) claiming total cure from various stages of prostate disorder tells me the herb must be doing its work" (Hemmes, 1995, 39). She also recommends it for urinary tract infections, cystitis, and kidney and bladder problems in both men and women.

TASTE:

astringent, mucilaginous

TISSUE STATES:

relaxation, atrophy

SPECIFIC INDICATIONS:

MIND, SENSES, NERVES, EMOTIONS, PERSONALITY
- Balances will power and anger; helps to master the will; wild, angry, overactive children are sedated, timid, shy children are strengthened, and angry, willful adults are tempered (flower essence).

RESPIRATION
- Inflammations of the ears, nose, and throat (external).
- Sore throat, laryngitis.
- Whooping cough, asthma, spasmodic coughing.

DIGESTION
- Gastritis, gastric ulcer, colitis.
- Diarrhea of a watery character; with colicky pain.
- Feculent discharges with straining.
- Chronic diarrhea with harsh, dirty appearing, and contracted skin.
- Cholera infantum, with greenish discharges.

- Chronic candidiasis.
- Diarrhea of typhoid fever.

KIDNEYS AND BLADDER
- *Cystitis.*

MALE
- *Swollen prostate, inflamed prostate.*

MUSCULAR AND SKELETAL
- Tight muscles from unexpressed anger (flower essence).
- Arthritis.
- Bruises, boils, burns (external).

SKIN
- Harsh, dry skin; psoriasis, eczema, acne.

PREPARATION AND DOSAGE:

Infusion of the dried leaves, 2 ounces to a quart of water, or a heaping teaspoon to a cup of boiling water. Steep, 3–5 minutes. Dose: 2 ounces every 4–6 hours or 1 ounce an hour. Tincture, fluid extract, usual dose, 10–20 drops, up to 3x/day (Rogers, Fyfe).

LITERATURE:

Traditional, John Scudder, John William Fyfe (6–9, 11), Rolla Thomas (6–8, 16), Maria Treben (13), Hilde Hemmes (12, 13), Michael Moore, Julia Graves (14), Robert Dale Rogers (2–5, 10, 15–17), Flower Essence Society (1).

Erechtites hieracifolius. Fireweed.

Fireweed is a representative of the willow herb family, closely akin to epilobium, native to recent burns in pine forests on the Canadian shield. It has properties similar to epilobium. Although little used in the past or present, it is widely available and ought to be more frequently contemplated. William Cook (1869, 413) writes: "The leaves and flowers are somewhat pungent and disagreeably bitter in taste, leaving behind a mild astringency. They act chiefly upon mucous membranes, to which they are astringent and stimulant tonics. Their principal use is in relaxed and insensitive conditions of those tissues, with too free mucous discharges, as in some cases of chronic diarrhea, leucorrhea, and catarrhal coughs. In the 'relax' (not acute) dysentery of children they are truly excellent." They are also used in relaxation of the bowels in children (chronic diarrhea, not dysentery), atonic dyspepsia, hemorrhages from the lungs, bowels, kidneys, and uterus, ulcerations of the digestive tract, with bloody, purulent discharges, without inflammation (low-grade, septic infections). The leaves are used externally in ulcers of a "half indolent grade," poorly healing sores, to promote granulation, and on "recent burns." These uses are similar to those for the epilobiums.

Erigeron canadensis. Canada Fleabane, Daisy Fleabane.

The fleabanes are widely distributed in the fields of temperate North America. They are an old Indian remedy. Edwin Hale (1875, 1:281) records the name "cocosh," evidence of the Native origins of the medicine. Erigeron is one of the most pepperish medicines in North America and certainly would not have been missed by a people observant in woodlore. Constantine Rafinesque (1828) introduced Erigeron spp. into the medical literature. It is a member of the aster family, containing flavonoids, bitters, tannins, and volatile oils.

Erigeron is a very intense stimulant that increases the action of the kidneys, removing gravelly, earthen deposits. It is also used to stop excessive flow of urine from the kidneys (diabetes insipidus). Likewise, it is well established as a stimulant to stop bleeding—stimulants open up the peripheral circulation, make the capillary bed into a big sponge, and deprive a local area of the excessive blood lost in a hemorrhage.

William LeSassier recommended erigeron in profuse diarrhea where a microorganism is related to the cause. Stimulants directly oppose these organisms by increasing tissue life in the host and decreasing the depressed environment the organism makes for itself by lacing the tissues with exotoxins. The volatile oils found in stimulants are often antimicrobial.

Dr. John Eberle (1834, 2:369), of Philadelphia, writes, "In this city it has been a good deal employed, within a few years past, in nephritic and gravely affections. Dr. Physic employed it in a case of dysury, attended with great pain and irritability of the bladder, with much relief to the patient." Dr. Wistar used it in "gout and hydrothorax," or water on the chest. "I have been much in the habit of prescribing this plant in gravely and hydropic [dropsical] disease. It has seldom failed to produce a pretty copious diuresis in my practice." Dr. Eberle notes in addition that "it will in general lie easy on the stomach, and has no tendency to weaken the digestive powers. Some of my patients have even found an increase of appetite from its use."

"This old remedy," writes John William Fyfe (1909), "constitutes a valuable medicament in many wrongs of life. In diseases of the kidneys and bladder, especially when a tonic and stimulant action is desired, it is used with gratifying results. In albuminuria much benefit is derived from its employment, and in diabetes insipidus it exercises a restraining influence. In painful diseases of the kidneys and bladder its action is decidedly corrective, and in chronic nephritis and chronic cystitis it is deemed a remedial agent of great value. It is also a favorite remedy in the later stages of gonorrhea, gleet and urethritis. In dysuria of the child or adult erigeron affords much relief, and in chronic catarrhal affections of the genitourinary organs of the female, especially where there is a profuse discharge, it is often useful. In chronic cough with much expectoration it exercises a quieting influence, and its astringency is of marked benefit in diarrhea and dysentery, as well as in cholera infantum."

The oil of erigeron was especially employed late in the nineteenth and early twentieth centuries as a hemostatic in "passive hemorrhage," which usually means a darker, slower flow, from the nose, mouth, uterus, or urinary tract. Finley Ellingwood made a particularly effective postpartum antihemorrhagic from oils of erigeron and cinnamon. Stimulants increase peripheral circulation, reducing the amount of fluid flowing out through a particular opening. In the eighteenth and nineteenth centuries the usual "scientific" explanation for staunching bleeding was that a plant contained tannins, which bind tissue, but many of the best hemostatics were stimulants, with or without tannins. Shepherd's purse is another stimulant used to stop bleeding that the "scientists" of the era discounted because it did not contain tannins. Yarrow, one of the superlative hemostatics, is both a stimulant and an astringent. Cinnamon is another such example.

I asked traditional Appalachian herbalist Phyllis Light how fleabane was used to kill fleas. "According to my grandfather, you put the whole plants in the box where the dog sleeps." Other sources say it is the smoke from the burning plant that drives away fleas.

TASTE:

pungent

TISSUE STATE:

depression

SPECIFIC INDICATIONS:

RESPIRATION
- Conjunctivitis.
- Chronic cough with profuse mucoid discharge; chronic bronchitis; tuberculosis.

DIGESTION
- Lack of appetite.
- Chronic diarrhea; bacterial diarrhea; dysentery; cholera; typhus; prolapsed rectum.

KIDNEYS AND BLADDER
- Chronic, painful nephritis, with edema, gravel, albuminuria.
- Profuse urination (diabetes insipidus).
- Chronic cystitis, urethritis; painful, gonorrheal discharges; profuse catarrhal discharges; in women.

FEMALE
- Suppressed or painful menstruation.
- Postpartum: severe bleeding (oil, more effective).

MUSCULAR AND SKELETAL
- Rheumatism (external liniment).
- Gout.

SKIN AND MUCOSA

- Passive hemorrhage from any surface (oil); nosebleed; tuberculosis; dysentery, bloody vomiting; excessive menstruation; postpartum bleeding.
- "Active hemorrhage, with strong and not very frequent pulse" (1–5 drops of the oil) (Rolla Thomas).

PREPARATION AND DOSAGE:

The plant is collected when in flower (Eberle), which is easily half the summer. Fluid extract, 5–60 drops (Fyfe).

LITERATURE:

Traditional, Constantine Rafinesque (4, 6, 7, 8), John Eberle (3, 5, 11), John Scudder, John William Fyfe (2, 6, 7), Finley Ellingwood (7, 9, 12), William LeSassier (4), Rolla Thomas (13).

Eriodictyon californicum. Yerba Santa.

"Sacred herb" is a resinous desert plant that has long been used in respiratory therapy. "This remedy has been highly recommended as a stimulant to the respiratory tract. In pharyngitis, chronic laryngitis and bronchitis it has often been used with great advantage, and in broncho-pneumonic catarrhal affections it has yielded very satisfactory results. In chronic humid asthma, with profuse expectoration, thickened bronchial membrane and impaired digestion, it is of some value, and in coughs characterized by copious and easy expectoration it is a good remedial agent. It also exerts a favorable influence in catarrhal gastritis" (Fyfe, 1909, 521). Yerba santa is specific for a slightly moist cough where the cough reflexes are exhausted and too weak to bring up the phlegm, the voice is weak, the throat is raw, and there is a general lack of strength.

A useful trick I have learned about this medicine: it is valuable when symptoms are obscure and it is difficult to understand what is going on. After a dose the picture may become more focused and the solution clear. This is especially the case where there is some sort of psychic interference.

TASTE:

sweet, pungent • warm • resinous, moist

TISSUE STATES:

depression, atrophy

SPECIFIC INDICATIONS:

- Grief with lung affections (flower essence).
- Eyes dry and lusterless.
- Throat raw.
- Voice weak.
- *Chronic, exhaustive, weak cough, sticky, damp mucus.*
- Exhaustion.
- Obscure disease; brings the disease out of hiding and makes its nature more evident.
- Alcoholism.

PREPARATION AND DOSAGE:

The gummy, resinous leaves are picked at the end of the first year (before they collect dust). Dose of the fluid extract, 5–60 drops (Fyfe).

LITERATURE:

Traditional, Matthew Wood (7, 8).

Eryngium yuccifolium. Rattlesnake Master.

Rattlesnake master is one of the most powerful "snake medicines" known to the Eastern Woodland Indian people. As they emerge from the ground in the spring, the young shoots look like a snake's jaws opening wide to bite! The first time I noticed this I was almost shocked by the intensity of the picture presented—as if one is looking into the jaws of a rattlesnake. The old authors testified that Eryngium *is the most important remedy for the bite of the rattlesnake. Constantine Rafinesque (1828–30) says it is unsurpassed in the treatment of rattlesnake bite (used externally and*

*internally). Beal P. Downing (1851), after a lifetime wandering in the
American wilderness, gives no other medicine for this complaint. On the
other hand, the method of the early Virginia planter William Byrd (1729)
seems wise: he always traveled with "3 Kinds of Rattle-Snake Root ...
in case of Need" (Moss, 1999, 201).*

The snake medicines are suited to conditions of depression. They are
almost all used for snake bite, or where tissues have been killed by poison.
They are also widely used in skin rashes where the outbreak recedes and
the poisons inflict themselves on interior organs. "I have found a warm
infusion of it quite valuable to promote the tardy eruption in scarlatina,
small pox, and other exanthemas" (Cook, 1869, 415).

"Eryngium is a general stimulant, being diaphoretic and diuretic, with
a special affinity for the mucous membranes. It has been given in infusion as a diaphoretic, in dropsy, gravel and jaundice, and in the com-
mencing stage of catarrhal inflammation, such as occurs in the upper air
passages in epidemic influenza. It must be given early in acute cases as a
diaphoretic" (Ellingwood, 1918).

"Eryngium is another so-called diuretic which has very little diuretic
action, but the remedy is one of our best agents for irritation of the neck
of the bladder, whether this arises from inflammation, gravel, gonorrhea,
or nonspecific urethritis. Eryngium is indicated by burning and itching
in the urethra, with frequent micturition. It may be given with confidence
in this condition, and the size of the dose gradually increased until results
follow, which is always a good rule in specific medication" (Lyman
Watkins, 1901).

I find that Eryngium is *an absolute specific when swellings are hard.*
This usually occurs due to the infiltration of blood proteins into the lymph.
I have used this indication in humans and in horses. The latter not uncom-
monly have hard swellings on the legs—from old bruises, I suppose.
Eryngium has a salty taste, indicating that it is an emollient, or softening
agent.

TASTE:

salty

TISSUE STATES:

depression, atrophy

SPECIFIC INDICATIONS:

GENERAL SYMPTOMS
- *Swollen tissues are hard from infiltration of protein into the lymph;* either cold or hot.
- Chronic inflammation of the mucosa, loss of tone, free secretion.

RESPIRATORY
- Scrofulous ophthalmia.
- Chronic laryngitis.
- Chronic disease of the respiratory organs, with relaxed mucosa and profuse expectoration; bronchitis; tuberculosis.

DIGESTION
- Weak appetite and digestion, with general debility, in convalescence from fevers.
- Mucus diarrhea, epidemic influenza.
- Hemorrhoids and anal prolapse from excessive diarrhea.

SEXUAL AND URINARY
- Atonic dropsy, gravel, chronic nephritis.
- Irritation of the bladder and urethra.
- Urinary tract inflammation, pain.
- Loss of tone of mucosa with free secretion; gonorrheal discharges, stricture; chronic gonorrhea.
- Urinary incontinence.
- Confusion of urinary and sexual impulses.
- Nymphomania and satyriasis.

OTHER
- *Bee stings, insect bites, snake bites; where the tissue is hard and swollen.*

PREPARATION AND DOSAGE:

The roots are described as officinal in nineteenth-century literature, but I have been assured by a Cherokee medicine woman that the leaves are just as serviceable and are preferable. Dosage: 1–10 drops, internally or externally, as needed.

LITERATURE:

Traditional, Matthew Wood (1), Gideon Lincecum, Constantine Rafinesque, Beal P. Downing, William Boericke, Julia Graves (8), H. Inberg (*Ellingwood's Therapeutist*, 1908, 2, 7, 29) (13), Frederick Locke (16).

Eschscholzia californica. California Poppy.

Like other members of the poppy family, this plant is a sedative, but it is not as depressing or narcotic in effect. It is a bitter that (like skullcap, bugleweed, and motherwort) sedates partly because it increases fluids and lubrication. Daniel Gagnon, of Santa Fe, has worked out many of the specific indications.

TASTE:

bitter

TISSUE STATES:

atrophy, irritation

SPECIFIC INDICATIONS:

- Susceptibility to glamour (flower essence).
- Sleepless, frenetic children.
- Nervousness, inflammation of the skin.
- Sleep is not deep enough; waking during the night or too early in the morning.
- Sleep is too deep; children who sleep through the impulse to wake up and go to the bathroom (cf. *Verbascum, Aquilegia*).
- Tinnitus from listening to rock music.

PREPARATION AND DOSAGE:

Tincture made from the fresh plant in flower. "Take 20–40 drops one hour before sleep and again just before bedtime. For bed wetting, in children over five years old, use with horsetail, 10 drops of each twice a day" (Daniel Gagnon, 2000, 69).

CAUTIONS:

It is contraindicated during pregnancy, or while on an MAO inhibitor (Gagnon, 2000).

LITERATURE:

Traditional, Flower Essence Society (1), Daniel Gagnon (2–5), Matthew Wood (6).

Euonymus atropurpureus. Wahoo.

The name "wahoo" attests to the American Indian origins of the medicinal use of this plant. Beal P. Downing, who graduated from Dartmouth in 1805 and traveled extensively with the Indians of the "West" (that is, the Midwest), records it under a perhaps more original name, "wa-ahoo." It is a small bush, native to the Midwestern forests of North America, a member of the Celastraceae family (a kin to the great Indian blood purifier, bittersweet vine). A cousin, E. americana, *is better known in horticulture for its red leaves and is called "burning bush."*

Wahoo is one of the many plants that filled an important niche in nineteenth-century America as a remedy for the hepatic side effects of malaria (cf. *Chelone, Chionanthus, Podophyllum, Juglans,* etc.) but that is little used today. Our late friend, William LeSassier, esteemed it highly in liver affections, so it is still worth considering at the present time, though such affections arise from different causes. It contains some impressive chemicals—sterols, alkaloids, digitaloids, tannins, and volatile oils. The sterols probably stimulate the liver to greater activity, while the tannins check this mildly; thus, euonymus is known as a slow-acting laxative.

"This root bark is very largely relaxant, and moderately stimulant," writes William Cook (1869, 416), "quite slow in action, but very positive and reliable in its influence. Its principal power is expended upon the gall-ducts and liver, and from these upon the bowels; but it also exerts a gentle influence upon the stomach and the secretion of the kidneys. It is especially valued for its influence on the hepatic apparatus, for which (in its own kind) it has few equals and no superiors in the whole Materia Medica. It secures a persistent and not excessive discharge of bile, and leaves behind a very gentle tonic impression upon these organs" (from the presence of the tannins). "It is thus available in all cases of biliousness, chronic liver complaints, persistent constipation, and eruptions of the skin, where a slow and laxative hepatic is indicated." One would not normally use astringents in constipation. It "forms an excellent agent for the intermediate treatment of agues," or malaria, "and is valuable for its action on the biliary apparatus in dropsies, and many other actions where torpor and tension of the liver is a prominent trouble." As a slow evacuant it is "best suited for sub-acute and chronic cases" and is frequently combined with more stimulating agents such as hydrastis and gentiana.

Euonymus ought to have a cardiac impression, with its digitaloids. Indeed, Cherokee author J. T. Garrett (2003) records that it is an East Medicine, thus associated with the heart, and that it corrects irregular beats. An elder warned him that caution is necessary in the administration of wahoo, because of its cardiac activity, and that the seeds and fruits are poisonous.

TASTE:

bitter

TISSUE STATE:

stagnation

SPECIFIC INDICATIONS:

- Hepatic torpor—that is, sluggish biliary function with constipation, indigestion, coexistent lung and kidney ailments.
- Headache with indisposition to work, dark spots before the eyes, complexion muddy, urine dark.
- Tongue coated yellow; bad taste.
- Cough associated with biliousness, hepatic torpor.
- Loss of appetite, indigestion, and constipation dependent on hepatic torpor.
- Malaria with indigestion, biliousness, constipation, hepatic enlargement, jaundice.
- Habitual constipation from poor bile secretion (combine with *Juglans*).
- Edema, albuminuria.

- Rheumatism.
- Skin disorders.
- Breast complaints *(E. americana)*.

PREPARATION AND DOSAGE:

The Native American preference for the root bark is observed in the traditional application of this plant. The root bark is used by decoction, tincture, or fluid extract, administered in small doses, as large ones are irritating to the intestines; 1/2 fluid ounce of the decoction, 2–3x/day or 10–40 drops of the tincture; combine with ginger for hepatic torpor (Christopher, 1996, 220).

LITERATURE:

Traditional, William Cook, John Christopher, J. T. Garrett (11).

Eupatorium fistulosum, E. maculatum, E. purpureum. Gravel Root, Joe Pye Weed, Queen of the Meadow.

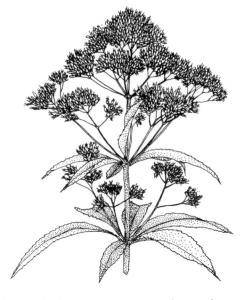

Gravel root is an Asteraceae native to low meadows, swamps, and the margins of waterways in eastern North America. It also grows on gravelly soil near such locations. I have seen it growing on the shores of stormy Lake Superior, its interwoven roots keeping the soil from washing away. It grows at the intersection of water and land, like all the great kidney stone remedies (gravel root, hydrangea, smartweed, marshmallow). Very often there will be calcifications on and around the roots. This caused it to be called gravel root and suggested its most famous use—gravel. It has properties similar to the European hemp agrimony (Eupatorium cannabinum), *which it resembles markedly in appearance*

and flavor. It also has bone-healing properties in common with its cousin boneset and antiseptic properties like white snake root. Indeed, it is an extraordinary antiseptic.

The habitat of gravel root suggests its major property: it is a superlative remedy for balancing liquids and solids. It keeps minerals from precipitating out of solution to produce arthritic deposits and kidney stones, but it also controls processes where the water gets out of control and there is excessive flux of water, blood, and even pus. Gravel root is an extremely important remedy for the kidneys, helping to maintain the balance between liquids and solids. It is said to dissolve calcareous matter and promote diuresis to pass the gravel. It protects the kidney membranes against passage of crystals through them, thus in diabetes mellitus it preserves or improves the function of the kidneys. As a warming stimulant it probably also mildly increases cellular activity and therefore uptake of blood sugar, thus reducing the effects of type II diabetes symptoms. In this disease it should be compared to *Rhus typhina* (sumach). It also maintains the balance between the liquids and solids in the menstrual sphere, suitable when there is excess bleeding with or between the periods.

Gravel root is supposed to have been first introduced to colonial American settlers by Joe Pye, an Indian medicine man, who used it as a specific for typhoid and "typhus fever" (low-grade, putrefactive fever). There was a time when nearly every New England homestead had gravel root in the garden for medicinal use. Its use in putrid conditions of the intestines and elsewhere is well established in the tradition, but this application has been largely forgotten in favor of the kidney applications. I have seen it stop Crohn's disease that was in the deadly, last phase where the intestine was abscessing and pus was already in the peritoneal fluids. In one case the surgeon commented on the fact that the abscess on the intestine had broken open but there was no peritonitis. Gravel root is the great enemy of pus. It may seem extraordinary to claim that any agent of any kind could act on peritonitis, but I have seen this repeatedly. And then, I found the indication given by John Skelton (1878, 97). I asked an experienced nurse how this was possible and she said, "I have been in a lot of operating rooms and I can tell you that the peritoneum has a powerful ability to flush itself and could be healed sometimes by natural means."

"Queen of the Meadow is useful in all ills of the joints, influencing aching or sprained back," writes Louise Tenney (1983, 104). "It is used for all strains and sprains and pulled liagments and tendons." It can free up a frozen joint. I believe it facilitates the flow of interstitial fluid out of the capillaries to lubricate the joints, tendons, muscles, and bones. As it makes them more supple it also decalcifies. In a sense, the liquid/solid balance it maintains in the renal sphere extends to the muscular and skeletal system. It breaks up calcification in the bones, yet heals broken bones like its cousin boneset *(Eupatorium perfoliatum)*. It is an old remedy for arthritis (cf. *Eupatorium cannabinum*). Its action on the female system is accounted for by its ability to tone the attachments to the uterus; improvement in the position of the uterus accounts for its importance in restoring fertility (indications from Darrell Martin, Biloxi, Mississippi).

The exclusively southern species, *Eupatorium fistulosum* (Queen of the Meadow), is used on the same indications as *E. purpureum*. "The root is a most powerful diuretic, and is the only part that I have ever used. For the suppression of urine and in the dropsy, I have found it beneficial" (Samuel Henry, 1814, 219).

The disparate uses of gravel root as a renal diuretic, a cleanser of the peritoneum, and a bone and joint healing remedy are all united by the fact that it increases the flushing action of porous tissue inside the body (it is not, however, used as a diaphoretic for the skin). It helps stiff joints and it should be considered in deterioration of the hip joint, since this flexure has a poorer circulation than most of the other joints of the body.

TASTE:

pungent, bitter

TISSUE STATES:

atrophy, depression, stagnation

SPECIFIC INDICATIONS:

MIND, SENSES, NERVES, EMOTIONS, PERSONALITY

- Fears related to loneliness; inability to form relationships (flower essence).
- Lack of will power; too easily dominated.

HEAD

- Headache, neuralgia.
- Ears; loss of hearing from calcification.

RESPIRATION

- Chronic cough, unduly prolonged whooping cough, asthma; with weak peripheral circulation.

DIGESTION

- *Enteritis, Crohn's disease, colitis, typhoid, peritonitis; even after the formation of pus and putrescence.*

LIVER AND GALLBLADDER

- Gallstones.

PANCREAS

- Diabetes mellitus, type II; preserves the kidneys, improves the uptake of sugar in the cells, invigorates, and prevents putrefaction.

KIDNEYS AND BLADDER

- *The remedy of choice* (with hydrangea and smartweed) *for passage of kidney stones* (hot decoction).
- *Preserves the filters of the kidneys under the stress of the passage of sugar crystals through the membranes.*
- Pain in the region of the kidneys; lower back pain from kidney troubles.
- Diabetes insipidus.
- Renal dropsy; edema following scarlatina.
- Albuminuria.
- Difficult and painful urination, the urine scanty and passing a few drops at a time; smarting and burning in the urethra; heat in the region of the kidneys; urine cloudy, loaded with mucus.
- Irritability of the bladder during pregnancy; constant desire to void urine, with urine passing with coughing.
- Urine scanty, dark, or mixed with blood and solids.

FEMALE
- *Uterine atony; prolapsus, retroversion; infertility, threatened miscarriage; spotting during the period, excessive flow.*
- Vaginitis with discharges and debility.

MALE
- Swollen prostate, impotence.

FEVER
- Fever with hot, dry, constricted skin.

MUSCULAR AND SKELETAL
- *Arthritis*, rheumatism, gout, *bursitis.*
- "All the ills of the joints, including aching or sprained back" (Louise Tenney).
- Bone weakness, broken bones (cf. *Eupatorium perfoliatum*).
- Frozen joint.

OTHER
- Poisoning by vapor inhalation.
- Spider bites, snake bites (cf. *Eupatorium rugosum*).
- Pus formation, putrefaction, peritonitis, typhoid, sepsis.
- *Ringworm.*

PREPARATION AND DOSAGE:

Fluid extract, 5–60 drops; decoction, hourly (Fyfe).

CAUTIONS:

Gravel root can cause kidney stones to pass in people who did not know they had them (Terry Willard). Prolonged doses can pump out the kidneys (Edwin Hale).

LITERATURE:

Traditional (9, 22), David Dalton (1), Frederick Locke (3, 11–21), Darrell Martin (18), Matthew Wood (2, 4–10, 23, 24, 25, 27, 28), John Skelton (28), Brent Davis (26), Jack Ritchason (5), Louise Tenney (3, 7, 8, 9, 11, 13, 20, 21, 22, 23, 29), Rolla Thomas (21).

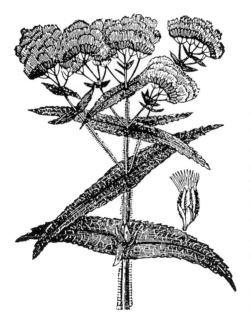

Eupatorium perfoliatum.
Boneset.

This is an important old Indian remedy native to North America but naturalized in Europe. The original Indian names translate into English as "agueweed" and "bone-repair" or "boneset." Eupatorium perfoliatum *was first introduced into professional medicine in 1810 by Dr. Anderson, physician at the New York City poorhouse, who used it as a substitute for quinine. It is widely stated in ethnobotanical literature that boneset was never used for bone setting, despite the name, but rather for fever with pain in the bones. However, boneset is widely used among the Indian people for setting bones.*

Boneset is indispensable in the northern climes for influenza. It is particularly suited to cases where there are marked chills intermitting with fever, with achiness in the bones. It is also appropriate where there is achiness but the chills are not marked and it is difficult to tell whether something is coming on, or one is really sick. Boneset brings the chill to a head and flushes it out of the system, whether it is well marked or not.

In the old days boneset was used not only for influenza but for the more severe chills of malaria. It was also used for the severe debility and exhaustion that set in after people had suffered a long time with the chills of malaria—the shaking running through the autonomic nervous system would wear out the constitution. It was also used for digestive debility in the elderly. In these cases, debility of the innervations and secretions of the gallbladder and digestive tract is particularly developed. Boneset stimulates deficient secretions from the gastrointestinal tract and liver, also making it mildly laxative. It is also useful for acne (Donald Law), a condition associated with liver stress. Boneset also gets secretion going in the lungs, when mucus is stuck and is not moving out.

Herbalist Matthew Becker says that boneset is useful for viral infections at the beginning, before the characteristic bone pains and periodic chills appear. He also uses it to slowly flush the liver and reduce the anger often associated with a congested liver. Boneset is suitable when there are vague fevers and chills, achiness and discomfort, where it is hard to tell whether one is sick or not. Herbalist Jennifer Tucker comments, "It is a wonderful herb for chilly, skinny-types. It is warming, a tonic, and they feel the influence on their digestion, and their bones and muscles feel stronger, and less achy."

Some self-appointed expert in the nineteenth century declared that boneset was not for setting bones, despite the name, but this is not true. It is one of the most important remedies for bone-setting in Native practice. I have ascertained this fact from members of a half dozen different Indian groups. Once when I was teaching at White Earth Reservation in northern Minnesota I noticed a picture of boneset with the English, Latin, and Anishinabe names. I asked what the Anishinabe name meant and one of the elders (a member of the Warren family) said, "Bone . . . to repair." At that moment I thought, "Yeah, sure, it's not for setting bones!" I gathered this traditional application from a retired Minnesota Supreme Court Justice, who grew up on the Kansas-Oklahoma border, so this usage is deeply established and widely spread in folk medicine.

In practice, boneset has turned out to be a superlative remedy for bone repair. Comfrey will seal bones together even when they are not correctly set and in the wrong place, but boneset will help bring them together into the right place and then set them from the inside out. When bones are broken they secrete chemicals that draw the pieces back together and there can be little doubt that boneset stimulates this process. A woman who had shattered the ball of the humerus, but not the socket, was told by the emergency room staff that they might have to amputate her arm at the shoulder. She took boneset for two weeks, plus Reiki energy healing, and a dose of comfrey before the operation. The fragments came back together perfectly. In addition to my own case histories, many more could be cited from Richard Reardon, a holistic practitioner in Pasadena, California.

The overall picture presented by boneset shows that it is almost certainly a remedy that normalizes androgen imbalance, especially on the excess side. This hormone heightens the immune response, stimulates bone growth, stresses the liver (hence producing anger), and often causes acne.

Boneset is a cousin of white snake root *(Eupatorium rugosum)* and like that remedy may be used to treat the bites of "venomous animals."

Samuel Henry (1814, 37) recounts, "As I was travelling from the Creek nation of Indians, a young man had been bit by a rattlesnake's pilot; and after walking a little distance his leg began to pain him and swell. He was ordered to pound the leaves of boneset and apply it over the wound, and to drink a gill of the juice of the herb, which cured him in the space of two hours. He went to a ball the same night, and felt no inconvenience from the exercise of dancing."

When I can't get white snake root I use boneset or gravel root for spider bites. I paid back my Anishinabe friends at White Earth Reservation who taught me about the true origin of the name boneset by recommending they use boneset, gravel root, St. John's wort, and plantain on a spider bite that was poisoning the blood—the wound turned purple and red streaks were running up the arm. By morning only a small spot was left.

TASTE:

bitter, acrid • aromatic

TISSUE STATES:

depression, constriction

SPECIFIC INDICATIONS:

MIND, SENSES, NERVES, EMOTIONS, PERSONALITY
- Anger; tantrums; changeable, fickle moods.

HEAD
- Acne.

RESPIRATION
- Old bronchial catarrh settled in the lungs, with atonic mucosa and lack of cough reflex; especially in old people, debilitated cases.

DIGESTION
- Indigestion in old people.

LIVER AND GALLBLADDER
- Biliousness, jaundice, acid reflux, indigestion, exhaustion; *after malaria.*

MUSCULAR AND SKELETAL
- *Crushing pains in the bones;* aches in the muscles.
- *Broken bones, crushed bones;* damage to connective tissue.
- *Osteoporosis, osteomalachia;* recalcifies bone.
- Multiple sclerosis; rebuilds the myelin sheaths.

FEVER
- *Influenza; chill returning at regular intervals with crushing, aching pain in the bones.*
- *Influenza; chills very indistinct; can't tell if sick or not; beginning of the illness.*
- Measles, mumps, scarlet fever, yellow fever, typhoid fever, Rocky Mountain spotted fever.
- "Full pulse, full skin, tendency to perspiration even during the fever" (Rolla Thomas).

PREPARATION AND DOSAGE:

Warm or tepid infusion for fever and chill. Pour 1 pint of boiling water over a handful of fresh roots, set until cool. Go to bed and sweat (Ralph Russell). Cold infusion as a bitter tonic. Tincture, 1–25 drops.

LITERATURE:

Traditional (3–7, 11–13), homeopathic provings and clinical use (3, 5, 6, 7, 8, 11, 12), Matthew Becker (1, 13), Richard Reardon (1, 7–9), Donald Law (2), Louise Tenney (3, 4, 5, 10, 12), Matthew Wood (6, 7, 10, 11), Phyllis Light (7), Keewaydinoquay (7), Tommie Bass (7), Paul Red Elk (1, 7), Sondra Boyd (7), Rolla Thomas (13).

Fraxinus americana. American Ash, White Ash.

Fraxinus americana suddenly appears in the writings of Dr. Compton Burnett (1840–1901) with no introduction and to this day no one is sure where he got the remedy. I did find that the burnt ash of white ash was successfully used by Thomas Palmer, of Middleborough, Massachusetts, for prolapsed uterus before 1696 (this was probably a Native American remedy), but his medical notes were not published until seventy-five years after Compton Burnett died.

Compton Burnett's case is rather dramatic. A woman is brought to see him for a "hugely hypertrophied uterus, that was so much in excess of the space Nature had for its storage, that the unfortunate lady could do nothing whatever, and it was hardly possible to even keep the immense mass somewhat propped up with the aid of a very large pessary." Surgery was planned, but Compton Burnett talked the woman out of the procedure. He gave *Fraxinus* in 5-, 6-, and 7-drop doses, and her uterus slowly shrank back to its normal size. "In seven weeks the patient could, and actually did, go to Scotland ... and was running about on the Scottish moors, rejoicing in her new-found liberty." "Nobody can understand it," commented a relative.

"An infusion of white ash bark has been much used in cases where an astringent tonic was deemed necessary; it also proves cathartic, and has been found useful in constipation, especially of dropsical subjects." That would be cases where the water is building up and is not being evacuated. "It has received much praise in mastitis, and enlargement of the spleen, as well as in some forms of eczema, and in gouty affections. There is a belief extant in the South that the seeds prevent accumulation of fat" (Millspaugh, 1892, 549).

"It is highly recommended as a remedy in uterine engorgements, and in bad cases of subinvolution and prolapsus of the uterus," in plethoric (full) conditions of the uterus, congestive dysmenorrhea, "in conditions characterized by heavy, dragging sensations in the lower part of the abdomen, and a feeling as if the uterus would fall out of the pelvis," when the uterus is "large, soft, and doughy, and a slight touch causes sharp pain," in irregularity of the menses, "and in wrongs in which there is constant headache, with soreness in a circumscribed spot on the head, and which feels hot" (Fyfe, 1909, 545).

TISSUE STATES:

relaxation, atrophy

SPECIFIC INDICATIONS:

- General debility and cachectic conditions.
- Dropsical conditions.
- Enlargement of the spleen.
- Constipation due to retention of water in the tissues.
- Dyspepsia, atonic.
- Uterus; prolapsed, enormously swollen, hemorrhaging; with backache.
- Uterus; atonic, enlarged, soft, doughy, prolapsed, subinvolution; heavy, dragging sensations in the lower abdomen; sharp pain on touch; feeling as if the uterus would fall out of the pelvis, or actual protrusion.

PREPARATION AND DOSAGE:

In small doses it is tonic, alterative, and astringent, whereas in large ones it is purgative. This, of course, depends on the sensitivity of the patient. Dosage: 5–30 drops of the fluid extract (Fyfe).

LITERATURE:

James Compton Burnett (1, 6), Charles Millspaugh (2, 3, 4), John William Fyfe (1–5, 7), John Hauser (6-confirmed).

Geranium maculatum.
Wild Geranium, Crane's Bill.

Wild geranium is native to the forests of eastern North America. The root is intensely astringent.

Crane's bill is a powerful astringent. It not only checks excessive secretion from the mucosa, but it improves the quality of the secretion. It acts strongly on the mucosa of the mouth, stomach, large intestine, lungs, and sexual-urinary

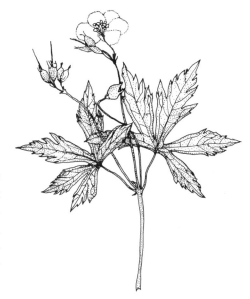

tract. It is perhaps the archetypal remedy for catarrhal gastritis. "A very efficient medicament in all cases characterized by profuse fluxes, whether of mucus, blood or serum. These often occur in chronic or sub-acute diseases. It is a most excellent remedial agent in many cases of diarrhea, especially when there is frequent watery stools and a constant desire to evacuate the bowels" (Fyfe, 1909, 551).

TASTE:

extremely styptic or astringent

TISSUE STATE:

relaxation

SPECIFIC INDICATIONS:

CONSTITUTION, COMPLEXION, CHARACTERISTIC SYMPTOMS

- People who have lost a part of their essence; people who depend on prescription or recreational drugs to function and have lost the ability to function on their own; people in recovery from drug addiction.
- Helps to separate people who have been closely connected after the failure of a marriage, relationship, or friendship.
- Helps mothers separate themselves from children.
- Children who fail to thrive due to a wet, mucusy stomach that impedes digestion.
- *Relaxed membranes with profuse discharges, usually with much mucus.*

RESPIRATION

- Nosebleed; nasal polypi (external).
- Relaxation of the mucosa of the throat; canker sores; tongue coated white and moist.
- Tuberculosis with profuse expectoration, teasing cough, bloody sputum and night sweats.

DIGESTION

- Dampness in the stomach; swishing and watery sounds.
- Peptic and duodenal ulcers with excess mucus discharge, with or without passive bleeding; lessens the vomiting in gastric ulcer.
- Catarrhal gastritis with profuse secretion, tendency to ulceration and passive hemorrhage.
- Acute and chronic diarrhea and dysentery, cholera infantum; after the fever has subsided but the tone of the intestines allows frequent, profuse, and debilitating stool with mucus discharges.
- *Constant desire to go to stool, with inability to pass anything for some time; with chronic diarrhea, with offensive mucus; constipation.*
- Hemorrhoids; prolapsus ani (internal and external).

KIDNEYS AND BLADDER

- Restores the essence of the kidneys (external).
- Urine loaded with mucus and blood.

FEMALE

- Uterine bleeding; menorrhagia, metrorrhagia; postpartum hemorrhage.
- Pelvic atonicity with leucorrhea, gleet.

SKIN AND WOUNDS

- Externally on bruises of various kind, especially "black eyes."
- Ulcers and bedsores (external; dilute 1:10 in olive oil).
- Passive hemorrhages from the lungs, stomach, colon, bladder, uterus.

PREPARATION AND DOSAGE:

The root is used; the stems and leaves have a different taste and properties.

LITERATURE:

Traditional, Rolla Thomas (13), Matthew Wood (1, 2, 4, 9), Julia Graves (3, 15), Yadubir Sinha (6, 14, 20).

Geum rivale, G. virginianum.
Water Avens, Chocolate Root.

These two avens cousins are native to low ground in eastern North America. They contain clove oil in the root, like the European "city avens" (see the Old World volume of The Earthwise Herbal*), and have almost identical properties to that plant, as a review of the American and British sources indicates.*

William Cook (1869, 449) points out that water avens or chocolate root has a unique niche in the pharmacopoeia that is apt to be overlooked. "Its action on the duodenum and mesenteries fits it for a class of cases to which few articles are applicable; and I am decidedly of the opinion that it will be found useful in tabes mesenterica, and in those forms of scrofulous looseness of the bowels which are dependent upon defective assimilation, and which often pass roughly as chronic diarrhea. This distinction between tonics to the digestive and to the assimilative apparatus, is one that has not heretofore been made; but it is one of importance, and those which act on the assimilative organs are so few as to deserve especial notice."

The root is a mild astringent, but it is "not so drying as it is strengthening to the mucous membranes." It is used in the inactive stage of dysentery and diarrhea, following active infection, where a tonic is needed (see Samuel Henry's use under *Geum urbanum* in the Old World volume of *The Earthwise Herbal*), and in similar conditions such as leucorrhea, mucus in the urine, spitting of blood, passive menstrual bleeding, and canker sores. "In those forms of indigestion which arise from debility of the duodenum, pancreas, and mesenteries—connected with pains and laxity of the bowels, curdy stools, and slow loss of flesh."

Samuel Henry (1814, 26) learned of a secret remedy for consumption from "Mrs. Shaw" called "Indian chocolate." "Powders of avens root, two ounces, arum root [*Arum triphylum*], skunk cabbage, American ginseng, and masterwort [*Angelica atropurpurea*], each half an ounce, sugar, one ounce. Mix one tablespoonful and boil in one quart of water and one pint of new milk for an hour." "In debilitating complaints, or beginning consumptions, the patient may take two tea-cups of this chocolate, morning and evening, sweetened with loaf sugar, and ride out every day, for two hours, before dinner," an activity that stimulates the lymphatics. "Thus I have made public a secret, with some valuable additions, which will be of great utility to the community."

Geum triflorum. Prairie Smoke, Prairie Avens.

Avens is a genus in the rose family. In North America we have three major representatives: clove root or city avens (naturalized on overused and urbanized land), water avens (native to moist woods), and prairie smoke (native to the western and northern prairies). All three of them have the distinctive clove flavor due to the presence of eugenol. They have properties similar to their cousins agrimony and potentilla as astringents for pain and torsion. The roots contain phenols, tannins, and essential oils (including eugenol). Prairie smoke and water avens have an affinity to the female system; the latter for stagnant blood (Francis Bonaldo).

The leaves and flowers of the beautiful little prairie avens are used by Native American people for inflammation and torsion of the ovary (Paul Red Elk, Yako Tahnahgah). One can hardly look at the mature red flower hanging down without thinking of an inflamed ovary! The root in decoction was used by other Native people for washing sore and inflamed eyes, sore throats, sore nipples from nursing, coughs, saddle sores, children's cankers, chapped lips, chicken pox, diarrhea, loss of flesh (convalescence), externally to stop bleeding, and on stiff, sore muscles and joints. The root decocted in water, with a little bit of vinegar, produces the oil of cloves smell (Robert Dale Rogers, 2000, 52).

Gillenia trifoliata. Bowman's Root.

This is an unusual member of the rose family because it is emetic and cathartic. It was used by the Indians for this purpose, hence the name "Indian physic." It grows in the Alleghenies and westwards, so it probably entered American folk practice about the beginning of the eighteenth century. It became well established among the common people as a "physic." Samuel Henry (1814) used Gillenia *and it was put to use by other professional physicians in the early to mid-nineteenth century. It was largely forgotten by the end of the century. It is not generally used today, so constituents have not been isolated.*

Gillenia was primarily used as an emetic. Vomiting was followed by free perspiration, which was relieving in the presence of fever. It was also used as a purgative in sluggish disposition of the bowels. As an emetic, it was especially used in the beginnings of fever, colds, pneumonia, asthma, and whooping cough, like *Lobelia* or the emetics of Ayurvedic practice. Dr.

William Cook (1869, 449) reports that large doses (20–25 grains) cause catharsis, larger doses (30 grains) bring on vomiting, while small doses (2–5 grains) promote digestion. The "vomiting induced by it is followed by free and warm perspiration, distinct softening of the pulse, and often by mild catharsis; and it may be used in this way to advantage in recent colds, catarrhal fever, and at the commencement of bilious fever, and pneumonia."

Cook notes that the root is "relaxing and stimulating, acting rather promptly; and chiefly influencing the skin and mucous membranes." It "acts favorably on the skin in securing diaphoresis, when small quantities are given in warm infusion with asclepias and zingiber; and its relaxing qualities make such an employment of it good in securing relief from congestion and arterial excitement in most forms of fever."

Samuel Henry (1814, 59) recommended *Gillenia* in asthmatic coughs, difficulty breathing, and the whooping cough of children.

SPECIFIC INDICATIONS:

- Incipient colds.
- Respiratory congestion with phlegm and fever (cf. *Lilium longiflorum*).
- Asthmatic coughs and difficulty breathing (cf. *Agrimonia*, a botanical cousin).
- Whooping cough in children.
- Incipient pneumonia.
- Indigestion; sluggish bowels.
- Fever; congestion of blood and arterial excitement; lack of perspiration; rapid, high, hard pulse.
- Commencement of bilious fever (that is, indigestion with chills and fever).

PREPARATION AND DOSAGE:

See Cook, above.

LITERATURE:

Traditional, William Cook (1, 2, 5, 6, 7, 8), Samuel Henry (3, 4).

Gnaphalium obtusifolium.
Sweet Everlasting, Rabbit Tobacco.

The properties of most of the everlastings (Gnaphalium spp., Antennaria spp., Anaphalis spp., Helichrysum spp.) seem to be relatively similar, except for Gnaphalium dioecum *(also known as* Antennaria dioica*). They are aromatic astringents with a slight bitterness, whereas the last is predominantly bitter. Members of the composite family, they have been used to a small extent in western European medicine since the time of Dioscorides and Plinius, but more widely in the traditional practice and modern medicine of Russia. The most prominent American species is* Gnaphalium obtusifolium. *It has the most beautiful aroma of any of the American everlastings. Known as sweet everlasting or rabbit tobacco, it has long held a place of great respect in North American Indian medicine. It entered into pioneer American folk medicine but has by now been largely forgotten. Properties are similar to marsh everlasting, the species used in Russian medicine.*

Rabbit tobacco was used by the Indians of the eastern seaboard and quickly passed into the knowledge of the early colonial settlers as a remedy for injuries and as a sweet-scented posy to be placed around the house. It is still an important Cherokee medicine. It is said that rabbit discovered the medicinal properties of this plant when he got tangled up in a briar in the mountains. He learned that it was good for sprains, strains, cuts, and wounds. Another observation is that the skin of a rabbit is thin and easily damaged. If a rabbit is chased by a big dog, even for a short distance, the skin can tear and bleed. Yet another story is that the old people noticed that the rabbits liked to congregate where rabbit tobacco grew, so they realized it was their tobacco for contacting the Creator. It is used by some as a tobacco (inadvisedly say others) and as a lung remedy.

Another name for rabbit tobacco is owl's crown. This derives from the pale, brown, tawny colors of the plant and the tufts of flowers, which have the color of an owl and the appearance of tufts on an owl's head. The name also recognizes the relationship between owl and one of its most important food sources, rabbit. More deeply, it refers to the relationship that this plant has with the dead—owl, messenger of the Underworld. Rabbit tobacco is specifically used when the dead have a message for the living and cannot get through. It is a "walker between the worlds" (Paul Red Elk). It will release both the living and the dead from an unfinished relationship. In more materialistic terms it is an important remedy, in my experience, for congenital or inherited problems. It is also for people who are too open to psychic or emotional vibes from others. On a purely physiological level it opens and normalizes the pores of the skin and internal membranes.

As a remedy, rabbit tobacco is especially suited to lifelong and congenital asthmatics. It is almost always indicated in respiratory disease when the complexion is pale, from lack of oxygen, and also often a little tawny or slightly brown. It opens up the lung passages and helps these people to feel like they are getting enough oxygen. As one of them said, "I feel half dead, like I am not totally in my body." It helps them come more fully into incarnation in the world and also soothes the fear associated with exposure to the world. As another asthmatic said, "It soothes my small animal self."

I first learned about rabbit tobacco from a woman in Virginia who had been raised on a mountain farm in the days when doctors were unaffordable. She had asthma from birth to age seven. A kindly neighboring man picked some rabbit tobacco and his wife sewed it into a pillow. They gave it to her to be her very own—a child in a big family on a mountain farm doesn't grow up with much of her own. She slept with it for a year until it was in tatters. At that time she was completely cured. Knowing the difficulty in curing asthma from birth, I considered this to be a remarkable case history and began to use rabbit tobacco in chronic and lifelong asthmatic patients. It is far more than an expectorant, as some sources relate, because it opens up and deepens the respiration.

More recently, I have found this remedy very soothing for celiac sprue, another congenital condition, and for autoimmune excess conditions, which are very often from birth or near birth. Proven by iritis.

TASTE:

sweet, pungent • warm, dry • aromatic

TISSUE STATES:

depression, atrophy

SPECIFIC INDICATIONS:

- *Pale, dark, gray, yellowish, tawny complexion.*
- *Nervous, fearful, though not readily perceptible.*
- Headache; specific for migraine.
- Sinusitis.
- Quinsy, tonsillitis.
- *Asthma.*
- Lack of appetite.
- Gastrointestinal problems with colic and spasms; internal bleeding from intestine; celiac sprue.
- Diarrhea, dysentery.
- Kidneys; loss of fluids; diabetes.
- Impotence.
- Excessive menstrual bleeding.
- Sciatica.
- Fresh cuts with profuse bleeding.
- Strains and sprains.

PREPARATION AND DOSAGE:

Rabbit tobacco is one of the only plants picked after the season is over and the plant is dead. The flower tops retain their sweet aroma. An infusion, smoking tobacco, or tincture can be made from them. The chemical properties are not fully developed until after the plant dies, according to a spectro-chromatograph study by Alabama herbalist Dwight Collier.

LITERATURE:

Traditional American Indian use (2–15), Matthew Wood (1, 2, 6, 8, 9), Tommie Bass (3–6), homeopathic provings and clinical experience (7, 10, 11, 13), Dwight Collier (4, 5, 6).

Grindelia robusta. Gumweed.

The various gumweeds are native to California and the Great Plains, east to about the Mississippi River. They prefer the heavily alkaline soils found in the West. The common name refers to the sticky resin that coats the green parts of the plant and protects it against water loss and insects. The picture of stickiness is reinforced by the hooks on the underside of the corolla. The grindelias are used for sticky, dried phlegm. They also have produced (and cured) symptoms of respiratory arrest. Hence, they are used in bronchitis, asthma, and sleep apnea. G. robusta is native to California. It is the original plant introduced into settler medicine from Indian usage as an antidote for poison oak. G. squarrosa grows as far east as the Mississippi. It has similar uses. They are members of the aster family.

Grindelia is resinous, and like most such remedies it brings up mucus and acts as an expectorant; in this case it has been used for dried-out, sticky phlegm. In addition it acts on the nerves of respiration, first to depress them in toxic doses, and then to stimulate them in moderate ones. It is not very toxic, but in cases that have terminated fatally from overdoses of *Grindelia robusta* "respiration becomes slower, jerky, and death results from arrest of respiration" (Petersen, 1905, 100). These must have been overdoses caused by the use of gumweed as a medicine, since no one would eat it in large amounts—it tastes like a petroleum distillate, or some kind of "sweet turpentine."

To continue with Petersen: "In full and frequent doses it is an excellent remedy in asthmatic breathing, producing expectoration, and its continued use in smaller doses will remove the entire train of symptoms. May be combined with other indicated remedies such as lobelia, yerba santa, or stramonium to advantage. Its influence on asthmatic breathing is more permanent than any other agent. It is not indicated in spasmodic asthma with complete relief between the attacks," for which lobelia would be more appropriate.

"Applied locally and used internally it is a fine remedy in rhus tox poisoning. Locally applied to old, indolent ulcers it gives good results." I remember a terrible case of red, itching, burning rash all over the torso and arms that was relieved by grindelia tincture, externally and internally. The waves of heat coming off the body after giving the medicine were noticeable. The young man was grateful as he was to be married in a week!

TASTE:

warm • stimulating, resinous

SPECIFIC INDICATIONS:

RESPIRATION
- Acute bronchitis leaving behind dried-out, sticky phlegm, difficult to raise.
- Chronic bronchial cough of spasmodic nature.
- *Asthma; labored respiration with dusky flushing of face, in plethoric (full) persons* (1 dram to 2 ounces of syrup).
- Irregular heart action if accompanying chronic coughs; pneumonia; and chronic coughs that often follow pneumonia.

OTHER
- Vaginitis, applied locally.
- Poison ivy, applied locally.
- Old atonic ulcers; tissues full (1–2 drams in 4 ounces water, as a local application).

PREPARATION AND DOSAGE:

Infusion: dried flower tops, 1 teaspoon to 1 cup of boiling water, cover and steep until cool (Rogers). Tincture: 5 drops every 15–30 minutes during coughing paroxysms until the spasm is relieved (Yadubir Sinha; Ralph M. Russell). Three times/day when the cough is less intense (Sinha).

LITERATURE:

Traditional (see Kelly Kinsher for California Indian uses), Frederick Petersen (1, 2, 4, 5, 6), Rolla Thomas (3, 7).

Grindelia squarrosa. Gumweed.

Indications for *Grindelia squarrosa* are similar to those for *G. robusta*. Toxicologically, "interruption of respiration takes place, so that it can sometimes only be carried on by will power," noted Petersen (1905, 101). (Hence, this has been used as a remedy for sleep apnea in homeopathy.) "It is the remedy for chronic or old cases of malaria, malarial cachexia, splenic hypertrophy, stomach troubles, neuralgia, irritable coughs with nervous erethism, the result of malaria. It must be continued for some time to effect a cure. In sore and painful eyes, pain worse on movement from cold, it is of value. Locally in skin disease it may be used with glycerine." It is certainly effective in poison ivy, like its cousin.

SPECIFIC INDICATIONS:

- "A pale, puffy appearance of tissue, pain in the right or left hypochondriac region, enlarged spleen or liver, chills and fever, pain in the eyes, dull pain in the head, determination of the blood to the head, in fact any of these conditions if caused by malarial poison" (Petersen).
- "Pain in hepatic and splenic regions, especially effective in enlarged spleen; puffiness of the tissues, and pallidity of skin and mucous membranes" (Rolla Thomas).
- Sleep apnea.
- Skin lesions, wounds, cuts, abrasions, etc. (equal to *Calendula;* Michael Moore).
- Poison ivy (external).

LITERATURE:

Frederick Petersen, Rolla Thomas, Finley Ellingwood, William Boericke.

Guaiacum officinale. Guaiac Bark.

The bark of this large tree, native to the West Indies and Central America, early passed from indigenous use into trade as a medicine for arthritic complaints. It was widely used in allopathy and herbal medicine until fairly recently. The wood is exceptionally hard—ship propellers were made from it. The chips of the wood and the resin have been used, the former acting more slowly than the latter, but in a similar manner. Dorothy Hall likens the hard wood to the hard arthritic joints for which this plant is remedial.

Guaiacum is especially useful for persons suffering from cold, damp, inactive extremities with arthritis or fibromyalgia (formerly called rheumatism). When given warm, or with warmth, it arouses a gentle, outward circulation to the capillaries and opens the pores of the skin; given cold, it runs through the kidneys and influences the womb in chronic obstructive conditions.

William Cook (1869, 458) specifies the conditions and persons in which it is indicated and contraindicated: "The resin is an active stimulant, quite local in action, exciting to the stomach and slowly so to the remote circulation, and elevating all the secretory organs by increasing their sensibility and capillary flow. Such qualities at once interdict its use in any case of irritated stomach or bowels, acute forms of dyspepsia, and febrile or inflammatory conditions. Nor is it an agent that should be resorted to for sensitive or plethoric persons, nor for those inclined to pulmonary or uterine hemorrhage. It is best fitted for phlegmatic and leuco-phlegmatic patients [heavy, damp, cold, *kapha*-type constitutions], and for maladies where the stomach is depressed and the general activity of the system much reduced [cold, depressive]."

"Acute tonsillitis, and in amenorrhea and dysmenorrhea when due to atony of the pelvic viscera—20 drops to 1 dram in 4 ounces water" (Rolla Thomas, 1903).

Hamamelis virginiana. Witch Hazel.

Witch hazel is a beautiful small tree or large shrub native to eastern North America, but widely planted elsewhere because it flowers in November, when every other plant has given up. The bark contains an astringent that entered into use in the colonial era and is still widely utilized. It addition it contains saponins and flavonoids. The sticks are used for "witching water."

Witch hazel is usually classified as a mild astringent used to soothe and tone varicose veins, hemorrhoids, and skin problems. John William Fyfe (1909, 562) writes that it "exerts a special influence upon the veins, facilitating the flow of blood toward the heart. It causes contraction of the veins, and is employed in diseases characterized by venous dilatation. In hemorrhoids, when there is fullness of the part with heaviness and downward pressure." If the return venous circulation from the mucosa is stagnant, the mucous membranes can become swollen and relaxed. Therefore, witch hazel "is a valuable remedy where we have an enfeebled mucous surface, indicated by the relaxed, swollen, and thickened surface, evidencing feeble vitality and sluggish circulation. Hence, it is an admirable remedy in acute catarrh when secretion is established; in chronic catarrh, chronic pharyngitis and tonsillitis, when the child's voice is husky or flat; in chronic bronchitis, with free secretion; in mucus diarrhea, abundant urine, but painful micturition; in hemorrhoids, prolapsus ani, otorrhea, sprains, bruises, atonic inflammations, etc. Remembering that it strengthens and improves the venous circulation, freeing parts from congestion and giving them tone, we can hardly go astray in its use."

Witch hazel flowers in November, out of season, hence the use as a flower essence for feeling out of sync (Julia Graves). Some cardiovascular conditions are characterized by a lack of sync between the arterial and venous circulation. Dorothy Hall (1988, 261) addresses this problem in her discussion of rue. "Ideally, when any circulatory adjustment is called for, it is advisable to balance both veins and arteries together to avoid change in one causing uneven rhythms in the other." Sluggish venous circulation may put a burden on the kidneys and heart, she continues, and this is even more troublesome if there is a circulatory fault in the arterial side as well. "One half of the blood going too fast and the other half too slowly means that pressure 'walls' will occur, with risk of rupture of vessels both minor and major."

TASTE:

astringent, slightly sweet, slightly sour • cooling, drying

TISSUE STATE:

relaxation

SPECIFIC INDICATIONS:

CONSTITUTION, COMPLEXION, CHARACTERISTIC SYMPTOMS

- Relaxation, pallor and fullness of the mucosa; abundant mucus discharge; acute catarrh, ozena, pharyngitis, laryngitis, bronchitis, tonsillitis, when the tissues are relaxed and the discharges are copious.
- Veins full, feeble, inclined to dilation, varicosities and passive hemorrhage hemoptysis, hematuria, epistaxis, excessive menstrual bleeding, puerperal hemorrhage.
- "Thickening of mucous membranes, with enfeebled circulation and increased secretion, either mucus or muco-purulent" (Scudder).
- Tissues soft, feeble, relaxed, swollen.

MIND, SENSES, NERVES, EMOTIONS, PERSONALITY
- Out of sync with people, places, and things; jet lag, recent household moves, culture shock (flower essence).

RESPIRATION
- Swollen tonsils, spongy throat, mucus discharge from nose.

DIGESTION
- Ulceration of the stomach and intestines.
- Gastrointestinal irritability in the later stages of tuberculosis.
- Abraded and inflamed mucosa.
- Child persistently throws up food, mixed with mucus.
- Diarrhea, with large, light-colored discharges, and prolapsus ani.
- *Hemorrhoids, when the venous circulation is enfeebled.*
- Abdomen full and doughy, with relaxation of the perineum, prolapse of the bowels; fullness about the anus, prolapsus ani, difficult evacuation of feces; swelling of vulva or prepuce.

SEXUAL
- Pain in the testicles and ovaries, produced by congestion.
- Hot flashes.

LOWER EXTREMITIES
- Edema of legs.

SKIN
- Locally for various forms of eczema and other skin diseases; bruises and wounds, hemorrhoids, varicose veins, aphthous sore mouth.

PREPARATION AND DOSAGE:

The bark has long been used, but Samuel Thomson, who was acquainted with this remedy from childhood, used the leaves. Organizes and directs other herbs in a formula (herbalist Ginny LoJacono of Virginia).

LITERATURE:

Traditional, John Scudder (3), Julia Graves (5), Dan Kenner and Yves Requena (15).

Hedeoma pulegioides. American Pennyroyal.

This is the American pennyroyal, in distinction to the European penny-royal (Mentha pulegium), *which has similar properties. They possess tannins, bitters, and volatile oils (including pulegone, borneol, camphor, and limonene).*

From the presence of limonene, pennyroyal tea has a sort of tart flavor, which speaks of its cooling or refrigerant properties. It is also slightly bitter and astringent, and diffusively stimulating, like other *Menthas.* Thus, it is somewhat similar to peppermint, both warming and cooling, antispasmodic and diaphoretic—but more active on the female system. Pulegone is a uterine vasodilator. As a diaphoretic, it brings rashes to the surface (scarlatina, measles, smallpox), and cools fever with intermittent chills. It relaxes the lungs, settles cough, brings up mucus, settles the digestive tract, soothes nausea and vomiting, relaxes the intestine, helps pass urinary calculi, and relaxes the uterus.

Michael Moore (2003, 191) describes the actions in the female sphere. He recommends "larger quantities of the tea—from a generous tablespoon to one-half ounce of the dried herb, steeped in an appropriate amount of water." This is a "sure and safe menstrual stimulant, particularly when the period has been delayed several days" with sensations of bloating, or when it becomes scanty and painful. "When there is a short and inadequate progesterone phase (many causes, even a cold), the secretory glands whose maturation it stimulates may be unable to invest menses with anticoagulants, antimicrobial enzymes, and simple mucus volume." This results in clots, slow onset, and cramps. The tea or tincture helps the uterine lining "liquefy and flow." In short, "pennyroyal is for the Period-from-Hell."

The oil was formerly used as an abortifacient, and proved dangerous enough to have established a record of mortality among woman (see John H. Clarke, 1962, for accounts of mortal poisonings). Michael Moore (2003) believes, from observational data, that pennyroyal herb is not an abortifacient, but merely a remedy for delayed menses. Pennyroyal should never be used, either in concentrated or in small doses, as an abortifacient. Nor should it be taken during pregnancy. It can, on the other hand, be used for delayed menses. And it can be taken at birthing time to stimulate and regulate healthy contractions—a cup or two.

TASTE:

sour • cool, dry • diffusive, astringent, bitter

TISSUE STATE:

constriction

SPECIFIC INDICATIONS:

HEAD
- Toothache (palliative).
- Earache.

RESPIRATION
- Colds, catarrh, bronchitis, pneumonia, pleurisy, tuberculosis.
- Cold with fever and chills (tea at the start).

DIGESTION
- Lack of appetite.
- Stomach; colic or ache in small children (tea).
- Indigestion, nausea, vomiting, intestinal spasm.
- Splenitis.

FEMALE
- Cervical ulceration, genital itch.
- PMS.
- Cold delaying menses.
- Menstruation: delayed, with bloating, scanty flow, and pain.
- Menstruation: slow onset, clots, cramps.
- Uterine fibroids.

FEVER AND SKIN
- Influenza; alternating chills and fever.
- Fever; brings out a sweat (tea of the whole plant).
- Brings rashes to the surface (scarlatina, measles, smallpox).
- Insect repellent.

PREPARATION AND DOSAGE:

Herb (aerial parts) as an infusion; 2–4 ounces, up to 5x/day. Tincture of the fresh plant, 1:2: even a few drops will cause diaphoresis, though the standard dosage is 20–60 drops in hot water (Michael Moore, 2003).

CONTRAINDICATIONS:

Not to be taken during pregnancy. Not to be taken as an abortifacient. Not to be taken for chronic menstrual cramping or irregularity, but rather for occasional incidents (Michael Moore, 2003).

LITERATURE:

Traditional, Michael Moore (4, 6, 11, 12, 13, 15, 16).

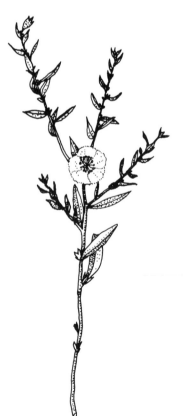

Helianthemum canadense, Cistus canadense. Frostweed, Scrofulawort, Rock Rose.

This little plant is seldom used today but was formerly an important remedy in the treatment of lymphatic conditions. It is generally known as rock rose in horticulture. The name frostweed refers to the fact that frost crystals form on the stalk and spread outward. The name scrofulawort is perhaps most important for us; it reflects the folk medical usage in lymphatic conditions. It is classified as Cistus canadense *in the homeopathic materia medica. In addition to being an important remedy for scrofula it is also important for what we would call compromised immunity (cf.* Scrophularia*).*

"This new discovered plant grows in the woods on Long-Island, and plentifully in New-Jersey," writes Samuel Henry (1814, 126). And indeed, in my copy of William

Buchan's *Domestic Medicine* dated 1779, belonging to my ancestors, Edmund Prior and Thomas Pearsall, of Oyster Bay, Long Island, is a recipe for using "frostwort" to make a salve for scrofula.

"Its principal employment is in those forms of scrofula where there is a tendency to diarrhea, with impurities dependent upon the absorption of ill-vitalized nutriment," writes William Cook (1869, 463), and "in chronic diarrhea, epithelial ulceration of the bowels, and aphthous sores of a light grade, it is a serviceable agent."

Jethro Kloss refers to *Helianthemum* as a valuable remedy long used in scrofula, taken both internally and externally. It is an "excellent gargle for cankered sore throat and scarlatina. Good for diarrhea, syphilis and gonorrhea. Superior remedy for cancer" (Kloss). *Helianthemum* is suited to putrid, septic conditions of the glands of the neck, poisoned wounds, bites, and putrid ulceration and is considered a specific in mononucleosis (William Boericke).

Since diarrhea is most commonly associated with relaxation, syphilis with atrophy, gonorrhea with torpor, and pus production with depression, frostweed is suited to a combination of the most deteriorated and run-down tissue conditions.

Juliette de Bairacli Levy (1973, 121) writes that rock rose *(Helianthemum canadense)* is "considered good for infants, to cure their fears and give them courage." She adds that "for children (and for adults, if desired) an ancient remedy for timidity involves steeping flowers of rock rose in sunlight and moonlight for two or three days, using preferably a shallow glass dish. At early morning and before bedtime, a teaspoonful of the dish's contents is taken." This bears close resemblance to Dr. Bach's use of rock rose flower essence for extreme fear. If this is an "ancient remedy," then the reference would be to an Old World rock rose.

TISSUE STATES:

depression, torpor, relaxation

SPECIFIC INDICATIONS:

CONSTITUTION, COMPLEXION, CHARACTERISTIC SYMPTOMS
- Nervous, with stomach trouble.

MIND, SENSES, NERVES, EMOTIONS, PERSONALITY
- Fear, terror, and timidity.

- Shock (flowers in sweet, red wine).

HEAD AND FACE
- Itching, burning, and crusts on the cheekbone; lupus of the face, caries of the facial bones; open, bleeding cancer of the face; small, painful pimples.

RESPIRATION
- Colds center in the posterior nose, sniffling, watery, fetid, purulent discharge from the ears; tetter, herpes around the ears; putrid breath and gums; hurts to protrude the tongue; breath, mouth, tongue, and throat feel cold.
- Tonsils swollen, hawking of mucus, swelling and suppuration of glands of the throat; dryness, heat, itching in throat; neck studded with swollen glands; indurated breast lumps.

DIGESTION
- Cold feeling in stomach, abdomen; cold hands and feet; aggravation from exposure to cold air.
- Putrid vaginal discharge.
- Skin of hands hard, thick, dry, fissured; deep cracks; general itching of skin preventing sleep.
- Tetter, herpes on extremities.

LITERATURE:

Traditional, Jethro Kloss, Edward Bach (2, 3), William Cook, William Boericke, Juliette de Bairacli Levy (1, 2, 3).

Helianthus annuus. Sunflower.

The seed of the sunflower, native to the prairies of North America, is used as a food but also has utility as a medicine. It is high in unsaturated fatty acids. The root is brown and furry and the plant is one of the half dozen or so "bear medicines" associated with the prairie and western environment. Like other such medicines, sunflower seeds contain oils that build up the adrenals and kidney function. One of the few references for it in the old American literature is William Cook (1869). He says it was first introduced by Dr. Horton Howard (d. 1833).

Sunflower seeds are oily and moistening. They rehydrate the skin and mucosa, lessen irritation in the throat and lungs, and act "efficiently upon the kidneys—promoting the flow of urine, and soothing inflamed and irritable conditions both of the kidneys and the bladder" (Cook, 1869, 464). A warm decoction "gently promotes the action of the oil glands upon the surface, perhaps more efficiently than is done by the seeds of the burdock; and this fact renders it useful in scarlet fever." Cook considered burdock, sunflower, and *Celastrus scandens* to be the only remedies that increase the sebaceous sweat from the skin. Dr. Henry Nowell also spoke of the positive effect of sunflower seed in stimulating the sebaceous secretion from the skin.

Despite such encouraging information about sunflower, its use as an herb has not developed very far, except as a detoxificant in Ayurveda (see below). The followed observations show that it possesses many possible applications, but they are only scattered snapshots.

I was once plagued by an irritable cough for about six months. I went to visit an herbalist friend in southern Minnesota, Denese Ullom. She asked if I wanted her to do some "shamanic drumming" for me. "Sure," I replied, not certain what she meant. She had me lie down and she started drumming. All of a sudden I saw a professorial Bear standing on his two hind legs, directing my attention with a rubber-tipped pointer to a blackboard where a picture of a sunflower was inscribed in chalk. I understood immediately, even though I hadn't asked about my cough, what Bear was saying: "Sunflower is a medicine for the chest because Bear has a big chest." I went down to the convenience store, bought some sunflower seeds, ate them, and the problem disappeared for five years. A month later Denese called seeking help for an irritable cough and flooding of the lungs. "You need the remedy you taught me," I told her. Sure enough, sunflower seeds cured her. Five years later I was sick with an irritable cough in the throat that plagued me for three or four months. One of my students, who'd heard the story, said, "I looked over and saw an enormous sunflower superimposed on you." I was feeling exhausted, just like symptom number 1, below. Again, sunflower seed promptly cured my cough.

Sunflower seeds have been used to make a cough syrup. Dr. Leonard Thresher (1871, 338) gives one such formula for "coughs, colds, bronchitis, and consumption of the lungs" in an incipient stage. It also contained white hoarhound, bloodroot, comfrey root, liquorice, honey, and gin.

J. I. Rodale, of organic fame, discovered that sunflower seeds are beneficial to the eyesight. It helped him see in bright, snowy weather. He wrote about this discovery in *Prevention* magazine and many readers reported improvement in eyesight. Several got rid of reading glasses or lessened their prescriptions (Richard Lucas, 1972, 59).

Sunflower is extremely detoxifying. It was planted near Chernobyl to take up radioactive residue. It did this so successfully that the sunflowers that grew on the plot had to be placed in nuclear waste sites. Other scientific studies have shown that it detoxifies heavy metals, bacteria, and viruses. In Ayurveda, sunflower oil is used for detoxification. It is held under the tongue for 20 minutes then spit out. My friend Sondra Boyd says this is also an old Cherokee recipe for alcohol poisoning. One recipe has the person hold the sunflower oil under the tongue for 15–20 minutes; another has one swish it around the mouth 10–15 minutes, until it emulsifies. Follow by rinsing the mouth out and brushing the teeth to remove the film of toxins.

When I heard about using sunflower oil for a detoxification program I wasn't in a hurry to try it, but it came to mind in a difficult case. I had a client who was poisoned by dental work. She had been in shock for three weeks (see the rest of this case history in the Old World volume of *The Earthwise Herbal,* under *Carthamus tinctorius,* safflower). I had her use sunflower oil, held under the tongue, 3x/day or more, as possible. Although the oil tasted normal at first, within 10 minutes it was burning—the same effect caused by the dental materials—and she spit it out. We continued with this method until the oil stopped burning. Slowly, she tapered off and recovered.

TASTE:

(seed, oil) sweet • moist • oily

TISSUE STATE:

atrophy

SPECIFIC INDICATIONS:

CONSTITUTION
- Weak and stressed nervous system; adrenal exhaustion; dry skin and mucosa.

MIND, SENSES, NERVES, EMOTIONS, PERSONALITY
- Strengthen the sense of self, especially when there is conflict with authorities and "father" figures; useful in children (flower essence).

HEAD AND EYES
- Lusterless hair.
- Improves eyesight.

RESPIRATION
- Colds and flus; particularly during the winter.
- Chronic dry cough.
- Coughs, bronchitis, early tuberculosis (seeds/syrup).

DIGESTION
- Pulls toxins out through the mouth and tongue (dietary oil held in the mouth for 15 minutes); good for the gums.
- Indigestion (dietary oil is mildly soothing).
- Constipation (seeds; lubricating, bile-stimulating, and fibrous).

CARDIOVASCULAR
- Atherosclerosis (dietary oil).

KIDNEYS AND BLADDER
- Kidneys and bladder, inflamed and irritable conditions.

SEXUAL
- Sexual neurasthenia.

MUSCULAR AND SKELETAL
- Arthritis, rheumatism, fibromyalgia (American Indian).

SKIN
- Dry skin.

WOUNDS
- Snake bite (American Indian; part used not specified).

FEVER
- Malaria, intermittent chills/fever.

- Fever with dry skin; scarlet fever.

PREPARATION AND DOSAGE:

The fresh seeds, even the roasted seeds, or the cold pressed oil from the seeds.

LITERATURE:

Traditional, Flower Essence Society (2), Julia Graves (1, 2-confirmed, 5), J. I. Rodale (3, 4), William Cook (5, 10, 12, 15, 18), Matthew Wood (1, 6), Rose Elliot and Carlo de Paoli (5, 6, 10), Alma Hutchins (6, 11, 13, 16), Henry Nowell (15), Leonard Thresher (7).

Helonias luteum, Chamaelirium luteum. False Unicorn Root.

The false and true unicorn root (Aletris farinosa) *are easily confused. They have similar properties and appearance; both are members of the lily family used by the Indians and pioneers as female reproductive medicines.*

The most marked effect of *Helonias* is upon the uterus, and it is especially called for in cases where there is a loss of tone. "In sterility from uterine atony it is without doubt the most efficient remedy known. It many times prevents miscarriage through its tonic action on the uterus and the general system" (John William Fyfe, 1909). *Helonias* also has a general tonic influence through the digestive tract, increasing digestion and assimilation. It is especially of value in dyspepsia of atonic origin.

"Remember it for women with prolapsus from atony, enervated by indolence and luxury (better when attention is engaged—hence when the doctor comes), or for those worn out with hard work; tired, strained muscles burn and ache; sleepless" (William Boericke, 1927).

TASTE:

bitter

TISSUE STATE:

atrophy

SPECIFIC INDICATIONS:

CONSTITUTION, COMPLEXION, CHARACTERISTIC SYMPTOMS
- "Phosphatic diathesis."

MIND, SENSES, NERVES, EMOTIONS, PERSONALITY
- *Mental depression and irritability associated with chronic problems in the female reproductive tract.*
- Profound melancholia; better from engaging the mind in some activity and from exercise.
- Irritable, cannot endure contradiction.

DIGESTION
- Nervous dyspepsia, loss of appetite, irritable digestion, anemia.

LIVER
- "Albuminuria, where the liver is at fault."

FEMALE
- Nipples sensitive, tender, painful; breasts swollen; pressure of cloth intolerable.
- "Bearing down sensation throughout the floor of the pelvis; a feeling as if parts were about to fall out, consequently a tendency to hold up or support the extreme lower abdomen and its contents."
- Consciousness of the womb, of the kidneys.
- Uterus; prolapse, malposition; uterus lying low down, fundus tilted forward.
- Dragging sensations in the extreme lower abdomen, due to uterine trouble in women or cystic atonicity in men.
- Tired, backachy women; kidneys congested, full, menses suppressed.
- Amenorrhea, with abnormal condition of the digestive organs and anemia.
- Menorrhagia, due to weakness and atonicity of the reproductive tract.
- Nausea of pregnancy.

PREPARATION AND DOSAGE:

The same properties are attributed to it from the large to the small and even infinitesimal (i.e., homeopathic) doses.

CAUTIONS:

Since it is environmentally threatened, practitioners should consider the use of small doses. Recently cultivation of false unicorn root has brightened the ecological picture.

LITERATURE:

Traditional, Frederick Petersen (1, 6, 8), Rolla Thomas (2), William Boericke (3), Yadubir Sinha (5, 9).

Heracleum lanatum. Cow Parsnip.

This tall plant is a member of the Apiaceae family native to low, moist, open ground in North America. It was little used in herbal medicine in the nineteenth century, though a few practitioners spoke of it highly and a portrait of its properties was developed. Locally, it is used in the Southwest and has been reintroduced by herbalists practicing in that area, such as William LeSassier and Michael Moore. It must not be confused with wild parsnip, which produces a nasty dermatitis. Cow parsnip can also cause dermatitis, but less severe.

"The remedy has not received general attention," notes Finley Ellingwood (1918, 128). "But Dr. Vassar, of Ohio, has made some extended observations, which are worthy of note, and should be confirmed or disproved." The following account is from Dr. Vassar.

Heracleum "acts upon the nervous system as an antispasmodic. It produces, when taken in the mouth, a sensation of tingling, prickling, a benumbing sensation upon the throat, fauces, and tongue, similar to that of echinacea, aconite, and xanthoxylum." That would be the "diffusive" effect so desired by Samuel Thomson, indicative of a powerful, fast-moving effect on the nervous system and certainly justifying the use of the plant as a nerve relaxant. "It stimulates the pulse, and strengthens the capillary circulation. With the tingling and numbness of the throat, is difficult deglutition." Such stimulation will eventually, in excess, produce the low state with lack of reactivity of the tissues for which it is used. It is indicated where the tongue is heavily coated, the mucosa are bluish or leaden colored, bad breath, the pulse full and sluggish, patient drowsy, with general capillary stasis. "It exercises an influence upon the capillary circulation of the spinal cord, and upon the capillary circulation in general." Dr. Vassar compares its effects with echinacea, in blood toxicity or sepsis.

William LeSassier used this herb for its neurological applications. He passed on the observation that the seeds have a "revelatory aspect." Chewing a few "opens the third eye," heightens sensitivity to nature, and confers psychic benefits.

TISSUE STATE:

depression

SPECIFIC INDICATIONS:

- Trigeminal neuralgia; Bell's palsy; facial paralysis from cold winds (external application).
- Tonsillitis, diphtheria, ulcerated sore mouth.
- Glandular swellings with septic, necrotic tendencies; parts lifeless; foul and indolent ulcers.
- Sore mouth, gum disease, sore throat, erosions of the mucosa, with bad breath, cadaverous fetor, bad taste in the mouth.
- Tongue dirty and pasty, heavily coated or furred.
- Mucosa bluish or leaden.
- Membrane of the throat discolored, with very sluggish circulation, appearing as if they would slough tissue.
- Nervous dyspepsia; flatulence, decomposition of food in the stomach, offensive gases discharged after meals, excess acidity in the stomach or bowels (small doses).
- Hiatal hernia; in elderly women.
- Pulse slow; patient drowsy, general capillary stasis.
- Menstruation: amenorrhea, dysmenorrhea; pains severe, before or immediately when the flow starts.
- Uric acid diathesis.
- Convulsions, puerperal or childbed fever (30 drops of the tincture).

- Puerperal fever, temperature up to 106°F.
- Epilepsy.
- Blood poisoning.

PREPARATION AND DOSAGE:

The fresh stems, leaves, and roots can burn sensitive people. The decoction is usually prepared from the dried root. Dr. Vassar used a "good preparation of the green root." Dose of the tincture, 5 to 60 minims. Michael Moore (2003), on the other hand, recommends tincture from the dry root, 20–30 drops per dose.

LITERATURE:

Finley Ellingwood, Dr. Vassar, William LeSassier, Michael Moore (1, 9), 7Song.

Hydrangea arborescens. Seven Barks.

Hydrangea is an old Cherokee and Southern remedy that passed into widespread use in Western herbalism. It grows along streambeds in the South, holding onto the soil and not allowing it to be washed away—a signature demonstrating an affinity to the balance of water and solids (also see Eupatorium purpureum *in this volume and* Polygonum hydropiper *in the Old World volume). These three remedies all live on the water/solid edge and all are important in the removal of kidney stones. Some hydrangeas have leaves that turn blue or red, depending on the acid/alkaline balance of the soil—a remarkable kidney signature.*

Hydrangea acts efficiently on the urinary tract, especially to remove the tendency to the formation of gravel and stones, to dissolve them, and to hasten their passage. The late Tommie Bass had a formula for dissolving kidney stones in twenty-four hours: Hydrangea capsules hourly, and ten lemons in a gallon of water. Herbalist Thomas Easley, of Andalusia, Alabama, reports a case in which a kidney stone (watched on a medical imaging device) disappeared in five hours under this regimen.

Hydrangea relieves irritation of the urinary tract, improves nutrition of the mucosa, and invigorates the functional activity of the kidneys. It also exerts an influence upon the respiratory mucosa, relieving bronchial irritation. "Through its free action upon the kidneys, hydrangea is an excellent 'blood medicine.' It assists in washing out cutaneous, strumous, and perhaps tubercular disorders" (Scudder). Hydrangea contains cortisone-like compounds.

The fact that hydrangea acts on glands and contains steroidal compounds indicates an action in the sexual sphere. "In a case of enlarged prostate, where a surgical operation was declared imperative, *Hydrangea arb. o*, 6 drops, night and morning, effected a remarkable cure, and the patient was able to void his urine comfortably, and completely." This is reported by Dr. J. Compton Burnett, of London, who learned about the remedy from Dr. Henry Thomas, "who had elderly gentlemen coming to him from far and near for prostatic troubles and they mostly received *Hydr. arb.*" (quoted by Anshutz, 1900, 146).

A constitutional picture of the kind of personality for whom hydrangea is appropriate was developed by some nineteenth-century authors. "In the *Chicago Medical Times*, for December 1888, is an article upon a common trouble that has grown out of the fast life of the people of America." Symptoms include "nervous prostration, accompanied by symptoms of diabetes. The patients lose flesh and are unfit for business. When the urine is examined it is found loaded with phosphates, showing a great waste of nerve material. For this condition, the writer, an MD in good standing, recommended rest, change of habit, and a decotion of hydrangea, one tablespoonful, and five grains of citrate of lithia." This is recorded by herbalist James Neil, of New Zealand, who studied medicine in Chicago. He writes further, "We have tried it, and can recommend it to anyone suffering with the above symptoms" (Neil, original 1891, reprint 1998, 77).

Australian herbalist Dorothy Hall has developed a somewhat different, but not unrelated, understanding of hydrangea. She emphasizes a fixed, hard, bitter, willful, selfish personality. She also uses it for gallstones, whereas traditional texts limit its use to kidney stones.

Cortisol modifies both the thin, dry, nervous, weak constitution and the hard, bitter, willful type by promoting digestion and nutrition. Thus we see how both these constitutional types *(vata* and *pitta)* are helped by *Hydrangea.*

TASTE:

bitter

TISSUE STATES:

constriction, atrophy

SPECIFIC INDICATIONS:

MIND, SENSES, NERVES, EMOTIONS, PERSONALITY
- Resentful, bitter, argumentative; nothing is ever right.
- Willful, selfish, stubborn, cynical, rock-hard beliefs, can't let go.
- People who attempt to throw other people into doubt (cf. *Gentiana*).
- Nervous prostration, nervous wasting, loss of flesh, diabetes, phosphaturia.

HEAD
- Fixed facial expression.
- Twisted mouth.

RESPIRATION
- Bronchial irritation.

DIGESTION
- Irritation of the digestive mucosa.

LIVER AND GALLBLADDER
- Gallbladder spastic; gallstones, gallstone colic, lack of bile causing constipation.

KIDNEYS AND BLADDER
- Fluid retention.
- *Irritation associated with malnutrition of the urinary tract and mucosa.*
- Production of kidney stones.
- *Kidney stone colic,* sharp pains in the loins and back, bloody urine.
- Spasmodic stricture of the urethra with sediment.
- Painful urination, burning, frequent desire; urinary flow is hard to start.
- Catarrh of the bladder and urethra.

- Alkaline and phosphatic gravel; white precipitates.
- Enlarged prostate.
- Urinary problems with great thirst.
- Bedwetting in children.
- "Frequent urination, accompanied by a sense of burning and sharp, quick pain in the urethra."

MUSCULAR AND SKELETAL
- Severe arthritic pain, gout, rheumatism.
- "Aching in the back with irritation and partial suppression of urine."

OTHER
- Used as a substitute for cortisone.

PREPARATION AND DOSAGE:

Various kinds of ornamental hydrangea are reputed to substitute for the genuine species. Decoction. Fluid extract, 2 drops in a tablespoonful of water, 3x/day (Ralph M. Russell).

LITERATURE:

Traditional, John M. Scudder (11, 17), John William Fyfe (7, 12, 14, 16), Dorothy Hall (1–3, 5–6, 9–10), James Neil (4, 19), Frederick Petersen (11, 21, 23), Rolla Thomas (8), J. Compton Burnett (18).

Hydrastis canadensis. Goldenseal.

Goldenseal is a member of the buttercup family native to the rich forest floors of central North America. It was not widely known until the American pioneers crossed the Appalachian mountains in the late eighteenth century. Rafinesque (1828–30) is therefore one of the first sources on its use. "This plant is much used in Ohio, Kentucky, &c., for diseases of the eyes, the juice or an infusion are used as a wash, in sore or inflamed eyes. It is considered a specific by the Indians for that disorder; they also employ it for sore legs, and many external complaints. Internally it is used as a bitter tonic." In the early twentieth century goldenseal was recognized as what we would today call a "natural antibiotic." The substance that acts on

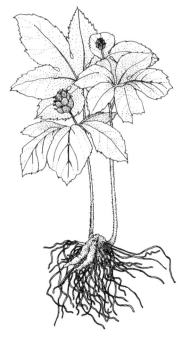

bacteria is berberine, also found in some other bitter plants. However, it was originally used in nineteenth-century medicine as a bitter tonic to stimulate digestion.

Goldenseal acts on the mucosa of the digestive and respiratory tracts, increasing tone, eliminating flabby, weak, debilitated, swollen, boggy, inactive tissues. It reduces unhealthy secretion (excessive, bloody, mucoid) and increases the positive digestive secretions, bile, and pancreatic enzymes. Hence, it is a normalizer of the secretion. It is indicated in cervicitis, sinusitis, and conjunctivitis. It promotes appetite, increases peristaltic action, and improves general muscular tone in the walls of the GI. It is indicated by a flat, atonic, apathetic tongue, dry toward the top and coated toward the back, indicating an apathetic digestion with poor secretion of healthy juices (dryness) but collection of mucoid secretion. The wall of the stomach is sometimes weak and collapsed, the stomach burdened by mucus, with nausea and inactive digestion. The signals to the pancreas and liver are probably lessened. It is suited to catarrhal congestion of the gallbladder ducts, gallstones, and congestion of the liver.

By increasing nutrition and through its own direct stimulating powers, hydrastis improves the general nervous and muscular tonus of the organism, especially the respiration and circulation. It imparts "tone and increased power to the heart's action, increasing arterial tension and capillary blood pressure. It stimulates normal fibrillar contractility and increased tonus, encouraging the nutrition of muscular structure. It inhibits the development of superfluous muscular tissue and abnormal growth within that structure. It is thus most valuable in altered conditions of the heart muscle. It stimulates muscular structure everywhere in the system in the same manner" (Ellingwood, 1918, 196; edited and condensed).

Goldenseal is currently lauded as a "natural antibiotic," but this is not a holistic use of the plant. Bacteria are usually scavengers who settle on sick tissues. To remove them without changing the condition that led to their appearance is therefore not competent practice but suppressive and will lead to side effects, since the large doses of goldenseal necessary to kill bacteria have an exhausting effect on the mucosa and nervous system. There are, of course, conditions where bacteria enter the system and cause disease—it is for these that we should save our antibiotics—but even when bacteria are the cause, tissue changes are the result, and need to be addressed. Used in small doses goldenseal is a mucous membrane tonic that removes the propensity for bacteria to flourish by strengthening the mucosa.

Goldenseal has been used to seal up wounds in the surface. It is so effective, however, that it can seal in pus, infection, splinters, and dirt, so it should only be used on a clean wound. A valuable property I have discovered that is analogous, is that goldenseal will seal internal tears like herniated disks in the spine, torn meniscus in the knee, torn bursa in the hip, and so on. Not only does it help the tissue directly (so long as there is not active inflammation making the union of the parts impossible), but I have found that weaknesses of this kind can indicate a constitutional need for goldenseal.

TASTE:

bitter with sweet aftertaste • stimulating • resinous

TISSUE STATES:

atrophy, torpor, depression

SPECIFIC INDICATIONS:

MIND, SENSES, NERVES, EMOTIONS, PERSONALITY

- Poor self-image; setbacks, disappointments, emotional shock; feels constantly drained, tired; with sore, tender spots on stomach, abdomen, and pelvic organs.
- *Torpor of the mucosa*, with lack of secretion and inactivity leading to pallor, swelling, ulceration, and the generation of a thick yellow mucus to cover the membrane, or a thin, runny discharge.
- *Chronic catarrhal conditions of atonic mucosa with secretion of profuse, thick, yellow or greenish-yellow and tenacious mucus.*

HEAD

- Cerebral congestion and engorgement.
- *Conjunctivitis;* mattering of the eye; styes; ocular ulceration; discharge from the ear.
- Crusted, sore nostrils (ointment).
- Nasal polypi with discharge (injected, snuff).
- *Tongue enlarged, scalloped, slightly dry toward the tip and slightly coated toward the back; sometimes ulcerated in the margins. "Apathetic tongue" indicating apathetic mucosa.*
- Gum disease, spongy, bleeding gingivae; sores, ulcers in the mouth.
- Sore throat, tonsillitis, hoarseness, diphtheria.
- Goiter of recent appearance.

DIGESTION

- *Torpid, atonic mucosa of the mouth, throat, and stomach; specific for gastric ulceration.*
- Lack of appetite.
- Atonic dyspepsia; catarrhal gastritis; stomach secretion underactive, mucosa atonic, lack of nerve sensibility; pancreas and liver underactive; fullness, nausea.
- Insulin resistance; may cause sudden drop in blood sugar level by stimulating cellular uptake; use cautiously with glycemic problems; diabetic ulcers (powder, external).
- Colitis, diarrhea.
- Imperfect recoveries from diarrhea and dysentery.
- *Liver, gallbladder;* congestion, catarrh of the bile ducts, jaundice, hepatitis, gallstones, constipation from lack of bile.
- Gallstones with catarrh of the bile ducts.
- *Constipation* habitual; with hemorrhoids; dependent on inertia or congestion of lower abdomen; sedentary habit; after purgatives; during and after pregnancy (5 minims in water before breakfast).
- Rectal prolapse; with ulceration, fissures, eczema (external).
- Digestive problems in chronic alcoholics (combine with capsicum; cf. *Brassica nigra*).

CARDIOVASCULAR

- *Heart muscle enfeebled;* irregular pulse, dyspnea, weight, oppression on the chest; valvular changes.

- *Weakness of nerves and muscles in general and of the heart in particular.*

BLADDER
- Bladder infection and catarrh; cystitis, urethritis.

MALE
- Prostate, swollen.

FEMALE
- Breasts; painful fullness during the period; benign tumors, hard and painful.
- "History of some chronic uterine disorder and where there is a pelvic fullness and weight and a feeling as though the parts are about to fall out"(10 drops every 3–4 hours) (Niederkorn).
- Vaginitis; *ulceration of the cervix,* leucorrhea.
- Uterus weak and atonic; excessive bleeding between or during the periods, irregularity, subinvolution of the womb after labor (cf. capsella).
- Uterine fibroids.
- Pregnancy: morning sickness.
- Partus: stimulates labor slowly.

OTHER
- Chicken pox, measles, ringworm, poison ivy (brings out the rash, cleanses the interior).
- Psoriasis, eczema, itching rashes, erysipelas, impetigo, infected sores, boils.
- The great remedy for *ulcers of all kinds;* internal and external; diabetic or not.
- *Torn disks in the spine;* acute injury; breakdown of disks is a constitutional tendency in the *Hydrastis* person.
- Intermittent fever.
- Exhaustive stage of fever, typhoid, dysentery, scarlatina, chicken pox.
- *Pulse; caliber diminished due to weakness.*
- Travel sickness; nauseous from all the turns while driving in the mountains.

PREPARATION AND DOSAGE:

As a tonic, goldenseal works best in small doses. I use 3 drops to a fraction of a drop, 3x/day. In some old notes from William LeSassier I found the following: "Goldenseal works on all mucous linings, but the body can develop a dependency so very small doses are recommended." The powder is used externally on lacerations and ulcers.

CAUTIONS:

Goldenseal can upset the liver, gallbladder, and small intestine, making people irritable (Ellingwood, Hall), and can cause a precipitous drop in the blood sugar levels (Christopher). Large doses can cause flabbiness of the tongue and mucosa, ulceration of the mucosa, and mucus discharges (Julia Graves).

LITERATURE:

Traditional (36), Constantine Rafinesque, William Cook (2, 3, 7, 9, 16, 17, 25, 26, 29, 35, 38–40), Finley Ellingwood (2, 3, 4, 11, 18, 20, 21, 22, 23, 24, 30, 31, 32, 34), Niederkorn (*Ellingwood's Therapeutist*, 1908, 2, 10, 28), John Christopher (15), Yadubir Sinha (7, 20, 21), Dorothy Hall (1, 6, 29, 36), William Boericke (5, 8), Matthew Wood (5, 8, 37, 40), Julia Graves (32, 41), George Royal (2, 3, 12, 14).

Iris versicolor. Blue Flag.

Iris is a native of freshwater ponds and swamps in eastern and northern North America. William Bartram noted that it was found in a pond near every Indian village in the southeast in the late eighteenth century. To judge from the folklore in the North, it was probably used by the southern Indians as an indicator for water quality. Also, snakes are said to be repelled by Iris, and a common North American Indian practice was (still sometimes is) to carry a piece of the root. Blue flag was used by the Indians as a purgative, just as the Old World Iris spp. was by the Europeans. However, it has much subtler properties. It contains tannins, resin, sterols, volatile oils (furfural, an irritant to the mucosa), and triterpenoid acids. The sterols make it active in the hormonal sphere. John Uri Lloyd insisted that it had to be picked north of the Ohio River to be effective.

Iris is an irritating bitter that provokes secretion from the mucosa, the glands in the mucosa of the gastrointestinal tract, the liver, and pancreas, increasing digestion, nutrition, metabolism, and elimination. It also acts on the endocrine system, especially the thyroid, which it regulates when there are precipitous up-and-down changes. It is called for when there are sudden flare-ups of sympathetic excess; also mood swings from high to low, according to Australian herbalist Dorothy Hall. One of her students recommended it in menopausal hot flashes. He had seen it work in more than a dozen cases. He characterized it as a remedy for a "pituitary gone crazy trying to stimulate the ovaries."

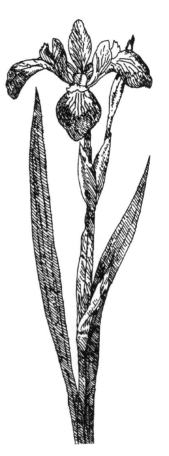

In large doses Iris increases salivation and stomach secretion, causing unpleasant burning, and purges the gallbladder, causing a yellowish, bilious diarrhea. In small, medicinal doses it is applicable in persons with lack of salivation, digestive secretion, enzyme and bile production, liver activity, and proper thyroid stimulation of metabolism. It is medicinal when the inner waters are contaminated and was used to remove "taint," as in supposed ancestral syphilis.

There is some history of use of the iris native to Europe. "Gordon, an old writer on physic, says, if a dropsy can be cured by the hand of man, this root will effect it. I have found it true in practice" (Hill, 1740, 181).

"An old eclectic once said that three drugs would cure many of the common ills of humanity, namely, *Irs. ver.* for skin diseases (especially syphilitic), *[Arctium] lappa* for rheumatism, especially of the joints, and *Rumex crispus* for the mucous membranes, such as catarrh" (Anshutz, 1900, 151).

TASTE:

pungent, bitter • warm

TISSUE STATES:

depression, atrophy, stagnation

SPECIFIC INDICATIONS:

MIND, SENSES, NERVES, EMOTIONS, PERSONALITY
- *Stuck artistic creativity.*
- *Extreme moods and energy levels follow each other closely.*
- *Excitement alternating with depression.*
- *Sympathetic excess alternating with exhaustion.*

HEAD
- Frontal headache; worse from not eating; better by moving about slowly.
- Mouth dry, scanty saliva.
- Tongue red, pointed, thin around the edges, coated in the middle.
- *Thyroid* output fluctuates wildly.
- Thyroid gland enlarges during sympathetic-excess episodes.
- Rash over the thyroid or thoracic duct, of nervous origin.
- *"Fullness of throat, enlargement of thyroid gland, fullness of throat with pulsation of arteries"* (10 drops in 5 ounces of water) (Rolla Thomas).
- *Loosens and straightens the neck; sensation of weight on the head, with depression.*

RESPIRATION
- Oppression of breathing.

DIGESTION, LIVER, AND PANCREAS
- Irritation of the mucosa of the digestive tract; pains burning like a hot wire.
- Pancreatic secretion deficient.
- *Pancreatitis.*
- Liver sore, swollen, painful.
- Duodenal catarrh; clay-colored stool, from lack of bile.
- *Gastrointestinal irritation and sensitivity,* with diarrhea, sometimes yellowish.

FEVER
- Fever alternating chills and heat; night sweats.

SKIN
- Sunburn, herpes, eczema, psoriasis. Locally, to prevent and cure sunburn.
- *Skin rashes.*

OTHER
- General toxic feeling.
- Hypoglycemia.

PREPARATION, CONTRAINDICATIONS, AND DOSAGE:

The root grown north of the Ohio River is harvested in the fall and dried for use by decoction or extracted fresh in alcohol. It is somewhat toxic and should not be used in large doses. Dose of the tincture: 1–3 drops, 1–3x/day. Also used in low homeopathic potencies. Moderate to large doses are unsettling.

LITERATURE:

Traditional, Flower Essence Society (1), Finley Ellingwood (6), Rolla Thomas (11), Julia Graves (12), Matthew Wood (12, 24), Dorothy Hall (2, 3, 4, 8–10, 18), William Boericke (5, 7, 8, 14, 15, 16, 17, 18, 19, 20, 21, 22).

Juglans cinerea. Butternut.

Butternut is a member of the Juglandaceae family. The oldest sources mention the use of the bark of the root, a preparative method that almost always indicates American Indian provenance. By the eighteenth century it had acquired the reputation of a specific for dysentery, according to Dr. Jacob Bigelow (1817–20, 119). It is "one of the most mild and efficacious laxatives we possess." Peter Smith (1812, 29), a backwoods doctor, is more specific. "This purge is preferable to any that I know of in a weak and debilitated state of the bowels." Smith gives a valuable account. The most careful account of the properties of butternut in the nineteenth-century literature, in my opinion, is the one by Dr. Edwin

Hale (1875, 2:361–66). He and other homeopaths picked up the use of Juglans cinerea from the eclectics and folk medicine. He documents the uses of butternut with extensive case histories, and he traces the effect of butternut through the usual applications for the intestines and skin.

Nineteenth-century practitioners uniformly preferred the butternut to its cousin, black walnut, but the roles reversed in the twentieth century. It appears that butternut and black walnut can be used fairly interchangeably. They both possess the naphthoquinone juglone, responsible for their distinctive powers as purgatives, antimicrobials, and parasite killers. Butternut was primarily used for constipation, diarrhea, parasites, and skin conditions associated with intestinal problems. Black walnut is also used for these same functions, but more subtle uses for toning the cardiovascular system and the thyroid were introduced. The former is more oily, so it would be better suited for stimulating the bile and purging the intestines, while the latter is more astringent and would reestablish tissue tone. They both contain flavonoids, bitters, tannins, naphthoquinones (similar to the purgative anthraquinones), juglone (kills low forms of life), and fixed and volatile oils.

Butternut bark is an oily purgative, exciting a discharge of bile from the gallbladder. Thus, it is used to remove gallstones, to correct constipation, and also to flush diarrhea due to bacteria. Samuel Thomson (1825, 2:127) used it himself in 1813 when he caught dysentery from one of his patients. "I was called to attend a woman with a relax," or severe diarrhea. He cured her in several visits but was called again after midnight on a false alarm by her family. On returning home he was "soon after taken in a violent manner with the same disease." He was so weak he couldn't attend to himself, his assistant failed, and finally he was forced to manage his own desperate case. He sent for some butternut bark, had a hot, strong tea decocted, and commenced recovery.

Peter Smith (1812, 29) writes that little balls or pellets of the bark "may be taken in as small quantities as you please, for if they do not purge immediately, they act the better as a stimulus and tonic to the system, and will produce a good habit of body by repeating them every night; and this may be done for a month together." Butternut bark "differs from all other purges that I know of—in this—that your doses may be less and less, but other physic must have more and more, or it will not purge. Other purges generally leave the body in a worse habit, but this in a better. Its general ease and safety, and its answering in almost every disease, so that I venture to say the trial of it will never be wrong, make it a far preferable medicine to salts or any other purge, where repeated applications are wanted."

Butternut bark stimulates and perhaps normalizes bile secretion. "Full doses produce large bilious evacuations, without much pain or griping," writes Finley Ellingwood (1918, 329). It is given in moderate doses when there is constipation from a lack of bile and the stool is "clay-colored and dry." It awakens a "torpid liver" or gallbladder, increasing secretion, and perhaps production of bile. It thus removes jaundice and the tendency to gallstone production but also coordinates with the digestive tract, which needs the correct amount of bile for healthy function. It removes "duodenal catarrh" in the upper intestine and tones the lower bowel. By maintaining a steady flow of bile it removes the tendency to chills, which is so often associated with liver and gallbladder malfunction. Hence it has some relationship to fever, chills, colds, and flu where the bilious apparatus is affected. In olden times it would have been curative in chills associated with malaria.

Prolonged overuse of butternut bark causes irritation and inflammation of the intestines, and even a single exposure will burn and raise blisters on the skin. Thus, as Edwin Hale points out, butternut is homeopathic to such conditions in the intestines: heat, bloody and bilious diarrhea, irritability, fullness, and inflammation. Here the dose is smaller.

These disorders of the intestines, in homeopathic provings or poisonings, were often followed by dermic outbreaks of all sorts. This includes eczema, herpes circinatus, acne, impetigo, pemphigus, rupia, lichen, and chronic scaly conditions. "In skin disorders named under dandelion, pustular and eczematous, it will act in the same manner as dandelion, and may be advantageously combined with that agent," reports Ellingwood.

Butternut also affects the mucosa in a manner similar to the skin, and is therefore indicated in chronic inflammation of the throat, enlargement of glands, congestion and irritation of the respiratory membranes, nursing sore mouth, ulcers in the mouth with constipation, and chronic, poorly healing ulcers. It has been used for rheumatism in the lower back, probably in connection with constipation.

There are some observations in the old literature about *Juglans cinerea* making an impression on general waste and nutrition. Dr. John Christopher (1996, 198) calls butternut a "valuable laxative remedy for the aged, middle-aged, and delicate children where no drastic" purgation is desirable. This suggests that it is nutritive. We must remember that the oily butternut and walnut are in fact highly nutritious. Dr. Shook and Phyllis Light bring out more about the nutritive capacities of black walnut that we will study under the following entry.

Butternut has the same mental indications that were worked out by Dr. Edward Bach for the Old World walnut *(Juglans regia)*: too much under the domination of another, needs the reassurance of a parental or guru-like figure. Butternut and the walnuts help to adjust the parent/child relationship. They are excellent when there is stress in the house due to separation, divorce, or parental death, where the child has separation anxieties. I have given it to such children, when they were constipated, and seen them run to the bathroom! Of course, we are interested in the deeper symptoms.

Here is an odd indication from Dr. Samuel Henry (1814, 111). "Pregnant women should always take a dose of butternut pills, a day or two previous to their falling in labor, which will prevent after pains." I have not verified this but it rather strangely agrees with my own use of the walnut clan for parent/child separation problems. This is probably another example of American Indian herbal midwifery.

TASTE:

sweet, nutty, slightly bitter • moist, cool • oily

TISSUE STATES:

atrophy, depression

SPECIFIC INDICATIONS:

CONSTITUTION, COMPLEXION, CHARACTERISTIC SYMPTOMS
- Delicate children, middle-aged or elderly person of delicate construction; with constipation.

MIND, SENSES, NERVES, EMOTIONS, PERSONALITY
- *Child/parent problems;* can't leave the nest or is precipitously tossed out.

HEAD
- Morning headaches or hangovers; associated with sluggish liver.

DIGESTION, LIVER, AND GALLBLADDER

- *Duodenal catarrh associated with lack of biliary secretion; dyspepsia; poor digestion of fats and oils; chronic constipation with dry, clay-colored stool.*
- *Torpid gallbladder, lack of secretion of bile, gallstones, obstructive jaundice, constipation, or diarrhea.*
- *The gallstone habit* (syrup of the green bark).
- *Intestinal parasites.*
- *Diarrhea;* bilious, bloody, with itching of the rectum (worms?) before and after.
- Hemorrhoids.

SKIN

- *Chronic skin eruptions of all sorts;* eczema, crusts, pustules, impetigo, patches, herpes, rupia, pemphigus, lichen, acne, ringworm, itching; following or associated with liver, gallbladder, and intestinal problems.
- Fevers, colds, flu.

PREPARATION AND DOSAGE:

The tree bark is collected in late winter, when the sap is running, and dried for more than a year to reduce the purgative properties. Used by decoction, capsules, and tincture. For constipation, the dose starts small (5 drops, 3x/day) and builds up by a drop a day, until purging sets in. Drop back slightly and keep the stool loose for a month. For diarrhea or parasites, 3 drops, 1–3x/day, hourly for acute diarrhea.

CAUTIONS:

Butternut has been almost exterminated throughout its range by a fungus.

LITERATURE:

Traditional, Samuel Thomson (8), Peter Smith (8), Edward Bach (1), John Christopher (2, 7, 9, 11), Edwin Hale (3, 8), Finley Ellingwood (4, 5, 7, 10), Eli Jones (6), Matthew Wood (3, 5, 10).

Juglans nigra. Black Walnut.

In the twentieth century, black walnut superseded its cousin butternut in importance. Dr. Edward Shook (c. 1945) seems to have been one of the first major authors to use black walnut rather than butternut. Dr. John Christopher gives the more prominent heading to butternut in The School of Natural Healing, *but he seems to have used black walnut hull more often in practice. Now* Juglans nigra *is the preferred representative of the family.*

Dr. Shook used black walnut leaves for their astringent properties; these are not found in butternut bark. Dr. Christopher, on the other hand, used black walnut hulls. Dr. Shook and, more recently, Hulda Clark, recommend the use of the green, unripe hulls, but the blackened, dried hulls have long been used in folk medicine. Fresh or dried, the hulls or husks will stain the hands for months and should be handled only with protective gloves. This stain is due to the presence of iodine, which hints at the use of black walnut for thyroid, an indication from contemporary herbalist Phyllis Light.

"Long experience has proved that a strong infusion of the leaves [of black walnut] is the ideal preparation for obtaining the best results," writes Shook (1978, 95) in his *Advanced Treatise.* The general indications for its use include "internal ulcerations, inflammations, mucus and hemorrhagic discharges, bleeding piles, leucorrhea, diarrhea, dysentery, relaxed and ballooned intestines; outwardly, for ulcers, tumors, cancers, abscesses, boils, acne, eczema, itch, shingles, and so forth. It is also used for sore throat, tonsillitis, aphthous sore mouth, relaxed uvula, epistaxis, nasal catarrh, falling hair, ringworm, hoarseness of the voice, and so forth." So far the indications are similar to butternut, but Shook soon follows another course.

"In relaxed and atonic conditions of the muscular structure of any organ, the astringing, contracting, and toning properties of walnut leaves or bark are most remarkable. Let us take, for instance, the ballooned condition of the intestines so frequently met with in our practices. A little knowledge will enable us to rectify this condition through the wonderful virtues of walnut. As we stated before, a simple infusion or decoction does not produce the best effects, but if we combine a strong decoction of walnut leaves with a mucilage of *Chondrus crispus*, we shall not only get the full effect of walnut, but also the effective virtues of *Chondrus*."

Shook goes on to provide his formula for "all atonic and prolapsed conditions": 6 parts walnut leaves, 4 bugleweed, 2 black cohosh, 4 hawthorn berries, 2 lily of the valley root, and 2 Irish moss *(Chondrus)*. This will be "found to be most effective for relaxed and atonic conditions of the walls of the intestines, veins, arteries, and the general tubular system, and also for various forms of dropsy, enlarged heart (variously named aneurisms), asthma, bronchitis, menorrhagia (excessive flow just before or at the time of the menopause), prolapsus ani, or any prolapsed condition in any part of the body."

"Do not get the impression that walnut alone will produce the spectacular and truly remarkable results that can be obtained by the use of this formula, but walnut is the principal *contracting* influence; however, without the other herbs, it would be only one-half as effective."

Phyllis Light says that in Southern folk medicine black walnut has an old reputation for removing fat deposition from the arteries. This usage may owe something to Shook; he is the first author I am aware of who used black walnut to "tone" the arteries.

Christopher Menzies-Trull (2003, 665) makes a statement (under *Juglans cinerea* and *J. regia*) that follows well on these observations. "Vasocompression is the term used [by Dr. Joseph Thurston] to describe the ability of a medicine to constrict the tissue, thereby supporting improved muscle tone, mucous membrane, and blood vessel. Compressing tissue improves blood vessel tone and ultimately blood supply to that organ." These remedies are therefore suited to inflammatory conditions of the mucosa, vessels, and skin, chronic inflammation of the throat from intestinal toxemia (tonsillitis), and dry, congested, and irritated mucosa. *Juglans* spp. "gently tones the intestinal wall if given over time. Stimulates lower bowel clearance, this encourages the portal system to decongest. Chronic constipation, waterbrash, and flatulence." The term "vasocompression," introduced by Thurston, is a complicated way of describing what usually amounts to astringence. Let us return to Dr. Shook.

"The green husk of the unripe kernel contains potassium iodide, a recognized remedy for scrofula, syphilis, and other forms of bad blood. The husk and brown skin covering the inner kernel or nut when it is green or unripe have powerful antiseptic, germicide, vermicide, and parasiticide properties. No insect will touch the leaves or husks of the walnut tree. The brown stain, found principally in the green husk, contains organic iodine which is much more antiseptic and healing than the usual poisonous iodine, so commonly used to put on infections, cuts, and so forth."

"A strong infusion of the powdered bark . . . is either gently laxative, or purgative according to dose. A wineglassful can be given to start with, and then increased or decreased, so as to bring about a soft, molded stool twice or three times a day. Diarrhea, or watery stool should always be avoided, except in dropsy or when it is urgent to quickly empty the colon. Then, of course, there is nothing that is more quickly effective than a properly administered colonic."

Black walnut not only cleanses and tones the colon, but according to Shook it prevents the uptake of toxins from constipated bowels, a process that the old physicians called "autointoxication" or "toxemia," and which is today referred to as "leaky bowel syndrome" or "dysbiosis." It also treats the opposite condition: malabsorption from a closed gut, notes Phyllis Light. She says it helps the assimilation of nutrients, especially fats and proteins, and reduces unhealthy fatty acids in the bloodstream. Thus, it tones the vascular system and the heart, both of which are subject to damage from bad-quality lipids. This alterative/nutritive property complements the astringency mentioned above.

Apropos of this nutritive content, we might quote Dr. John Christopher (1996, 200), who writes of the inner bark of black walnut, "Besides being cathartic, [it] is a fibrin solvent (potassium sulphate), muscle and nerve food (magnesium sulphate), and food for hair, nails, skin, nerve sheath, and periosteum (silica)."

Perhaps the most valuable insight into black walnut passed on by Phyllis Light is its use as a thyroid medication. She says the black hulls (not the green) are a traditional remedy in the South for goiter. She has used it much for hypothyroidism (often combined with chickweed). "Bad blood" is believed to be caused by toxemia or closure of the channels of elimination or a faulty liver, but it is also caused by low cellular metabolism from thyroid, and it very often is cured by the use of thyroid medication (Broda Barnes, *Hypothyroidism*, 1976). Black walnut is a superlative remedy for hypothyroid. I have confirmed this usage in my own practice many times and in severe, lifelong, and hereditary cases. Prior to this, I did not know of any remedy that consistently cured hypothyroidism, but black walnut hull has not disappointed me.

One of the old theories about the thyroid, which we find in alternative medicine back into the 1930s at least, is the idea that the healthy thyroid disperses a small amount of iodine out into the carotids, which run by the thyroid. This explains the curious placement of the thyroid. Thus, the antiseptic powers of iodine are used to keep the blood going to the brain clean and pure. This is very important, since the hypothalamus can be confused by "dirty blood" and can't read the hormonal feedback signals correctly or send out good hormonal advice. This clean, iodized blood would also keep the sinuses in good health.

A number of herbalists have introduced black walnut hull as a remedy for sinusitis. Herbalist Daniel Gagnon points out that recent research indicates that most chronic sinusitis infections are associated with fungal infections in the upper respiratory tract and that black walnut, as a known antifungal and antimicrobial is thus indicated in many such conditions. He has proved this in his own practice. He recommends: boil ¼ teaspoon of salt in a cup of water, add 30 drops of black walnut hull tincture, let sit 25 minutes, and run it through the sinus passages with a neti pot. Independent testimony on the use of black walnut in sinus problems comes from herbalist Thomas Easley, of Andalusia, Alabama. It might also be pointed out that precipitation of mucopolysaccharides in the internal waters of the body, in other words catarrh, is a typical production of low thyroid.

The old authors sometimes speak of the use of butternut and black walnut for rheumatism and arthritis. We might especially expect them to be available in the ache of the lower back that accompanies constipation. However, fibromyalgia (as rheumatism is called today) is a characteristic symptom of many people with hypothyroidism. Phyllis Light and others have indeed used black walnut for this common condition.

Iodine is concentrated in and secreted by the breasts, and essential for breast health. Deficiency is believed to cause fibrocystic breast disease and breast cancer (David Brownstein, MD).

Finally, there is hardly an herbalist who would travel to areas where diarrhea is likely to be picked up, who would not include black walnut hull (nowadays green hull) in the first-aid kit.

TASTE:

fragrant bitter • astringent

TISSUE STATES:

depression, relaxation, torpor

SPECIFIC INDICATIONS:

(leaves)
- Canker sores; tonsillitis, sore throat, relaxed uvula, diphtheria; hoarseness.
- Epistaxis, nasal catarrh.
- Internal ulcerations, inflammations, mucus and hemorrhagic discharges.
- Diarrhea, dysentery; relaxed and ballooned intestines.
- Bleeding hemorrhoids.
- Arteriosclerosis, fatty deposits, venous congestion.
- Leucorrhea.
- *Ringworm, falling hair, eczema, itch, shingles, tumors, cancers, abscesses, boils, acne* (external).
- Moist skin disease, bleeding (powdered leaves).

(hulls)
- Conditions where there is a combination of intestinal and skin problems suggesting the participation of low forms of life.
- Too much under the influence of another person, thought, or scheme.
- *Low thyroid, low metabolism, "bad blood."*
- Swellings on the thyroid—that is, goiter.
- Irritation of the mucosa.
- Scrofulous enlargement of glands (ulcerating, chronic, suppurative).
- Jaundice; pain around the liver and right scapula.
- Duodenal catarrh, with torpid liver and jaundice.
- Congestion of the gallbladder; gallstones.
- *Diarrhea, constipation, parasites.*
- Irritability and inflammation of the intestines; *worms.*
- *Skin conditions; impetigo, eczema, herpes, shingles, cold sores, acne, pemphigus, rupia, athlete's foot, lichen, ringworm, rashes, chronic scaly skin conditions,* especially when associated with intestinal disorder (external).
- Skin eruptions red, like the flush of scarlatina or erysipelas (cf. Stellaria).
- Abscesses, boils (external).
- Electric shock.
- Valley fever.

- Diarrhea from drinking bad water (combine with *Capsicum*).
- *Fibromyalgia,* arthritis, swollen hands.
- Cancer.

PREPARATION AND DOSAGE:

I use small doses, 1–3 drops, 1–3x/day.

LITERATURE:

Traditional, Edward Shook (1–9), Phyllis Light (6, 12, 13, 14, 25), Brent Davis, Edward Bach (11), John Christopher (9), Jack Ritchason (12, 24, 25), Otto Wolff (15).

Juniperus communis. Juniper.

Juniperus is a low shrub native to open territory in North America, Europe, and Asia. It is a member of the cypress family. The berries are used in gin and in herbal healing. It contains volatile oils (1–4%), sugar (15–30%), resin (10%), juniperin (yellow bitter principle), proteins (4%), tannins, fat, wax, flavonoids, malates, vitamin C, formic and acetic acids, and minerals (sulfur, copper, cobalt, tin, and aluminum).

Juniper berries are a traditional diuretic. They contain volatile oils, which irritate the membranes, so they are classified as an irritating diuretic. That means they are indicated in depressed tissue states while very much contraindicated in acute, hot, and irritable states. In Greek medicine they are considered suitable to cold, damp, and wind. Sir John Hill (1740, 221) writes, "They have two excellent qualities, they dispel wind, and rock by urine, for which reason they are excellent in those cholics which arise from the gravel and stone."

The volatile oils dilate the glomeruli of the kidneys, so juniper is used in chronic renal congestion and swelling, with backache. The irritating effect of juniper oil causes mucus discharges from the membranes, which resemble the gleety discharges of gonorrhea. In appropriate doses it therefore removes mucus from the genitourinary tract. Juniper berries also act on the mucosa of the digestive tract and lungs.

Dorothy Hall has developed a picture of the classic juniperus person. They have water-logged kidneys with generalized retention of water in the body, especially in the lower parts of the body. The thighs may become water-logged, causing a waddling gait, spreading apart the legs, with the rear end "waggling like a duck." The legs can be as thick as trees; there is little definition between the ankles and feet, which may overflow the shoes. Every step becomes an effort. Conditions include diabetes insipidus (continual, clear, copious urine); incontinence; deterioration of ureters, kidneys, and bladder; fluid retention in upper arms, face, and chin; and weight gain around the hips in later life. Diabetes mellitus, type II, may cause the condition or may develop.

Juniper is one of the simples favored by William Salmon (1692, 23, 677; 1710). He describes it as a remedy for cold, damp, phlegmatic conditions. It is also for wind or spasm, sometimes associated with an acute attack of cold resulting in chills, tension, and spasm. Salmon gives a fairly comprehensive account of the organs and systems upon which juniper acts. It is for "cold and moist diseases of the brain, as old pituitous headachs, megrims, the apoplexy, falling sickness, convulsion, cramp, lethargy, carus, vertigo, etc., by outwardly bathing the head or parts afflicted therewith, and also taking them inwardly." Dr. Christopher (1996, 273) adds that it is "a strengthener of the brain, memory, and optic nerve."

Juniper likewise acts on cold, damp, mucus, and spasm in the lungs, reports Salmon. "Asthmas, coughs, difficulty breathing, wheezing, shortness of breath, hoarseness, and other the like cold and moist diseases of the lungs." It acts on the digestive tract and is "prevalent against all diseases proceeding from wind in the stomach or bowels." He also mentions the traditional uses for sand, gravel, and slime in the urine.

Salmon gives an extensive account of the properties of juniper berries in female conditions. "They are good against fits of the mother [PMS, cramps], facilitate both birth and after-birth, and repress vapors from the womb [PMS, hormonal moods], cleansing, warming, and strengthening that part, and causing fruitfulness. Inwardly taken and outwardly applyed, they give present ease in after-pains, and wholly remove them." They stimulate circulation to the extremities, increase diuresis, and remove edema in the legs. "Outwardly being bathed therewith, they help coldness of the limbs, cramps, watery swellings in the hands and legs, numbness, palsies, weakness of the nerves and muscles, as also old aches and pains, proceeding from cold, bruises, or strains, &c. though never so vehement."

TASTE:

pungent, bitter, acrid, sweet • warm, dry • oily, stimulating, aromatic, antiseptic

TISSUE STATES:

depression, stagnation, constriction

SPECIFIC INDICATIONS:

CONSTITUTION, COMPLEXION, CHARACTERISTIC SYMPTOMS

- Exhausted kidneys, resulting in extensive edema, with nervous system weakness, incontinence, and heart symptoms.

HEAD

- Headache, migraine, vertigo (oil on temples, bathe the head).
- Gums, bleeding.

RESPIRATION

- Respiratory congestion; bronchitis, coughs, chest infections, *colds;* with scanty, dark urine.
- "Asthmas, coughs, difficult of breathing, wheezing, shortness of breath, hoarseness."

CARDIOVASCULAR

- Heart burdened by edema; "passive congestion of the kidneys resulting from heart problems" (Christopher).

DIGESTION

- Loss of appetite, poor digestion, dyspepsia, flatulence, intestinal pain; especially in the elderly.
- "Wind in the stomach or bowels"; colic, griping of the guts, flatulence.
- Typhoid fever.
- Hemorrhoids.

PANCREAS

- Pancreas, sharp pain, pancreatitis; with depression.
- Diabetes mellitus, adult onset, in diabetics with water retention, renal problems.

KIDNEYS AND BLADDER

- *Edema without active inflammation; uric acid buildup.*
- Feeble or aged persons with persistent dragging or weight across the kidneys.
- Old people, with poor digestion and scanty secretion of urine.
- After acute renal inflammation has subsided and there is renal swelling and nephritis and high blood pressure.
- *Chronic renal congestion and swelling, pyelitis, pyelonephritis;* aching through the back and loins.
- Chronic catarrhal affections of the urinary tract; often associated with gonorrhea.
- *Urine; retained,* amber colored.
- Clear, copious urine (diabetes insipidus).
- Cystitis, strangury.
- Sand, gravel, and slime in the urine.

FEMALE

- Menstruation; sudden suppression from exposure to cold; accompanied by nervousness.
- Dysmenorrhea, cramps (feet in hot water with juniper oil).
- Amenorrhea, atonic.
- Leucorrhea.
- Infertility.
- Parturition: facilitate labor and expel the afterbirth (contraindicated earlier in pregnancy).

MUSCULAR AND SKELETAL

- Arthritis, swollen joints, lumbago, sciatica, muscular rheumatism; associated with poor peripheral circulation, cold and damp (the oil externally).
- Stiff, contracted, cramped, chilled muscles (gin, external oil, salve, or bath).
- Edema of the hands and legs.
- Nerves and muscles; numb, shaking.
- "Old aches and pains, proceeding from cold, bruises, or strains, &c. though never so vehement."

SKIN

- Moist eczema, psoriasis, herpes, lichen, porrigo (oil externally).

FEVER
- Intermittent fever, ague.

OTHER
- Snake bites, insect bites.
- Sores.

PREPARATION AND DOSAGE:

Collect only the second-year berries, which are dark, almost a deep purple, not the green first-year berries (Christopher, 1996, 278). "Best form is the infusion. One ounce to a pint of boiling water. Dose, one-half to two ounces, or tincture, one to ten drops" (Boericke). Spagyric tincture, 20–50 drops, or more, "according to the age, strength, and urgency of the occasion" (Salmon, 1692, 677).

CONTRAINDICATIONS:

Avoid when there is acute inflammation, blood in the urine, proteinuria, nephritis, large stones in the kidneys, damaged nephrons, neuritis. Contraindicated in pregnancy; stimulates uterine contractions.

LITERATURE:

Traditional, Phyllis Light (11, 12), William Cook (17, 18, 19, 21), Dorothy Hall (1, 6, 12, 20), William Boericke (16), Finley Ellingwood (16, 18), A. W. Kuts-Cheraux (7, 19), Christopher Menzies-Trull (2, 3, 7, 24, 25), John Christopher (6), Edwin Hale (3), Louise Tenney (3, 4, 8, 9, 10, 11, 17, 19, 23, 26, 30, 31, 32, 35–37), William Salmon (2, 5, 8, 22, 24, 27–33).

Larrea divaricata. Chaparral, Creosote Bush.

Chaparral is a shrub native to the deserts of Arizona. It is used extensively by the Indian people. It entered the literature of Western herbalism in the early twentieth century. It is a stimulant, antiseptic, and alterative. It contains bitter terpenes, placing it in the category of herbs useful for depression and toxicity. The terpenes stimulate secretion and cleansing of the mucosa and tissues. They are antibiotic and antifungal. There are also saponins (soaps), which bind and remove oils. Chaparral contains volatile oils, which are released after a desert rain, making the air smell fresh and invigorating. It also contains a specific "active ingredient" called nordihydroguaiaretic acid (NDGA), which has been shown to possess anti-cancer potential, especially in tumors and leukemia.

Chaparral is used especially for people who have been poisoned by chronic exposure to drugs or chemicals or tissue breakdown, as in severe acute poisoning, chronic venereal taint, or acute or chronic medical and recreational drug and alcohol overdose. It is suited to the destructive tissue states—depression, torpor, and atrophy. As with basil and dandelion, there is thickened, polluted fluids, or "humors in the blood." It kills low forms of life that thrive when the tissues are depressed.

All the channels of elimination—lungs, skin, kidneys, colon, menses—can be affected as toxins get caught in them. The lymph/immune function is depressed and the liver is compromised. Chaparral counteracts these problems. So strong is the action of *Larrea* on the liver that large doses have induced a toxic hepatitis, leading the FDA to put chaparral on the list of suspicious plants. This indicates a homeopathic relationship—what it causes it will cure. In appropriate doses chaparral improves liver function on both the catabolic and anabolic sides, so it is indicated when there is a need for tissue cleansing and building. It is called for when anemia is associated with impure blood.

Chaparral is indicated when the internal oils are polluted, as in the basil profile, perhaps because fats are used to store contaminants. It contains saponins, which remove toxic oils, and volatile oils, which stimulate lipid metabolism pathways.

People with a history of medical and recreational drug, alcohol, and caffeine use sometimes experience symptoms of detoxification while using *Larrea,* including headache, bodyache, and nausea. "Sometimes you may have nightmares, déjà vu's that never happened, all kinds of things that face you, all of your fears and everything else during" a twenty-one-day cleanse, comments Eva Graf (1978, 2).

Dr. Christopher, who used chaparral extensively, recommended alternating burdock tea and chaparral tea for arthritis. Both have an extremely good track record in this complaint separately. Take burdock tea, 1 cup, 3x/day for six weeks, then switch to chaparral, the same amount. Take one week off in between and alternate two or three times.

TASTE:

pungent • warm • antiseptic

TISSUE STATES:

depression, toxicity

SPECIFIC INDICATIONS:

CONSTITUTION, COMPLEXION, CHARACTERISTIC SYMPTOMS
- Chronic chemical poisoning, chronic use of allopathic or recreational drugs, alcoholism.

HEAD
- Scalp rash, eczema, lice, dandruff (external).
- "Toxic headache" (also caused as a side effect).
- Stye in the eye.

RESPIRATION
- Chronic mucus congestion, sinusitis, bronchitis; in people working with chemicals.
- Low immunity, allergies, fever, influenza, bodyache.

CARDIOVASCULAR AND BLOOD
- Anemia associated with impure blood (add slippery elm as a nutritive).
- Arteriosclerosis; amoebas, pinworms, parasites in the bowels.

DIGESTION
- Chronic indigestion, cramps, nausea.

KIDNEYS AND BLADDER
- Dissolves calcareous deposits; arthritis, kidney stones, gout, bursitis.
- Low-grade, ongoing kidney and bladder infections, kidney stones (combine with a mucilage).

FEMALE

- Female discomforts including chronic yeast infection, vaginitis, irregular menstruation, cysts, uterine fibroids, pelvic inflammatory disease, venereal warts, gonorrhea, abnormal cervical tissue, leucorrhea, dysmenorrhea, prolapsed uterus; cancer.
- Uterine prolapse, leucorrhea, amenorrhea, dysmenorrhea.

SKIN

- Skin fungus, athlete's foot, nail fungus; skin mites, ringworm, scabies, chiggers; herpes simplex, shingles; poison ivy; insect and snake bites; inflamed splinters, impetigo, staph infection, acne, blackheads, whiteheads, liver spots, psoriasis, eczema; abscesses and boils (combine with slippery elm and poultice).

MUSCULAR AND SKELETAL

- Arthritis.

OTHER

- "Essential in the treatment of cancer" (traditional, quotation from Brent Davis).
- Preventative of cancer from radiation exposure.

PREPARATION, CONTRAINDICATIONS, AND DOSAGE:

Because of the bad taste, many people prefer to use the capsules or a tincture, but the tea is considered to be the most effective preparation. Eva Graf (1978) learned from a Native American practitioner in the Southwest how to prepare this powerful medicine. It was emphasized to her that many people do not get the results they want because they use chaparral incorrectly. The correct method is called the "twenty-one-day cleanse." Put 1 teaspoonful of chaparral leaf in a cup. Add 1 cup of very warm, but not hot or boiling, water. Cover (to preserve the volatile oils) and let stand overnight. Strain and drink on an empty stomach, in the morning. Take the same chaparral and put it in another cup. Pour warm water over it and let it stand overnight. Strain and drink in the morning. Again, take the same chaparral and repeat. On the fourth day, put the old chaparral out under a tree. Take a new pinch of chaparral, a teaspoonful, and start the process over. Repeat seven times for a total of twenty-one days. This method provides a slow, steady cleansing that avoids unnecessarily intense and unhealthy detoxification. It often brings up emotions connected with the liver, such as anger, but slow enough so that they can be handled appropriately. Dr. Christopher (1996, 79) gives a formula for a nonbitter chaparral tea: 8 parts chaparral, 6 parts elder flowers, 2 parts peppermint. It is not recommended for infants under two, or pregnant or nursing mothers. Lalitha Thomas (1996, 77) suggests that when detoxifying a particular organ with chaparral one may in addition place a stimulating poultice on the part.

TOXICITY:

Excessive doses have caused symptoms of hepatitis.

LITERATURE:

Traditional (1, 2, 5, 6, 15, 16), John Christopher (1, 2, 3, 5, 6, 15), Brent Davis (4, 6, 16), Eva Graf, Lalitha Thomas, Richard Lucas (15), Ute Indian (17).

Ledum groenlandicum, L. palustre. Labrador Tea, Marsh Tea.

This genus of the heath family is widespread in boreal regions, where it separates into two closely related species, L. groenlandicum *in North America and* L. palustre *in Europe. They can probably be used interchangeably. However, they have not been deeply explored in Western herbalism. Marsh tea is slightly warming, oily, and astringent. The European* Ledum *is best known as a homeopathic remedy, most famous for puncture wounds.*

The former is a popular fall tonic and cold remedy among the Indians of the Canadian shield and northern Minnesota. It is used as a strengthening tonic after loss of fluids from participating in the sweat lodge. It is also used in the fall to stop excessive sweating, in preparation for winter, and is one of the most important Anishinabe Ojibwe cold and flu remedies in northern Minnesota. It is traditionally used for excessive urination and diabetes mellitus. A general tonic is made in the spring with fresh, hot maple sap. "It is wonderful" (Clara NiiSka).

PREPARATION AND DOSAGE:

Tincture, 4–5 drops in water (W. T. Fernie, 1917, 435).

CAUTIONS:

Used as a beverage and commonly considered safe.

LITERATURE:

Traditional, homeopathy.

Leptandra virginica, Veronicastrum virginicum Culver's Root, Black Root, Bowman's Root.

This member of the veronica family is native to moist ground in eastern North America. It was used much in the colonial period as a purgative with an affinity to the liver and typhoid fever. It was at this time that it acquired the names Culver's root, Bowman's root, and Tinker's root from its use by various doctors. Peter Smith (1812, 1, 26) writes that his father, Hezekiah Smith, was "a home old man" or "Indian Doctor" who "for the cure of the pleurisy practised long with the root, and used to cure the pleurisy with amazing speed." Culver's root contains volatile oils, saponins, mannitol, dextrose, and tannins.

Culver's root is an old purgative, adopted from the Indians by the American colonists. It operates through the liver and gallbladder, forcefully expelling bile, which decongests those organs, lubricates the intestines, and moves the stool. Dr. Ralph Russell (1911, 315) puts it correctly when he says it "makes the liver act." It was widely used by the eclectics and nineteenth-century physicians for congestion of the liver and gallbladder, constipation, and irritation of the intestines. It was also highly valued in typhoid fever. The homeopathic provings produced the black, tarry stools associated with blood from the small intestine, typical of this disease.

Leptandra in very small doses "augments bile flow, removes catarrhal and granular detritus from the biliary passages and increases intestinal peristalsis. In delicate constitutions it does not diminish autonomic tone as do harsh laxatives such as cascara, buckthorn, rhubarb, etc. It is indicated in atony of the gallbladder, common bile duct, and intestines" (Brent

Davis, DC). When the bile releases, it is more sticky and darker; leptandra improves the outflow of this material without causing irritation of the intestines (Christopher Menzies-Trull).

TASTE:

bitter, acrid

TISSUE STATES:

constriction, atrophy, torpor

SPECIFIC INDICATIONS:

CONSTITUTION, COMPLEXION, CHARACTERISTIC SYMPTOMS
- People with gastrointestinal distress who are frustrated and discouraged from inability to actualize goals; also works more broadly when characteristic mental indications are not present.

MIND, SENSES, NERVES, EMOTIONS, PERSONALITY
- Hopeless, despondent, drowsy, with hepatic affections.
- Anxiety felt at the stomach; distress, unsatisfied with oneself, one's progress in life, current situation.

RESPIRATION
- Pleurisy.

DIGESTION
- Dyspepsia due to faulty digestion of fats and proteins.
- Nervous stomach, with cutting, shifting pains and dark stools.
- Food poisoning.
- Fullness in the abdomen; chronic diarrhea.
- Distress in the stomach and intestines.
- Black stool in typhoid.
- Intestinal ulceration, enteritis, typhoid.

LIVER AND GALLBLADDER
- Dull, heavy pain in the right hypochondrium.
- Hepatic congestion, soreness.
- Acute hepatitis, acute gallstone colic; with pain, jaundice, depression, bitter taste, flatulent colic, clay-colored stool.

- Atony of the gallbladder, common bile duct, and intestines.
- Constricted bile duct, associated with chronic emotional stress, chronic hepatic congestion.
- Constipation associated with poor bile flow and atrophy of the intestines, inactivity of intestinal secretion, thirst, lack of appetite, headache.
- Portal obstruction with edema, ascites.

FEVER
- Intermittent fevers with biliousness, malarial, typhoid.
- Fever in early stages.

SKIN
- Skin disease.

PREPARATION AND DOSAGE:

Dried rhizome and roots are used, never fresh (like many purgatives). Tincture, let stand in the alcohol four days (Ralph Russell). It works best in small, repeated doses, over a long time, and can be borne for long duration, but is cathartic and disturbing in large doses.

CAUTIONS:

Nontoxic, but purgative, even in small doses.

LITERATURE:

Traditional, homeopathic indications (2), Finley Ellingwood, Brent Davis (1, 5), Peter Smith (4), Christopher Menzies-Trull, William LeSassier.

Ligusticum porteri. Osha Root.

The name "osha" is from the Spanish oso *for bear. This is a very important Native American bear medicine. The oily, spicy, brown, furry root is typical of the bear medicines that stimulate the adrenals (cf. angelica, spikenard, lomatium, sunflower, balsam root, American liquorice, etc.). The American Indian esteem for this plant passed over to the culture of Spanish New Mexico, where this is perhaps the most highly regarded medicinal plant. It is native to the southern Rocky Mountains above 6,000 feet. Ligusticum is a member of the Apiaceae family somewhat akin to angelica in properties. It contains bitters, glycosides, volatile oils, resins, and silicon.*

Osha is used like the analogous angelicas, but is more potent and probably somewhat different in action. The warm, spicy root is tonifying to the glucocorticoid side of the adrenal cortex—that is, to the cortisone-building side; hence it is anti-inflammatory, promotes digestion and nutrition, and settles the nervous system. Therefore, it is carminative to the stomach (see Cook, below). The resins stimulate expectoration and clear the lungs, while reducing inflammation. It is excellent when the cough reflexes are exhausted, in old cases. "Expends the greater portion of its influence on the respiratory passages," wrote William Cook (1898). "It is used mostly in coughs, proving expectorant and antispasmodic in a desirable degree, allaying tickling in the throat, averting paroxysms of coughing, and overcoming capillary congestion in bronchitis and catarrh." Brent Davis, DC, reports that "osha is a specific for relieving problems of milk and milk products (e.g. cheese) allergies; especially excess mucus production, congestion of the intestinal lymphatics, and sinus/ear congestion." He also says that it relaxes and drains a congested pancreas.

TASTE:

spicy • warm • oily, stimulating

TISSUE STATES:

atrophy, depression

SPECIFIC INDICATIONS:

- Mind and senses dull, with mucus congestion of the sinuses or bronchial tree.
- Old lingering bronchial cases, with heavy congestion, and weak cough reflexes.
- Milk allergies.
- Sinusitis, colds, influenza, pharyngitis, bronchitis, emphysema, tuberculosis, silicosis.

- Upper gastric spasm.
- Gastroenteritis, colitis.
- Amenorrhea, dysmenorrhea.
- Retained placenta.
- Measles.

PREPARATION AND DOSAGE:

The dried root is used by decoction or extracted in 87% alcohol (due to the high content of resins). The dose should be small to large, depending on the condition and needs. Brent Davis suggests 1–2 drops for upper gastric spasm, but increasing doses in respiratory conditions, until the patient can smell and taste the remedy.

CAUTIONS:

Pregnancy; like many members of the wild carrot family it is potentially abortifacient.

LITERATURE:

Traditional, William Cook, Brent Davis (2, 3), Michael Moore.

Liriodendron tulipifera. Tulip Tree, Yellow Poplar, Tulip Poplar, Whitewood.

This beautiful tree is native to the middle regions of the Eastern Woodland forest of North America, from New York to the Upper South, west to the Mississippi River. It is a member of the magnolia family and possesses beautiful, tulip-like flowers. It is an old American Indian remedy. The pioneers used it as an antimalarial for chills, fever, biliousness, and exhaustion from the disease. It contains a small amount of salicylates.

The bark of the tulip tree is sweet, acrid, and aromatic. It was used in the nineteenth century primarily as a substitute for quinine. It settles chills that wear out the autonomic nervous system and improves digestion and debility following malaria. It was particularly used to tonify people worn down by malarial chills. Francis Porcher (1863), the Confederate doctor, gives as an alternative to quinine bark the formula dogwood bark, tulip poplar bark, and wild cherry bark. The acrid constituent settles tension, while the sweetness builds up and restores when there is weakness.

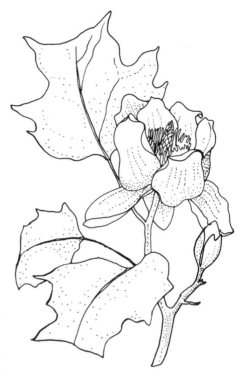

Liriodendron, though little known, is a valuable tonic because it unites properties that are often needed in combination—it is a sweet acrid bark suited to conditions where dry/atrophy unites with wind/tension. Such conditions are not uncommon, since nervous weakness can lead to tension, and vice versa. Hence, it is a tonic where there is weakness and a worn-out system from sympathetic excess and nervous tension. It is suited to neurasthenic types, where the system is worn down by tension and needs rebuilding. More specifically, liriodendron (1) relaxes and builds the stomach, (2) restores systems worn out by chills and fever or tension and debility, (3) calms the heart and strengthens the cardiovascular system, (4) moistens, nourishes, and strengthens muscles and joints to cure arthritis, and (5) gently tonifies the uterus.

Dr. Samuel Henry (1814, 304), who practiced in Florida, the South, New Jersey, and New York City, utilized tulip tree primarily as a carminative: it "creates a good appetite and strengthens the stomach." He combined it with orange peel and sometimes with gentian. This would resemble the construction of a European carminative. Daniel Cobb (1846, 2:60), a subsequent botanical doctor in New York, gave only a few keywords for the tree ("aromatic, antibilious, carminative, vermifuge") but these are enough to trace the direction of his thought. Cobb evidently saw liriodendron as an aromatic carminative that mildly warms and soothes the stomach, improves gastric tone, settles the symptoms of biliousness associated with malaria and chaotic digestion, and improves the health of the intestines to resist worms.

Tulip poplar is an old American Indian heart remedy. I first learned about it from the late Tis Mal Crow. He said it was the secret heart remedy of his mentor and would not discuss it until he confirmed that his teacher had passed on. Sondra Boyd, a Cherokee friend, confirmed that tulip poplar is a traditional heart tonic in her culture. It is also for use after a stroke. Alabama herbalist Phyllis Light considers tulip tree to be a tonic to the arteries and circulation, valuable in varicose veins and heart problems. In the South, it is an old remedy for thinning the blood.

The great eclectic pharmacist John Uri Lloyd (Lloyd and Lloyd, 1886–7, 7) suspected that liriodendron would make a heart medicine and recommended the study of it to a friend, Professor Roberts Bartholow. The latter administered a large dose of tulipiferine, an alkaloid extracted from the tree, to a frog. It caused convulsions followed by complete relaxation, until there were no movements or reactions in the voluntary musculature. Meanwhile, the heart muscle beat in a slow but stronger rhythm. "The alkaloid will, no doubt, be found useful whenever a tonic to the heart is required," concluded Bartholow. Sondra Boyd, herself now a cardiac researcher, laughed at this story. "That explains what happened when we were kids. We threw some poplar bark in a puddle and the frogs came up alive but unable to move. We were reprimanded for abusing a medicine."

William Cook (1869, 518) writes, "While it improves the appetite and digestion to a fair extent, and for this purpose is unsurpassed in convalescence, its most valuable action is upon the nervous system and uterus. In nervousness, nervous irritability, hysteria, and chronic pains through the womb, it is an agent of the greatest efficacy—both soothing and sustaining. The menses are not influenced by it; but it proves valuable in chronic dysmenorrhea, as well as in leucorrhea, prolapsus of a mild grade, and the uterine suffering incident to pregnancy. By its influence on the nervous system it sometimes promotes the flow of urine; and it favors greater freedom of the bowels, without being in any sense cathartic." For precision, Cook adds, "It is not an agent fitted to languid or sluggish conditions, or states of depression."

Darryl Patton, a student of the late Tommie Bass, noted that for his teacher yellow poplar was a substitute for its cousin, cucumber tree, which was Bass's favorite remedy for arthritis. It may be necessary to use liriodendron rather than its cousin, since the former is widespread and common whereas the latter has a limited range. Patton points out that tulip tree contains salicylates, explaining its use for arthritis, thinning the blood, strokes, and heart disease.

TASTE:

sweet, acrid, aromatic

TISSUE STATES:

atrophy, tension

SPECIFIC INDICATIONS:

- Debility and tension.
- Nervousness, nervous irritability, hysteria.
- Poor appetite.
- Gastric weakness and debility.
- Sluggish bowels; worms.
- Heart and circulation.
- Uterine weakness, debility, and tension.
- Leucorrhea.
- Postpartum uterine suffering.
- Chronic painful menses.
- Joints; arthritis.
- Stroke; to improve blood flow to the brain.
- Stroke paralysis; to strengthen the wasted tissues.
- Intermittent chills and fever; malaria; debility after malaria and fever.

PREPARATION AND DOSAGE:

William LeSassier points out that the bark is sweeter in the spring and more acrid in the fall. I have found this to be true.

CAUTIONS:

A mild, safe article.

LITERATURE:

Traditional, Samuel Henry (3, 4), Daniel Cobb (5), William Cook (2, 3, 4, 5, 7, 8, 9, 10), John Uri Lloyd (6), Sondra Boyd (6, 12, 13), Tis Mal

Crow (6, 12, 13), Phyllis Light (11), Darryl Patton (11), Matthew Wood (1), Francis Porcher (14).

Lobelia inflata. Indian Tobacco.

Lobelia is native to North America, as far west as the Mississippi River. It possesses alkaloids, bitter glycosides, resins, gums, and volatile oils. However, the "active ingredient" is lobeline, an alkaloid. It is a nicotine mimic. Thus, lobelia has an effect much like tobacco but also quite different. For one thing, it is not toxic when taken internally, though it has marked symptoms—usually vomiting.

This is the remedy that won Samuel Thomson such fame and infamy and it is to him that credit for its use in medicine must be given. Lobelia is an almost pure relaxant, and thus able to open obstructions to the skin, circulation, nervous system, muscles, and all internal organs that depend to any extent on nerve impulses.

Lobelia was most famous as an emetic—a large dose can easily provoke vomiting—and Thomson used it to "cleanse" the stomach. However, he also emphasized that it was not necessary to bring on emesis. Persistent small doses are relaxant to all structures and bring out latent tensions; in fact, continued small doses relax the entire frame to such an extent that the patient falls into a state of "suspended animation," as Thomson called it. The entire sympathetic nervous system is completely relaxed and the parasympathetic takes over, so that the patient, though awake, is incapable of movement. Several times patients were declared dead when they were simply incapable of movement. This allows free secretion, removal of all obstructions, and complete relaxation, so that the organism is free from offending substances. With this method Thomson and his early followers were able to expedite miraculous cures. It is not so used today, this being a less heroic age, and it is possible that the full healing powers of Lobelia are thus lost for the time being.

William Cook gives an extensive account of Lobelia. "It is a pure relaxant, possessing only the faintest moiety of stimulating property, and this of a transient character, expending itself upon the fauces, and the glands and mucous membrane of the mouth and respiratory organs. The quality for which it is so greatly valued, is its peculiar influence in relaxing the entire circuit of the organs and tissues—making prominent and diffusive impressions upon and through the nervous structures, but proving itself capable of reaching every portion of the body under the directing influence of the vital force.

"The circulation is materially equalized by its use, and the blood-vessels relieved from a condition of tension, whether the case be one of inflammation or fever. By relaxing the circulatory apparatus, it favors a full outward flow of blood, with diaphoresis; secures greater fullness and softness of the pulse, with a reduced excitability of the heart; and from the universality of this influence, expedites the re-establishment of the secretions of the skin, liver, and kidneys. Such extensive impressions fit it for the treatment of phrenitis, meningitis, pneumonia, pleurisy, hepatitis, peritonitis, and nephritis, and to inflammation of the periosteum—whether on the long bones, alveolar processes, about the ear, or other places. In some of these cases, as of pneumonia and pleurisy, this agent alone (especially in the form of tincture) is many times sufficient to cure acute cases, providing they have not yet passed into the stage of actual congestion—as congestion requires very little relaxation, and that always associated with an excess of stimulation. This action also qualifies it for almost universal use in synochial, catarrhal, bilious, rheumatic, typhoid, and other forms of fever. Its use in fever is valuable beyond any other remedy that has ever been introduced to the notice of the profession, and that without any reference to its emetic action; for it secures that sanguineous distribution, cardiac relief, and secernent activity which are so positively demanded in all such cases, and this in a manner at once powerful and harmless."

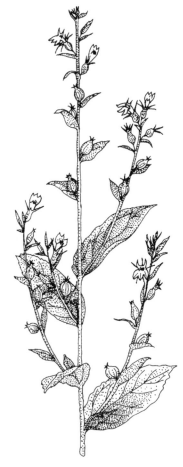

"The nervous system derives great benefit from it, as it is one of the most reliable articles to relieve all forms of suffering arising from tension and excitement of the tissues. Thus as a local application in external inflammation, over the seat of an abscess or a periostitis, on acute erysipelas or ophthalmia, and all other cases of the kind, it is of great efficacy; and internally in the suffering of acute rheumatism, or pleurisy, or periostitis, or meningitis, or neuralgia, it can be used to great advantage."

"Upon the muscular and fibrous tissues it expends its influence with a very direct and peculiar force. The nausea induced by it at the stomach, is the first manifestation of this, and the enlarging caliber of the pulse is from a similar influence upon the fibres of the blood-vessels. It is by this combined action upon both the nerves and muscles of the stomach, that small doses of weak lobelia infusion allay irritation of the stomach, and arrest spasmodic and even sympathetic vomiting."

"Its virtues are exhibited to the highest advantage in spasmodic and true membranous croups, hooping-cough, spasmodic asthma (but not the humid asthma, nor that form of difficult breathing accompanying heart disease), spasmodic strangury, subsultus tendinum, spasmodic occlusion of the gall-ducts (as in the paroxysms of suffering from the passage of gall stones), strangulated hernia, etc. So prompt and positive is its action in these several difficulties, that it may safely be set down as an absolute and reliable specific for them, so far as the excessive muscular contractility is concerned."

"This relaxing power over muscular structures is of great advantage not merely in the spasmodic affections above alluded to, but in spasmodic and convulsive troubles of the severest grades. Thus, in strangulated hernia, and in fits of hysteria and epilepsy, it is powerful in cutting short the clonic contractions."

Samuel Thomson writes (1825, 2:47): "It clears all obstructions to the extremities, without regard to the names of disease, until it produces an equilibrium in the system, and will be felt in the fingers and toes, producing a prickling feeling like that caused by a knock of the elbow; this symptom is alarming to those unacquainted with its operation; but is always favorable, being a certain indication of the turn of the disorder."

Lobelia is indicated in muscular spasm, torsion, in closure of the pores of the skin, and probably, in closure of the internal pores of the body. On the other hand, it will also close the pores if they are open, if there is profuse sweat. It acts in contradictory ways; in fact, it is impossible to predict its behavior and it will seldom (in my experience, never) act the same way twice. If given in excess it will produce excessive salivation or nausea, as the body tries to rid itself of this active agent. The tea is used as a stop smoking aid and was once USP officinal.

TASTE:

acrid • extremely diffusive

TISSUE STATE:

constriction

SPECIFIC INDICATIONS:

- *Unequal appearance of the tongue: coated on one side, not the other, red and swollen on one side, not the other, torqued to one side, etc.*
- *Never been well since giving up tobacco, bronchial spasm from exposure to tobacco.*
- *Muscular spasm causing torsion of the frame.*
- *Affinity to the vagus; hence for respiratory and gastric problems; heartburn.*
- *Spasmodic asthma; worse from cigarette smoke, exercise-induced asthma.*
- *Bronchial asthma, "pretzeling up of the tubes of the lungs," worse from exercise and exposure to tobacco smoke; old, stale smoke in furniture and clothing especially.*
- *Hiatal hernia, heartburn, nausea, feels the need to vomit but cannot.*
- Sudden, high fever with closed pores, with pores open and profuse sweating; puffiness under the skin from water retention.
- High fever with perspiration and exhaustion.
- Use 10 drops to relax before scopes down or up the gastrointestinal tract.
- "Tickle and tearing feeling in the throat, like you're going to throw up in front of everyone" (Jennifer Tucker).

PREPARATION AND DOSAGE:

The entire herb is picked while in seed and dried for use by infusion, or extracted fresh in alcohol. Lobelia works better when combined with other herbs (it likes to herd them around). Excessive doses cause salivation, nausea, and even vomiting, and it is often impossible to determine when the excessive dosage has been reached, but a small dose (1–2 drops) should be used. Discontinue when evidence of rejection by salivation or nausea appears.

LITERATURE:

Samuel Thomson, William Cook, Finley Ellingwood, Matthew Wood, Julia Graves (10), Jennifer Tucker (11).

Lycopus virginicus. Bugleweed.

This plant grows near water on low ground in the eastern part of North America. Its cousins L. americanus and L. europaeus can be used interchangeably. Bugleweed is one of the bitter mints that has a profoundly sedative effect (cf. Scutellaria, Leonurus). This genus contains flavonoids (cooling), bitters, tannins, and volatile oils.

Lycopus was introduced by Constantine Rafinesque as a remedy for conditions where the pulse is "rapid and tumultuous," indicating excitement of the heart and circulation. He used it for scarlet fever, irritable cough, and hemorrhage from the lungs. In the mid-nineteenth century it was a favorite hemostatic, even used in tuberculosis. Michael Moore (2003) recommends it as a general hemostatic. It is probably best indicated in conditions where there is fever with a rapid pulse rather than as a general hemostatic for any condition.

In the early twentieth century *Lycopus* was discovered to be an excellent remedy for hyperthyroidism and hyperadrenalism. It reduces the output of thyroid-stimulating hormone (TSH) from the pituitary, turning down the setting on the thyroid level. I find that it is indicated for the classic cases where the person has the staring, nervous eyes, "like a hunted animal." Michael Moore (2003) recommends it in late-pregnancy thyroid "storms."

I remember one woman who complained that she felt "all switched up." What did that mean? "At night sometimes I can't sleep, I'm totally awake, and my eyes are all bugged out." What's bothering her? "My husband is on disability. He follows me all around the house and tells me how to do the housework. I feel 'dogged.'" *Lycopus* tincture quickly controlled this case.

TASTE:

bitter

TISSUE STATES:

excitation, atrophy

SPECIFIC INDICATIONS:

MIND, SENSES, NERVES, EMOTIONS, PERSONALITY

- *Hyperthyroidism, hyperadrenalism; looks nervous, like a hunted animal; pulse rapid and tumultuous.*
- *Nervous, driven, fearful; like a hunted animal.*
- Wide, open, staring eyes; alert, unable to sleep; nervous fear, hyperthyroidism.

RESPIRATION

- Bronchial irritation, troublesome cough.
- Chronic cough, with rapid pulse, high range of temperature; hemorrhage.
- Asthma associated with hyperthyroidism; worse in summer heat, the metabolism is so high the person has to pant to get enough oxygen; not due to bronchial problems.

CIRCULATION AND FEVER

- Irregular, rapid, and labored, tumultuous action of the heart, with skin blanched, extremities cold.
- Hemorrhage, when the action of the heart is vigorous and the pulse is full and strong.
- Passive capillary congestion, involving either the lungs, with a tendency to spitting of blood; the kidneys, with profuse urination and the urine containing sugar; the liver, with various bilious symptoms; or the mucosa, with catarrhal conditions.
- Fever, scarlet fever; never well since; cardiac damage from fever.
- Rapid, tumultuous pulse.

DIGESTION

- Diarrhea and dysentery.

KIDNEYS
- Albuminuria, with frequent pulse.

PREPARATION AND DOSAGE:

Hard to identify until in flower, but better if taken earlier. Extract the fresh or dried herb in alcohol. Dose: 1–20 drops (Fyfe). Also used by infusion and in the low homeopathic potencies. Many of the properties are destroyed by hot water decoction (Michael Moore).

LITERATURE:

Constantine Rafinesque, John William Fyfe, William Boericke, George Royal, Rolla Thomas (5, 13), Matthew Wood (1, 2, 6), Michael Moore.

Magnolia acuminata. Cucumber Tree.

This interesting tree is native from the Gulf of Mexico to the northern shore of Lake Erie. It deserves attention as Tommie Bass's favorite remedy for arthritis and rheumatism. Members of the magnolia genus are old remedies for malaria and fever, both in the southern United States and China. The bitter taste increases the appetite and reduces anemia and debility. It increases secretion to cleanse the gallbladder, intestines, and kidneys. Decoct 1 tablespoon of the dried root bark in a cup of boiling water. Two cups a day. The cold tea is more diuretic (Patton, 2004, 123).

If *Magnolia acuminata* is unavailable, its cousin, *Liriodendron tulipifera*, may be used as a substitute. "The use of this native magnolia bark in bitters for rheumatism was similar to use of the related tulip tree" in Southern folk medicine (Moss, 1999, 180).

Melilotus officinalis. Melilot.

Melilot is a member of the clover family native to North America. It has a taste similar to its cousins red clover and alfalfa, but possesses more of the sweet vanilla flavor indicating the presence of even higher levels of coumarins. It contains flavonoids, tannins, mucilage, and glycosides that dry to form coumarin.

This member of the clover family is probably the highest in natural coumarins, so high that it has caused bleeding in cattle. It is a natural blood thinner and has been used to relieve congestions, as in headaches from congestion of blood to the head. Some of the Lakotas call it "sunstroke medicine"; it thins the blood to relieve congestion in the head.

Menispermum canadense. Moonseed, Yellow Parilla.

This curious plant is a vine native to the Eastern Woodland region of North America. It has its own family, the Menispermaceae. It has a bitter, yellow inner bark, a classic signature for a purgative. Moonseed is superficially similar in appearance to the botanically unrelated Smilacaceae *(sarsaparilla, cat briar, etc.), so it was sometimes called "sarsaparilla" or "yellow parilla" in the old days. It was conceived in folk medicine to have analogous properties. That would make it a blood purifier or alterative with special action on the skin. For an account of the use of moonseed in traditional herbalism, refer to the late John Lee (below). In professional medicine* Menispermum *appears to have been thought of as a bitter tonic, alterative, and purgative, suited to conditions associated with malaria. In this capacity refer to William Cook and Edwin Hale. Moonseed contains resins, starch, and bitters—including berberine— making it a stimulant to the liver, gallbladder, and digestive tract. The homeopath Edwin Hale recorded many different symptoms that fit the properties associated with* Menispermum *in herbalism.*

Menispermum "influences the mucous membranes, stomach, gall-ducts, and liver, and makes a distinct alterative-tonic impression upon the secreting organs, and slightly increases the force of the general circulation. Its stimulating qualities fit it for cases of moderate depression; and it is not a suitable article for irritable and sensitive conditions. In small doses, its action is chiefly manifested upon the respiratory passages, where it increases expectoration and gives a feeling of stimulation to the lungs— an action which sometimes can be taken advantage of in the treatment of chronic and depressed pulmonary affections. The stomach is fairly improved by it, and the hepatic apparatus and smaller bowels distinctly influenced, whence it will lead to a free discharge of bile and to fair evacuations of the bowels. Such qualities fit it for use in biliousness, atonic indigestion with costiveness, agues, dropsy, and skin diseases" (William Cook, 1869, 561).

Menispermum is not widely used in modern North American herbalism. In order to get at the details of little-known or forgotten old remedies we sometimes need to find a single practitioner who used the dickens out of the remedy and really understood how it works. In this case our herbalist is the late Mr. John Lee, an African American practitioner in North Carolina. He used *Menispermum* under the name "sarsaparilla" for diabetes, high and low blood pressure, gout, arthritis (frequently with black cohosh), earache, prostate gland problems, kidney, bladder, and urinary tract problems, styes, boils, diarrhea, swellings, dandruff, sore or weak eyes, heart murmur, and loss of appetite. Lee's plant material was identified by Dr. James Duke (Arvilla Payne-Jackson, 1993, 92). Some of Mr. Lee's uses are not well explained by the usual conception of *Menispermum*.

SPECIFIC INDICATIONS:

MIND, SENSES, NERVES, EMOTIONS, PERSONALITY
- Low-spirited, absentminded, torpor of the mind.
- Surly, ill-natured, irritable, quick-tempered, stubborn.
- Sleep restless; sleeps late and heavy in the morning.

HEAD
- Dull, heavy headache, with feeling of fullness, congestion, to bursting.
- Eyes; sore, weak, styes.
- Earache.
- Nose, itching and soreness in the nostrils, followed by thick, yellow mucus.
- *Tongue coated at the base,* yellow, yellow-white; dry and parched; swollen; tip red.

DIGESTION
- Poor appetite, lack of saliva.
- Dyspepsia, inactive stomach.
- Diarrhea; constipation.
- Chronic congestive conditions of the viscera.
- Ague; malaria.

RESPIRATION
- Pulmonary congestion.

HEART
- High and low blood pressure.
- Heart murmur; poor circulation.

KIDNEYS, BLADDER, AND PROSTATE
- Kidneys and bladder; dropsy, with debility; scanty, dark urine; cloudy.
- Prostate congestion.

MUSCULAR AND SKELETAL
- Arthritis (with black cohosh).
- Gout (external).

OTHER
- Diabetes.
- Skin problems, acne, boils, swellings, dandruff (external).
- Fever.
- Worse in the morning.

PREPARATION AND DOSAGE:

Decoction. Tincture: the fresh root is extracted in water and alcohol.

LITERATURE:

Traditional, William Cook (10–14, 16), John Lee (5, 6, 9, 11, 15, 16, 17, 18, 19, 20, 21, 22), Maude Grieve (8–12, 14, 17, 19, 20, 22), Rolla Thomas (8), Edwin Hale (1–5, 7, 8, 13, 17, 21, 22, 23, 24).

Mitchella repens. Partridge Berry, Squawvine, Twin Berry.

Mitchella is a member of the Rubiaceae family, to which also belong such diverse agents as cleavers, dyer's madder, sweet woodruff, and coffee. An influence on the nerves is discernible from this list, which is borne out in the applications of mitchella.

Mitchella is an old Indian female medicine. In remarking on this fact, the nineteenth-century settlers named it "squawvine." Although this may well translate an Indian name or statement, it does not appear to have been the name chosen by Indians themselves. Richard Fulton (1948), a Cherokee practitioner, notes that this name was given to the plant by the white man. Today it is considered politically incorrect, but there is still debate about the etymology in some quarters—"squaw" seems to derive from the Algonquin *ekaw*. Better to be on the safe side. A name actually reflecting the Indian perspective is "partridge berry." Birds, especially crows, are fond of the berries, and in some Native groups or societies mitchella is known as "crow medicine." It is, however, preeminently a female medicine. In addition to having an influence on menstruation, infertility, and pregnancy it is used in some Indian cultures to "help a young woman understand her husband."

"It is par excellence the partus preparator," writes Finley Ellingwood (1918). "Erratic pains and unsatisfied longings are removed, the nervous system assumes a tranquil condition, reflex symptoms abate, the urinary function is performed normally, the bowels become regular, imperfect digestion is improved, and the appetite becomes natural. Labor approaches, devoid of the irritating, aggravating complications, the preparatory state is simple, the dilatation is completed quickly, the expulsive contractions are strong, unirritating, and effectual, and are much less painful than without the remedy; involution is rapid and perfect, there are no subsequent complicating conditions to contend with, the patient's strength is not abated, and the function of lactation is in its best condition." Even given on short notice during labor, "the bark of the fresh root in hot infusion given occasionally during the progress of labor when no previous care of the patient has been afforded the physician, will work wonders in some tedious aggravating cases."

Margi Flint uses Mitchella for infertility. It is especially suited to women who are thin, angular, often athletic (dancers, gymnasts), tall, dark-haired, *vata*. They are "too much in their minds," then "later in life they want to have a baby and the doctors give up on them." They have a history of irregular cycles. It seems likely that this is a remedy for progesterone deficiency.

TASTE:

slightly sweet

TISSUE STATE:

atrophy

SPECIFIC INDICATIONS:

CONSTITUTION, COMPLEXION, CHARACTERISTIC SYMPTOMS
- Women; thin, tall, angular, dark-haired, athletic, too much in their minds.

MIND, SENSES, NERVES, EMOTIONS, PERSONALITY
- Anxiety, insomnia, nervousness, inflammation.
- "Nervous feebleness and irritability of a chronic character."

EYES
- Eyes, sore (wash).

DIGESTION
- Diarrhea, hemorrhoids.

KIDNEYS AND BLADDER
- Gravel.
- Bladder: irritation.

FEMALE
- Leucorrhea, prolapsus of the uterus.
- Menstrual irregularity, swelling and pain, breast swelling and soreness, edema, puffiness over the kidneys, throughout the body, in the head; chronic menstrual pain.
- Congestion of the ovaries and uterus.
- Infertility.
- Childbearing: believed by the eclectics (Quigg, Ellingwood) to prevent birth defects.
- Parturition: preparative.
- Postpartum: depression.
- Lactation.

MALE
- Spermatorrhea (with althaea, celastrus, and uva ursi).

OTHER

- Muscle spasms, erratic.
- Varicose veins.
- Skin, wounds.

PREPARATION AND DOSAGE:

Infusion or tincture of the dried or fresh leaves. Ellingwood recommends 5–60 minims of an alcohol preparation, 1–2x/day for the sixth and seventh months, 3x/day in the eighth month, and larger doses in the final weeks. Margi Flint prefers to give teas during pregnancy.

LITERATURE:

Traditional, C. E. Quigg (*Ellingwood's Therapeutist*, 1908, 2, 8, 12), Finley Ellingwood, Margi Flint (1, 11), William Cook (2, 3, 8, 9, 16), Paul Red Elk (2), Alma Hutchins (7), Jack Ritchason.

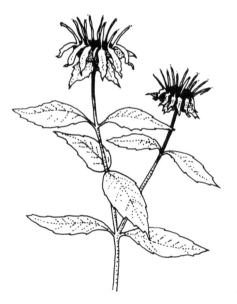

Monarda fistulosa. Sweet Leaf, Wild Bergamot, Bee Balm.

Although little used up to the present time, wild bergamot or sweet leaf is an excellent medicine that should be more widely used. It is a mint native to the New World, resembling the European oregano and used in a similar manner. It was and still is an important medicine used by Native American people. The first American author to use it was Samuel Henry (1814, 227), who calls it "rose balm." *He considered it more effectual in fevers than lemon balm* (Melissa), *but it did not catch on. This remedy is immensely popular among modern Indians in the United States and Canada. I first learned about it from a Native practitioner, Tis Mal Crow. A lengthy account is given in* The Book of Herbal Wisdom.

Monarda is a nervine, like most mints, but the hot, pungent taste indicates that it is also a stimulant. In addition, it is sweet and buttery or oily, so much so that it can move the gallbladder. It is suited to cases where the skin is moist and cool, or clammy, but fever is burning away inside the organism. It will drive the heat to the surface and retain the fluids in the inside to cool and lubricate, thus reducing fevers and conditions characterized by a cool, clammy skin. It especially acts on the kidneys and bladder, bringing heat to the surface in renal and cystic inflammatory conditions. It also has a powerful action on the bowel, not only cooling but correcting the internal ecology; it is an excellent remedy for candida. Here it acts identically to its cousin, oil of wild oregano *(Origanum vulgare)*. It also is beneficial in gallstone colic. Monarda is indicated for burns, fevers, digestive discomforts, gallbladder congestion, intestinal difficulties, diarrhea and constipation, urinary tract infections (acute and chronic), with burning and straining. It tones the pores of the large intestine; hence in leaky gut syndrome, systemic yeast. Monarda is one of the only curative agents in Ménière's disease and simple tinnitus. It has a deep, restorative action on the nervous system and tissues. It is an herbal "polychrest" or plant of many uses. Modern pharmacological studies show many interesting constituents.

TASTE:

pungent, sweet, slightly sour • hot • diffusive

TISSUE STATES:

paradoxical, irritation, constriction, relaxation, atrophy, depression

SPECIFIC INDICATIONS:

- Nervousness, anxiety.
- People who have difficulties with their passions.
- Deep nervous disorders.
- *A specific in tinnitus, Ménière's disease, poor hearing.*
- Bronchial asthma, with nervousness, cool, clammy skin.
- Nervous stomach.
- Gallstone colic; bloated, yellow complexion of gallbladder congestion; hangover.

- Diarrhea or constipation, with clammy skin, nervousness.
- Appendicitis.
- Urinary tract infections with cool, clammy skin.
- High blood pressure associated with anxiety, nervousness (cf. *Melissa*).
- *Yeast infection, with cool, clammy skin;* fungus, herpes.
- Leaky gut.
- Burns, sunburn (chew the flower tops, poultice on skin).
- *Cool, clammy skin.*
- Corpse sickness; from exposure to corpse.

PREPARATION AND DOSAGE:

Under the name "sweet leaf," "Indian perfume," etc., Native Americans refer to certain varieties of *Monarda fistulosa* and even *M. didyma* that have soft, oil-laden leaves and a sweet, pungent, burning taste. Avoid plants with harsh, dry leaves and a more bitter flavor. Pick at the height of flowering, about six inches above the root. Dry the entire plant for use by infusion. For burns, chew the flowers and use the saliva on the burn. For fevers, infuse the flower tops. For stomach and nerve problems, use the stems. It is also possible to extract the whole plant in alcohol. Dose: 1–3 drops, 1–3x/day.

CAUTIONS:

Combined with valerian can cause emesis. Very small doses of monarda combined with valerian operate as a stomach tonic.

LITERATURE:

Traditional, Tis Mal Crow (1, 5, 6, 7, 8, 9, 10, 12, 16), Paul Red Elk, Matthew Wood (1–16 confirmed).

Myrica cerifera. Bayberry.

Bayberry, most famous for the wax it provides to make scented candles, grows along the shores of the northeastern United States. The root bark was introduced into herbal practice by Samuel Thomson as a remedy for "canker," or thick, tenacious mucoid adhesions in the digestive tract, but

*the use of that particular part of the plant indicates American Indian ori-
gins. Indeed, Samuel Henry (1814, 35) records: "A gentleman in the city
of New York, informed me that some time since he had the king's evil,
and that several sores broke out on his neck. An Indian undertook to
cure him for a quart of rum" by applying the fresh bark, pounded, and
giving him a strong tea from the leaves. "The cure was completed in two
weeks." Myrica was primarily used by Thomson's followers. "Eclectics,
regulars, and homeopaths do not use this remedy very much, and it is
entirely unknown to many physicians," commented Dr. B. A. Burnett
(1906, 336) in an important article in the* Eclectic Medical Journal.
*"Myrica is essential to physio-medical practice, almost as much so as
lobelia and capsicum. It is a physio-medical polychrest, and a useful one.
I have used myrica ever since I began practice, and could hardly get along
without it. . . . It is my opinion that it would prove to be of value in most
all contagious diseases, and may act as a preventive." Myrica contains
flavonoids, tannins, and terpenoids. I use the local Myrica gale in place
of the officinal article with success.*

The old authors generally classified myrica as a stimulating astringent
suited to relaxed and depressed conditions where the mucosa was burdened by congealed phlegm and weak peripheral circulation. "It combines stimulating and astringing powers in about equal proportions,"
writes Dr. William Cook (1869, 571). "The entire circulation is slowly
but steadily elevated by it, and a good outward flow of blood secured;
and it leaves upon all the tissues of the body an astringing tonic impression," checking excessive discharge and secretion.

John William Fyfe (1909, 626) gives an extensive and knowledgeable
account of myrica. "The term 'canker' is commonly applied to the degenerate ulcerations of aphthae [canker sores]; and as this condition not
uncommonly extends through the entire alvine canal, and may exist in
the stomach and bowels quite independently of sores in the mouth, the
bayberry becomes valuable in all cases where such a state of the mucous
membranes exists."

"In warm infusion bayberry favors perspiration, followed by an increase
of arterial and capillary firmness and a general tension of the tissues." It
therefore combines well with the gentle diaphoretic *Asclepias tuberosa*
(pleurisy root).

"In flooding and excessive lochia, it has no superior, unless it is capsicum; and when combined with a limited portion of the latter agent, its

power in arresting such hemorrhages is so great as to be deserving of the word unfailing. And this article unquestionably exerts a direct stimulating influence on the uterus, leading to its firm contraction in cases of labor where the circulation is sluggish and the parts flaccid; whence it is a valuable parturient under such circumstances, and at the same time anticipating flooding. Used in cold preparations, it can be employed in chronic menorrhagia, and leucorrhea with prolapsus."

Myrica is also used in "degenerate scrofula," or swollen glands and wasting from poor nutrition. "In chronic diarrhea and dysentery, in colliquative discharges under all circumstances, and even in colliquative perspiration, it is valuable; and may be used to fine effect in the exhaustive discharges and hemorrhage from the bowels which occasionally set in during the latter stages of a typhus fever."

"This is somewhat extended praise to bestow on a single remedy, but this article fully deserves all here said of it. Its action can not fairly be judged of by comparing it to other stimulating astringents, as is commonly done; for it exerts a peculiar tonic influence throughout the frame, and has an especial use in the scrofulous and cachectic affections where it is customary to employ alterants [alteratives] alone."

"Yet there are many cases where bayberry should not be used, as for instance in typhoid fever, pneumonia, and similar acute maladies in their first and second stages, where it would be inadmissible to shut up the emunctories [secretory glands] and to dry the respiratory mucous membranes; in acute dysentery, vaginitis, irritable forms of leucorrhea, acute or chronic gastritis, irritable ulcers, dry sores of any grade, and similar conditions."

"Myrica possesses some antispasmodic power," writes B. A. Burnett (1906). "It acts on both nervous systems," the voluntary and involuntary. "It can be used with lobelia in puerperal convulsions, and with dioscorea for after pains, also with motherwort for suppressed lochia and menstruation, caused by taking cold." One of my friends, Chani Friedman, calls it "miracle" for its value in childbirth.

"The circulation in the surfaces and extremities is made perfect by the use of myrica. Its action in this respect is enhanced by the addition of capsicum and hydrastis." And "a combination of myrica and cactus makes a valuable heart tonic in many conditions. In cases where the blood is bad, poor digestion and nutrition, myrica will give good results." Michael Moore (2003, 49) explains, "It increases blood and lymph circulation and helps prevent the inefficient, poorly drained engorgements of sinus and stomach membranes many people are prone to."

TASTE:

pungent, earthen • astringent

TISSUE STATES:

relaxation, depression, torpor

SPECIFIC INDICATIONS:

CONSTITUTION, COMPLEXION, CHARACTERISTIC SYMPTOMS

- Low vitality, weakness, stagnation, inactivity of the mucous membranes and glands, with weak peripheral circulation, aching and soreness in the limbs, muscular soreness, dark membranes.
- Excessive secretion from the mucous membranes, which are full and relaxed.
- Imperfect circulation in the surfaces and in the extremities.

EYES

- Sore eyes (external wash).

MOUTH AND THROAT

- Chronic stomatitis (canker sores), with bad breath, slow, persistent ulceration, dark color to mucosa.
- Sore mouth, *spongy, bleeding gums;* thrush.
- "A cankerous or metallic taste in the mouth; it will appear to the patient that there is not enough saliva being secreted, and this is the fact" due to adhesive phlegm coating the mucosa (B. A. Burnett); but also in excessive secretion (combine with *Geranium*) (Ellingwood).
- Diphtheria (combine with *Hydrastis*).

RESPIRATION

- Colds, chronic or acute (with *Asclepias tuberosa, Capsicum, Zingiberis*).
- *Catarrhal affections of long standing, characterized by tenacious discharge,* often offensive and irritating.
- Nasal catarrh and polypi (with *Sanguinaria*).
- Croup (combine with *Lobelia*).

CARDIOVASCULAR

- Weak peripheral circulation; feeble capillary circulation; after giving a dose one almost always feels the pulse become stronger.

DIGESTION AND LYMPHATICS

- Foul stomach and breath, chronic ulceration, dark membranes.
- *Atonic and long-standing diarrhea; persistent and protracted loss of fluids with loss of tone of the membranes; dysentery* (follow with *Ulmus fulva*).
- Constipation with much mucus in the bowels.
- "Scrofula in a state of ulcer"—that is, suppurating, swollen glands (Beach).
- Hemorrhoids.

LIVER

- Jaundice due to catarrh blocking the outlets of the liver; yellow complexion; clay-colored stools; soreness in region of the liver; dull, frontal headache, worse in the morning; yellowishness of the eyes; scanty urine; tongue has dirty yellow coating, great muscular soreness and aching in the limbs, weakness.
- Neonatal jaundice (homeopathic 3x dilution).
- "Simple fevers, where the liver is torpid and general debility exists" (Boericke); (combine with *Leptandra, Asclepias*; B. A. Burnett).
- Congested liver, where mucus is passing in the bowels.

FEMALE

- Foul leucorrhea, chronic, deteriorative ulceration of the cervix (alone or with *Helonias* or *Trillium*).
- Menstruation: uterine hemorrhage (combine with *Capsicum* or *Trillium*).
- Uterine prolapse, amenorrhea (alone or with *Helonias*).
- Pregnancy: threatened miscarriage.
- Partus: delayed labor; false labor pains.
- Partus: delayed labor; breech birth; turns the baby right.
- Postpartum: severe hemorrhage (combine with *Capsicum*).

FEVER

- Very severe fevers, measles, scarlatina, epidemic dysentery; fever

with convulsions; with excessive and exhaustive perspiration.
- Measles, after the eruption has appeared but the fever is severe and unabated (combine with *Capsicum*).
- Perspiration insufficient.

EXTERNAL
- Foul *ulcers;* old, lingering wounds (external).

OTHER
- Shock, critical conditions, bleeding (combine with *Capsicum*).
- Diabetes; increases peripheral circulation and blood sugar uptake.
- Headache; worse in the morning; associated with liver problems.
- Tongue coated yellow; pulse slow; temperature subnormal.
- Unrefreshing sleep.

PREPARATION AND DOSAGE:

The bark of the root is traditional, but the leaves, bark, and berries have been used. It is usually dried and powdered for use as a tea. Steep a teaspoonful in a pan of boiling water for 30 minutes. Drink hot for colds and flus, warm for stomach and mucosa. B. A. Burnett (1906, 335) writes, "I find the Eclectic rule of giving small doses holds good when using this remedy. The average dose that I use is about two or three grains by infusion, or two or three drops of specific myrica. This can be repeated often."

I use *Myrica gale* (sweet gale) as a substitute, since it grows in northern Minnesota and is so sweet scented and lovely. It has never failed in any case in which *Myrica cerifera* was well indicated and I believe they are very similar in action. Sweet gale is used to flavor beer.

CAUTIONS:

Large doses, taken too frequently, can cause nausea (Gosling).

LITERATURE:

Traditional, Samuel Henry, Samuel Thomson, A. W. and L. R. Priest (3, 13), Wooster Beach (17), J. Compton Burnett (20), William Boericke (21), John Scudder (2), Finley Ellingwood (1, 2, 5, 6, 7, 10, 11, 13–15, 31, 32, 34, 37, 38), R. Swinburne Clymer, Chani Friedman (28-confirmed), John

William Fyfe (2, 15, 29, 30), H. M. Niazi (15, 18, 33, 34, 36, 37), Jethro Kloss, Daniel Cobb (4, 32), B. A. Burnett (6–12, 15, 16, 21–28, 31–32, 34), Matthew Wood (35).

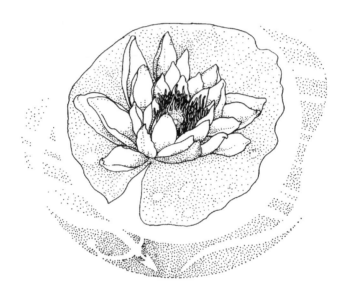

Nymphaea odorata. White Pond Lily, White Water Lily.

The water lilies, white or yellow, European or American, are used in Western herbal medicine. They are members of the lotus family. Nymphaea odorata *is the native North American species, used by the Indians, Samuel Thomson, the physiomedicalists, and the eclectics. Recently the theory has been advanced that water lilies are the famous "soma" of ancient Sanskrit literature. They possess alkaloids and have mild hallucinogenic or entheogenic properties. Similar traditions exist among the North American Indians, where the plant was associated with the Underwater Serpent and (thus) with seership. White water or pond lily root contains tannins, mucilage, resin, alkaloids, and earthen salts.*

White water lily is a mucilaginous astringent, so it both checks discharge and hydrates tissues. Consequently, it is a great "adjuster of fluids" in the body. This makes it suited to conditions where the fluids are running off through sweating, diarrhea, leucorrhea, and free expectoration. In addition, white water lily relaxes the parasympathetic system, in this way reducing excessive sexual preoccupation. Hence, it is useful for impotence, frigidity, and debility from sex and loss of fluid.

There is a long history of usage of the white water lily in Europe, preceding the invasion of North America. John Gerard (1633) mentions European white water lily for lascivious imagination, as a drying astringent for gonorrheal discharge, and as a moistening, cooling refrigerant in hectic fever with debility and fluid loss. William Salmon (1710, 635) writes that the leaves and flowers of the European white "water lillies are cold and moist in the end of the first degree; but the root and seed are cold and dry in the first degree." There are more tannins in the seed, according to nineteenth-century literature. "White water lily cools inflammations, abates the heat of fevers, procures rest, stops fluxes of blood or humors, whether of wounds or of the belly; cures the heat of urine, helps in a gonorrhea, stops the overflowing of the terms, and extinguishes venereal heats and desires."

Crossing the great water, we find similar uses of the American white water lily. "The roots, in decoction, were much esteemed by Indian squaws as an internal remedy, and injection or wash for the worst forms of leucorrhea, its properties in this direction being due to its great astringency. The macerated root was also used as an application in the form of a poultice to suppurating glands; its styptic properties were also fully known and utilized" (Millspaugh, 1892, 67). If he had written "suppurating wounds," the account would have been a little more accurate. Samuel Thomson introduced white water lily into white pioneer practice; it was his leading remedy for leucorrhea. It was used by the physiomedicalists and the eclectics for leucorrhea and suppurating wounds.

Here is an impressive case history from Dr. John King (quoted in Felter and Lloyd, 1898, 2:1318). "I recollect a lady, who, several years since, was pronounced by several physicians to have uterine cancer, which resisted all their treatment; she was permanently cured by a squaw, who gave her to drink freely of the decoction of a root, which proved to be that of the white pond-lily, as well as to inject it in the vagina." Herbalist Christopher Hobbs notes that there is a known anti-cancer compound in water lily.

Modern herbalist William LeSassier taught that the discharges associated with white water lily resemble "pastry starch" and it is an important remedy for candida, thrush, and leucorrhea. (The triumvirate of candida remedies in my practice is *Monarda fistulosa*, or its cousin, oil of wild oregano, yellow dock root, and white water lily.) From this indication I learned always to look for the white water lily when the tongue is coated white and is moist, indicating cold and damp. It is beneficial in bronchial cases, where the discharge is like pastry starch, or simply "white." I had a case that refused all the ordinary bronchial remedies; finally, white water lily cured the young girl.

As an astringent mucilage *Nymphaea* is well suited for external use on wounds. Samuel Henry (1814, 302) gives the following case history. "Cut the root and roast it in the ashes, rolled in wet brown paper: then mash the root, wet with water and apply it over the part." He treated a child who had run a nail into her foot. No lockjaw occurred and she was well in a week. Mrs. Lydia Child (1837, 125) recommends yellow pond lily as a poultice to bring swellings to a head, but white pond lily to close up proud flesh.

TASTE:

mucilaginous, astringent, slightly stimulating, earthen • cold and moist

TISSUE STATE:

relaxation

SPECIFIC INDICATIONS:

CONSTITUTION, COMPLEXION, CHARACTERISTIC SYMPTOMS
- Tendency to be thin, delicate, not a highly resilient constitution.

MIND, SENSES, NERVES, EMOTIONS, PERSONALITY
- Discouragement.
- Needy; lacks self-sufficiency (flower essence).

HEAD
- Conjunctivitis.
- Thrush, nursing sore mouth, *oral candida,* canker sores, pharyngitis, laryngitis.
- *Tongue with moist, white, thrush-like coating; candida.*

RESPIRATION
- Free secretion from the lungs, with irritable cough.

- Mucus like pastry starch.

DIGESTION
- Diarrhea, *candida*, colitis, enteritis; with backache, weakness of lower back.
- Morning diarrhea; with weakness of the back.
- Subacute diarrhea and dysentery.
- Weakness of the bowels and a tendency to curdy diarrhea.

KIDNEYS AND BLADDER
- Involuntary passage of urine, with feeling like it was not all expelled; enuresis.
- Gonorrheal discharges.

FEMALE AND MALE
- Excessive sexual desire, but weakness after the act.
- Impotence, loss of semen, involuntary emissions.
- Vaginal walls relaxed, weak; prolapse and *leucorrhea; curdy discharge.*
- Cervical ulceration and discharge.
- Prostatic enlargement with discharge.

MUSCULAR AND SKELETAL
- Weakness of the lower back and knees (cf. *Osmunda regalis*).

FEVER
- Fever with night sweats; general sweating with fluids loss; hectic fever.
- Brain fever; raving and frenzy.
- Putrefactive, septic fever.
- Fever; heat attacking the blood level; spitting, vomiting, purging, or urinating blood.

SKIN
- Ringworm, lice, scabbiness, sunburn.
- Ulcers, wounds, and fistulae, with discharges.
- Black-and-blue spots.
- "Yellowness of the face" (Salmon).

OTHER

- Weakness, restlessness, exhaustion; "watchings, pinings, wastings, and consumptions" (Salmon).
- Worse from cold and damp.

PREPARATION AND DOSAGE:

William Salmon (1710) lists many methods of preparation, reflecting European experience. He recommends the juice of the roots or rhizomes as the strongest representative of the plant, followed by the juice of the flowers. This can be preserved in a syrup, conserve, oil, or ointment. He makes no alcoholic preparation.

Dr. Cook (1869) reflects American Indian practice. He says that the fresh root or rhizome is gathered in the fall, sliced thin, and dried. "The form of infusion is the best for internal administration, in most cases; made by pouring a pint of boiling water on two drams of the root, of which one or two fluid ounces may be given every two hours." White water lily is still sliced into thin "buttons" and dried in American Indian herbalism.

Dr. Cook further relates that "no iron implement should be used while preparing" white water lily. In this the good doctor has unknowingly preserved a piece of Indian lore. Plants associated with the Underwater Panther or Underwater Serpent are not to be touched with iron. Water lilies are some of the most prominent plants associated with this creature. Native folklore warns that touching the Underwater Panther with iron, or shooting it with a bullet, will cause someone in your family to die before you get home.

The eclectics used the tincture, as I do. King (in Felter and Lloyd, 1898) recommends that a tincture be prepared from the root in 76% alcohol and given in doses of 1–10 drops. Many American herbalists associate low dosages with your author ("Wood doses"), but really they are just traditional posology in eclectic medicine.

LITERATURE:

Traditional, Ariel Rose (1), David Dalton (3), John Gerard (7, 9–11, 14–17, 20–21), Samuel Thomson (6, 9, 17), William LeSassier (8, 17), Julia Graves (1-confirmed, 2, 24), Matthew Wood (1, 6, 17-all confirmed),

Christopher Menzies-Trull (4, 5, 18–19), Lise Wolff (19-confirmed), homeopathic provings (25), William Salmon (15, 17, 20–29), Tis Mal Crow, John King.

Oenothera biennis. Evening Primrose.

Evening primrose is a prairie wildflower native to North America. It is used by the Indians. A beautiful Cherokee name is "falling sun rose" (Garrett, 2003). The seeds are high in fixed oils that yield essential fatty acids that are precursors to prostaglandins. It fits in the group with black currant, borage, and black cumin, the plants that provide nutritional supplementation of EFAs. However, each has its own personality. The bark, leaves, and twigs are used in herbal medicine. They are picked at the height of flowering, hence before the seeds appear. They contain flavonoids, mucilage, and tannins.

Frederick Pursh, the botanist, made an interesting comment. He had frequently observed that on a dark night, when no objects could be seen at a distance, the evening primrose in full flower was visible, "having a bright white appearance, which probably may arise from some phosphoric properties of the flowers" (King, quoted in Felter and Lloyd, 1898, 2:1320).

The oil is famous in commerce as a source of essential fatty acids, prostaglandins, and steroid precursors that are needed especially in women with hormonal imbalances. It is well suited to those who are dry and in need of lipid supplementation.

The plant is less commonly used. J. T. Garrett (2003) mentions its use in Cherokee medicine for premenstrual tension and breast tenderness. It did not pass into pioneer medicine to any great extent. "Its specific field of action seems none too well established," wrote John King (quoted in Felter and Lloyd, 1898, 2:1320). However, he quotes some specific indications from Dr. John Scudder. The latter used *Oenothera* for sallow, dirty, expressionless skin, stagnant lymphatics, torpor of the liver, spleen, mesenteries, and female organs.

In our times, William LeSassier used the stem, root, and leaves collected during flowering, before seed, for spastic colon, "crampiness" with the stool, tension in the lower pelvic area, spastic colon, bowel/ovarian pain, pain in the lower right quadrant from the ileocecal valve, and

gas. These are a different set of symptoms from those mentioned by
Scudder. The symptoms for the oil, as well as the symptoms for the herb,
are listed below.

TASTE:

(leaf) acrid • mucilaginous, astringent

TISSUE STATES:

torpor (Scudder), tension (LeSassier)

SPECIFIC INDICATIONS:

CONSTITUTION, COMPLEXION, CHARACTERISTIC SYMPTOMS
- "Sallow, dirty skin, with full and expressionless tissues, an
  expressionless face, an unnatural and large tongue, having the
  sallow, dirty hue of the skin, and the patient's mentality is of a
  gloomy and despondent character" (Scudder).
- "Face dull, apathetic" (King).
- Feeble innervation.

MIND, SENSES, NERVES, EMOTIONS, PERSONALITY
- Schizophrenia (oil).
- Dementia (oil).
- "Gloomy and despondent" (Scudder, King), depression (oil).
- Hyperactivity (oil).
- Memory loss (oil).
- Alzheimer's disease (oil).
- Restlessness at night.

RESPIRATION
- Asthma, chronic; with digestive disorder (oil; or a cough syrup
  made from the roots or tops, fresh or dried, in honey).
- Whooping cough (oil; cough syrup).
- Difficult respiration.

DIGESTION
- Dyspepsia; vomiting, distressing sensations after taking food,
  with desire for frequent urination.
- Irritable bowel syndrome (oil).

- Splenic and mesenteric glandular enlargements.
- Enteric fever, with destruction of Peyer's patches.
- Dysentery, with straining, bloody stools, cholera-like stools.

LIVER
- Hepatic torpor.

CARDIOVASCULAR
- Hypertension (oil).
- Excess cholesterol (oil).
- Excessive clotting (platelet aggregation) (oil).

URINARY
- Frequent desire to pass urine.

FEMALE
- "Torpor and pelvic fullness" (Scudder); "atonic reproductive wrongs of the female" (King).
- Endometriosis (oil).
- PMS (oil).
- Mastalgia (oil).
- Menopause (oil).

MUSCULAR AND SKELETAL
- Raynaud's disease (oil).
- Rheumatoid arthritis (oil).
- Sjögren's syndrome (oil).
- Chronic fatigue syndrome (oil).
- Multiple sclerosis (oil).
- Pain (oil).
- Neuralgia (oil).

SKIN
- Acne (oil).
- Dermatitis, eczema, scaly skin, psoriasis (ointment of herb, or oil).
- Wounds, bruises (oil).
- Brittle nails (oil).
- Ulcers (oil).

OTHER

- Carcinoma (oil).
- Omega-6 deficiency (oil).
- Diabetes; neuropathy (oil).

PREPARATION AND DOSAGE:

Commercial preparation of the EFAs from the expressed oil of the seed. The barks, twigs, and leaves are collected during flowering and used by infusion (King).

LITERATURE:

Traditional, John Scudder (1, 6, 24), Michael Moore (11, 12), John King (2, 3, 5, 6, 10, 12, 13, 14, 16, 17, 18, 19, 24, 37, 38), indications for the oil (4, 5, 7, 8, 9, 12, 15, 20–22, 25–43).

Osmorhiza longistylis. Sweet Cicely, Anise Root, Sweet Root.

This is the native American analog to European sweet cicely *(Myrrhis odorata)*. It possesses similar properties. It is an old Indian remedy for neurological disorders. Probably the sweetest root in the American forest, it also acts as a mucilage for irritable mucosa. *It is a specific for helping the cells pick up more blood sugar in type II diabetes* (Matthew Wood). Sweet cicely is indicated in peripheral neuropathy and retinopathy of diabetes.

TASTE:

sweet • moist • mucilaginous

TISSUE STATES:

atrophy, depression

SPECIFIC INDICATIONS:

- A reliable tonic for diabetes mellitus; reduces fluctuations of blood sugar, even in old cases, but does not cure, except adjunctively with dietary changes in recent, adult onset diabetes.
- Peripheral nerve debility, numbness, loss of sensation, pain.
- Repetitive coughing with exhaustion, irritation.

PREPARATION AND DOSAGE:

Must be distinguished from the almost identical *Osmorhiza claytonii*, with which it often grows. That plant lacks the sweet taste. Collect in the fall, dry for use per decoction, or tincture fresh in alcohol. Dose: 1–3 drops, 1–3x/day.

LITERATURE:

Traditional American Indian, Tis Mal Crow, Steven Foster and James Duke, David Winston, Matthew Wood.

Oxydendrum arboreum. Sourwood.

Sourwood is a small tree native to the South, the bark and leaves of which are intensely sour. This flavor usually indicates a coolant—which is confirmed by its uses. Sourwood is little used today. Phyllis Light brought this medicine to my attention; she had good success in a dangerous edema that had persisted for many months and was threatening the life of a man in Australia.

The naturalist William Bartram discovered sourwood or sorrel tree in the southern woods. Constantine Rafinesque (1828, 1:43) gave notice of its efficacy. "The leaves, and the wood, are a fine astringent acid, refreshing, cooling, allaying thirst, and antifebrile," he writes. "Clayton says that a decoction of the leaves mitigates the ardour of fever."

The following account, by Dr. E. C. Anderson, of Cleveland, Tennessee, appeared in an 1885 issue of the *Eclectic Medical Journal*. "This drug has really been long in use, especially among the mountain people of East Tennessee and North Carolina, who ascribe to it diuretic, tonic, and laxative properties. But its use as a remedy in dropsy, to which a number of articles in this *Journal* have lately referred, has led to its extensive use in this disease, and has placed it prominently among the vegetable diuretics.

"Having used sourwood for over two years I find that it possesses all the properties claimed for it as a diuretic, and not only is it serviceable in general dropsy, but it will remove other and lesser accumulations of water in different parts of the body. I think of a case of hydrocele, cured by this remedy, that has been reported, and its action in hydropericardium and pleuritic effusion is not to be forgotten. It does not seem to markedly increase the amount of solids in the urine, but augments the amount of water, and has a decided refrigerant effect—the mountain people, I am told, frequently using it in febrile complaints with the happiest results. The leaves and twigs are often added to whisky and used in the kidney and bladder affections of old men, and is said to not only increase the amount of water, but to relieve the unpleasant symptoms attending prostatic enlargement, stone in the bladder, and chronic irritation of the neck.

"I heard, not long ago, of another use of sourwood which is quite new to me. A hunter in the mountains of North Carolina had his thumb severely burned, and for want of something better, (as he supposed), wrapped the injured part with the bruised leaves of the sourwood. My informant stated that, much to his surprise the burned part 'did not even get sore,' but healed rapidly and without the slightest pain."

"In cases of urinary troubles accompanying ills of the prostate the *Oxydendrum arboreum o* [tincture], in doses of 5 drops, will often give relief; also in cystitis" (Anshutz, 1900, 145).

Panax quinquefolius. American Ginseng.

American ginseng is native to deep forests in eastern North America. It is sweet, nourishing, and moistening, whereas the Asian ginseng is more strongly warming and moistening.

American ginseng is moist, sweet, and bitter, making it an ideal "yin tonic" or moistener and rejuvenative for dry mucosa. It works slowly. The cultivated variety is traditionally used in Chinese herbalism for dryness in the respiratory tract and stomach. By increasing lubrication it is cooling, but deeper down in the endocrine system it has an activating effect, which is warming. Although American physicians did not much use their own ginseng, the same basic applications found in the Chinese pharmacopoeia were verified.

William Byrd (1729), an early Virginia settler, appreciated ginseng. "Its virtues are, that it gives an uncommon Warmth and Vigour to the Blood, and frisks the Spirits, beyond any other Cordial." He used it personally. "As a Help to bear Fatigue I us'd to chew a Root of Ginseng as I Walk't along" (quoted by Moss, 1999, 186).

Dr. Jacob Bigelow (1817–20, 95) records its use for moistening and nourishing the mucosa of the respiratory tract. "Dr. Fothergill tells us, that in tedious chronic coughs, incident to people in years, a decoction of it has been of service."

Dr. John Scudder (1870, 194) used American ginseng in the digestive sphere. He suffered from lack of saliva, which he cured with this plant. "We have laughed at the Chinese for their use of ginseng, which we have deemed inert," he writes. "But I am pretty well satisfied that in this, as in some other things, they have the advantage of us." He used it for lack of saliva and for dyspepsia associated with nervous exhaustion. "It is one of those remedies, however, that produces no marked improvement at first, and must be continued for weeks to obtain its good effects."

Samuel Henry (1814, 139) gives an unusually full account of the uses of ginseng. "This root is good in gravel and all debilitated habits, creates a good appetite, invigorates the system, and is an excellent restorative to those fatigued by travelling." It is more specific in the exhaustion that follows the loss of fluids. "In all weaknesses from excess in venery." (Henry treated a lot of New York sailors for syphilis.) Also in "pain in the bones from colds, and gravelly complaints, let the patient take a wine glass of this tincture" of ginseng in Jamaica rum, "three times a day, on an empty stomach." Pain in the bones is a frequent side effect of syphilis. "I knew a man in New-Jersey, who was so debilitated and afflicted with pains in his bones, that he expected nothing but death every day, who by taking the ginseng in rum was able to follow his business on the farm, and his pains entirely removed in a few days." People don't believe me (the author) when I recount cures that occurred in a few days, but I have seen such cases again and again—when the remedy is specifically indicated.

So much is written about ginseng that it is difficult to look at this plant with fresh eyes. However, while wildcrafting American ginseng I have noticed that it is perhaps the most soft and feminine plant in the woods.

TASTE:

bitter, sweet • moist • mucilaginous

TISSUE STATE:

atrophy

SPECIFIC INDICATIONS:

CONSTITUTION, COMPLEXION, CHARACTERISTIC SYMPTOMS
- Neurasthenia, nervous exhaustion, following loss of fluids, dry, atrophic, debilitated habits.

MIND, SENSES, NERVES, EMOTIONS, PERSONALITY
- Exhaustion of the brain or nervous system from overwork.
- Children who are too nervous to play.

DIGESTION
- Lack of saliva, loss of appetite, weak stomach.
- Dry, red tongue, sometimes with yellow coating and tooth decay.

KIDNEYS AND BLADDER
- Gravel, with weakness.

FEMALE
- Menopause (general tonic).

MUSCULAR AND SKELETAL
- Ligamentous looseness; easily injured, slow to heal.
- Pain in the bones; with weakness; worse from exposure to cold.
- Arthritis.
- Travel fatigue.

PREPARATION AND DOSAGE:

I use small doses of the tincture of the wild plant, 3–5 drops, 1–3x/day.

LITERATURE:

Traditional, J. T. Garrett (3), John M. Scudder (4), John William Fyfe (1, 2, 4), Christopher Hobbs (5), William LeSassier (8), Samuel Henry (1, 6, 9, 10, 11), Matthew Wood (7).

Parthenocissus quinquefolia. Virginia Creeper.

This plant was ubiquitous in the neighborhood in which I grew up and was always known to me as Virginia creeper, but it is sometimes known as American ivy. It was formerly called Ampelopsis. *It is a relative of the grape but has none of the edible properties of that plant, though it retains and amplifies the viny growth habit. It is an old, seldom used blood purifier, confirming Ben Charles Harris's observation that vines often are alterative (cf. sarsaparilla, yellow parilla, etc.). It is seldom used today.*

Grover Coe (1858, 155) wrote that the primary action of *Ampelopsis* is on the "absorbents," meaning the glands associated with the mesenteries and the digestive tract, and that it stimulates absorption throughout the body.

Parthenocissus is listed as a poison ivy remedy. Phyllis Light recommended it to me for this purpose. Strange to say, I have three times used it with success for eczema that looked like poison ivy rather than for the genuine article. It grows in amongst the poison ivy.

Dr. John Bastyr recommended ampelopsis for colds and persistent, nagging respiratory complaints. His dose was 10–20 drops of the tincture, 4x/day, or 2 tablespoons of a standard tea every 2 hours (Mitchell, 2003, 15).

TASTE:

acrid • mucilaginous (Hutchins)

TISSUE STATES:

tension, stagnation

SPECIFIC INDICATIONS:

- Colds.
- Persistent, nagging respiratory complaints; incipient tuberculosis.
- Bronchitis, whooping cough, asthma.
- Diarrhea.
- Hepatitis (with *Leptandra*).
- Dropsy.
- Poison ivy.
- Skin disease; eczema-like poison ivy (vesicles filled with fluid).
- Rheumatism (fibromyalgia).
- Scrofula.
- Alcoholism.

PREPARATION AND DOSAGE:

The bark from the vine and twigs is the part used. It is picked after the dark-blue berries ripen (though for poison ivy, take the vines and even the leaves at any time and rub on the skin). Decoction by boiling 1 teaspoonful in 1 cup water (Hutchins).

LITERATURE:

Grover Coe (2–6, 8–10), John Bastyr (1–2), Joseph E. Meyers (11), Phyllis Light (7), Matthew Wood (8).

Passiflora incarnata. Passionflower.

Passionflower is native from the southern United States to Guatemala. It is an old traditional remedy for the nervous system, insomnia, tension, spasms, and restlessness. It contains flavonoids, including rutin (cooling), indole alkaloids, fatty acids, and sterols.

Passiflora is suited to conditions of nervous and cerebral overstimulation, excitement, and irritation. It is also suited to spasms, convulsions, and tremors that follow nervous overstimulation. It is a sedative of considerable power, but with no side effects, except in children four and under, who become overexcited from a large dose—it causes what it cures. Early experimentation indicated that it calms the cerebral cortex and has a special affinity to the medulla oblongata, the area of the brain stem that oversees sleep, temporary blood pressure fluctuations related to stress, and the vagus nerve—hiccough, vomiting, and respiration. These are the areas to which it is particularly suited. With passiflora, herbalist Daniel Gagnon cured two people with hiccoughing lasting more than a year.

Passionflower is one of the most important remedies for insomnia from overstimulation of the mind, excessive thinking, and chatter in the brain. It increases concentration during waking, by cutting out excessive internal chatter, but will not induce drowsiness. "It is wonderful for the headstrong individual, the thinker and the chronic worrier" (Daniel Gagnon). It is specific for insomnia caused by inability to stop mental chatter, but not caused by pain. On the other hand, it will reduce pain due to overstimulation. The sleep produced is normal.

Passionflower acts also on the nerve centers controlling respiration and blood pressure, so it is suited to conditions where there is spasmodic cough and temporary high blood pressure induced by overstimulation, tension, and stress. It has been used in whooping cough and nervous asthma. It also settles digestive irritation related to nervous stimulation and tension: hiccough, vomiting, and indigestion.

TASTE:

sour, sweet

TISSUE STATES:

irritation, constriction

SPECIFIC INDICATIONS:

CONSTITUTION, COMPLEXION, CHARACTERISTIC SYMPTOMS

- "Nervous excitement, and irritation with muscular twitchings— evidences of approaching convulsions in children—with marked cerebral fullness."
- Convulsions of any character; mitigates spasms even when the irritating causes have not remained; epilepsy, tetanus, meningitis.
- Neuralgia of various kinds; facial neuralgia, facial erysipelas, menstrual cramps, ovarian irritation and congestion.

MIND, SENSES, NERVES, EMOTIONS, PERSONALITY

- *Wakefulness, sleeplessness, mental chatter, inability to turn off the internal dialogue; easily distracted and overstimulated during the day; can't fall asleep at night.*
- *Chatterboxes who talk all the time about themselves, family, and friends; or stoic persons who seldom talk about themselves.*
- Fretfulness of teething children.
- Sleeplessness, following the excessive use of alcohol.

HEAD

- Pain in the head, with sensation of great weight pressing upon the brain.
- Red-tipped tongue.
- Contraindicated by a "dirty and heavily coated tongue."

RESPIRATION

- Asthma and spasmodic cough, whooping cough (1 teaspoonful/dose).

CARDIOVASCULAR

- Insomnia with cardiac disturbance.

DIGESTION

- Hiccough, nausea, vomiting; pain in the stomach that comes on an hour or two after eating.
- Infantile diarrhea, with restlessness and spasmodic conditions.

FEMALE

- Pelvic engorgement attended with severe pain.
- Ovarian irritation, congestion, and pain; uterine congestion, spasm, painful menstrual cramping; cholera infantum, with restlessness and spasm; estrogen intolerance.
- Pregnancy: pains in the abdomen and pelvis; eclampsia.
- Partus: unbearable labor pains.

MUSCULAR AND SKELETAL

- Tetanus (1 dram in hot water every 15 minutes; then every 3 hours).

FEVER
• Fever with delirium and low muttering.

PREPARATION AND DOSAGE:

There is great variation in the medicinal properties of the wild plant. Fluid extract, 5–60 drops (Fyfe).

CAUTIONS:

Causes overexcitement and vomiting in children four and under (Gagnon, 2000).

LITERATURE:

Traditional, Daniel Gagnon (4), John William Fyfe, Darryl Patton, Tommie Bass, Christopher Hobbs (9), Frederick Petersen (10), Yadubir Sinha (17–18), Julia Graves (9), Finley Ellingwood (1, 2, 3, 4, 11, 13), Matthew Wood (5), David Winston (5).

Pedicularis spp. American Wood Betony.

This plant must be differentiated from the European wood betony. They are in different families (Scrophulariaceae, Lamiaceae), live in different parts of the world, but have a superficial physical resemblance and somewhat related medicinal properties. European wood betony (Stachys officinalis, Betonica officinalis) is a reliable nervine and sedative, whereas American wood betony is more of a powerful neuromuscular sedative and antispasmodic.

There are many different kinds of Pedicularis *found in North America. They are used fairly interchangeably. Generally, they are used more by Western herbalists—this probably due to the influence of herbalist Michael Moore, of Bisbee, Arizona.*

Cherokee herbalist Sondra Boyd speaks highly of *Pedicularis*. She uses it for neurovascular spasm, hence in stroke and syncope, to release tension in the blood vessels caused by particles that have caught in the arteries. She also considers it to be one of the few medicines that will act on grand mal and petit mal seizures.

Phytolacca decandra. Poke Root.

This native American plant was used by the Indians and pioneers as a spring green and tonic. The leaves are boiled twice and the water thrown off due to the toxicity. It is still widely eaten in the South today. The roots and seeds are also toxic, but the fruit (with seeds removed) is not. Medicinal preparations have been made from all three parts. Poke contains saponins, tannins, resin, and alkaloids.

Phytolacca is as profoundly acting as it is toxic. It has a special affinity for the glandular system. It is relevant when there are stagnant, swollen lymphatics, swollen sore throat, diphtheria, mastitis, or breast problems in general. As is common in remedies that affect the lymphatic glands, there is also a powerful influence on endocrine regulation. In addition, there are symptoms of toxic blood and blood stagnation (red and purple coloration and purple eruptions), and nervous symptoms such as shooting pains.

Poke root is especially suited to large, bulky persons, with large glands, large breasts, who are poky—they are continually exhausted and want to fling themselves down in a chair or bed. They come home, throw their tools or clothes on the floor, and lie apathetically; meanwhile their surroundings become a pigsty. There is a "lack of personal delicacy" (though sometimes the exact opposite—excessive delicacy). Such behavior is not uncommon in teenagers, going through hormonal and glandular development, and phytolacca is an excellent remedy for "lazy teenagers"—or for "lazy teenagers of any age." Poke root is indicated in fevers where the glands are involved and apathy and exhaustion take over, and in conditions where the glandular stasis is so great that the blood and nerves are blocked, resulting in lymphatic swelling, purple and red coloration, and acute nerve pain.

Dorothy Hall considered phytolacca to be the number one endocrine regulator. It enhances the environment through which hormones have to travel—that is, thinning fluids that are thick and stagnant. It has an especially strong influence on the pituitary and thyroid, but also on the adrenals and sex glands—that is, sterility, impotence, low sperm count, and prostate.

Dr. Horton Howard (1836, 2:154), an early physiomedicalist, introduced the use of phytolacca berries and cimicifuga in tea as a remedy for "rheumatism" (read "fibromyalgia"). This was a very popular remedy during the nineteenth century. It was sometimes augmented by the addition of prickly ash. This formula is listed still in Priest and Priest's *Herbal Medication* (1982).

TASTE:

pungent, bitter • irritating, burning, drying

TISSUE STATES:

torpor, depression

SPECIFIC INDICATIONS:

LYMPHATIC GLANDS AND ENDOCRINE GLANDS

- *Large, bulky persons with large glands, big breasts; teenagers in puberty, after glandular growth; lactating mothers; persons undergoing endocrine change.*
- *Lack of personal delicacy; disregard of surrounding objects; indifferent to life; sense of apathy and indifference, lives in a "pigsty" environment.*
- Excessive personal delicacy.
- Young children with persistent, relapsing head colds; poor immunity; "scrofula."
- Persons with lumpy lymphatic swelling, aches and pains, aggravated at times of hormonal change.
- Delayed puberty.
- *"Lazy teenagers of any age."*
- *Soreness of mouth, soreness of throat, with tendency to death of epithelium.*
- *Swollen throat; pain worse on sticking out the tongue; pain at the root of the tongue.*
- *Tonsils swollen, diphtheria, mumps.*
- *Diphtheritic deposits, fullness about the throat* (external).
- *Breast affections; mastitis, swollen breasts, sharp, shooting pains from the nipple, mammary abscess* (external).
- Breasts swollen, engorged before the period; at the estrogen to progesterone change (mid-period).
- Breast cancer, especially with purple coloration (external).

- Menopausal rheumatism (cf. cimicifuga).
- Constipation with lymphatic stagnation.
- Stagnation of lymphatics of the groin.
- Reproductive difficulties.

CIRCULATION
- High blood pressure.

MUSCULAR AND SKELETAL
- *Arthritis; especially when the endocrine system is out of order; rub thoroughly into the twisted, nodular joints* (external).
- *Aches and pains in muscles and joints.*

SKIN
- Skin rashes, purple, red, toxic quality, itch; scrofula.
- Skin breaks out at odd times.
- *Resistant symptoms due to ancestral taint; difficult to treat; slow recoveries.*
- *Disease of the skin or blood, with death of and imperfect reproduction of the epithelium.*

OTHER
- Pokiness in hot summer weather.

PREPARATION, TOXICITY, AND DOSAGE:

The leaves and roots are highly irritating to the mucosa, they are cathartic in large quantities, and in continuous dosage they are carcinogenic. Children have died from eating them unprepared. The root is more often used in herbal medicine. It is much milder when used dried, rather than fresh. Boil a tablespoonful in a pint of water for 10 minutes, strain; take no more than a teaspoon at a time for a dose (Tommie Bass). Tincture of the root: dilute one dropperful in an ounce of alcohol and use a small dose, 3 drops, once a day in chronic affections, hourly in acute fever (Matthew Wood). Oil or salve of the root is used externally in mastitis, itch, and arthritis. The less toxic berries are used for weight loss and rheumatoid arthritis (three berries a week).

LITERATURE:

Traditional, homeopathic authors (2), William Cook (berries), Matthew Wood (1, 2, 3, 7, 25), Tommie Bass (19), Lise Wolff (4), Dorothy Hall (4, 5, 6, 13, 15, 17, 18, 20, 21, 23, 24), Kathryn Thorngren (9), Rolla Thomas (10–13, 23).

Pinus strobus. White Pine.

White pine was widely used by the American Indians and adopted into practice by the early settlers and professional doctors of North America. The Indians used the bark, but the needles may be used for tea or tincture instead if one does not want to hurt the tree. In Europe, pine oil and pine products have been used since the Middle Ages. Pine sap from almost any kind of pine will have approximately the same properties. Pine contains flavonols, proanthocyanidins, resins, bitters, and volatile oils, so it is both stimulating and anti-inflammatory. This coincides with its use as a topical application in putrid wounds, or to prevent putrefaction.

White pine is a stimulating antiseptic indicated when there is inflammation with tendencies to poor oxygenation and tissue depression. The stimulation wakes up the system and increases the oxygenation. As a mild relaxant and stimulant a tea from the needles is sufficient. Thus, it is used in respiratory infections, where the phlegm is viscid, hardened, green (even bright green), and difficult to raise (Ben Charles Harris, 1972). The infection is often deep down in the bottom of the lungs, or sometimes in the sinuses. Pine's adhesive, antiseptic resins attach themselves to the mucus and draw it out. Therefore, it is better for pulmonary uses to make a strong tea by boiling the inner bark slowly to release the resins, or best of all, simply to chew the pitch (Michael Moore, 2003).

Pine is also traditionally used at the onset of the infection, in cold or flu, to stop the infection from going deeper. It also acts on the digestive tract, kidneys, and skin as an antiseptic.

The American Indians use pine sap as a sort of "patch" to keep a wound clean, disinfect it, and pull impurities up to the surface. Cadwallader Colden, in 1744, reported on its use by Native Americans, including for gunshot wounds (Erichsen-Brown, 1989, 2). A Navajo man told me he used sap of the pinyon pine to pull a bullet out of his horse. It kept the wound clean, and good skin formed afterward. As Golden explains, the

wound remains "a fresh & ruddy colour till it unites without digesting"—
that is, putrefying. Michael Moore (2003, 196) explains, "The abietic
resins stimulate topical circulation, increase inflammation, and notice-
ably speed up the foreign body response; pus and fluids build up much
more quickly than if unattended, and the splinter will usually pop out
the next day."

The antiseptic powers of pine were tapped through mere exposure for
the assistance of tubercular or consumptive cases. Lydia Child (1837,
112) explains, "Frequent morning walks in pine woods are very invigorating, particularly for consumptive people. It is even deemed healthy
to have these trees in the vicinity of dwellings. The bark of the twigs and
young trees is very mucilaginous. A decoction of it, when dried, is a gentle
and soothing laxative. In its green state it cannot be too highly praised
as a strengthening wash for weak joints, and healing and cleansing to
inflamed wounds and sores. The gum taken as pills is very physcial"—
that is, purgative.

Francis Densmore (1926, 334) treats us to an authentic formulation
from the Anishinabe Ojibwe Grand Medicine Society *(midewiwin)* used
for gangrene. It is made from the barks of white pine, wild cherry, and
wild plum.

The European pine or "Scotch pine," as we call it in America, is *Pinus
sylvestris*. It has similar properties to the white pine. Some mental indications for *Pinus sylvestris* are included below from Dr. Edward Bach
and Dorothy Hall. Bach used a decoction of the immature cone. *Pinus
montana* buds are used in gemmotherapy. They are trophorestorative to
bones and joints, cut down on wear and tear, and may prevent fractures
in the elderly (Tetau, 1998, 48).

Pine oil is used in aromatherapy. A fine portrait is rendered by Dr.
Dietrich Gümbel (1993, 196). It stimulates discharges from the outlets—
mouth and nose—down the tubes of the lungs to the alveoli, increasing
circulation in the capillary bed serving oxygen exchange. It increases
oxygen uptake in the cells, and carbon dioxide release, so it is vivifying
and cleansing. It clears out old mucus. He especially recommends it for
the gray, oxygen-poor skin seen in a smoker.

TASTE:

pungent • warm • adhesive

TISSUE STATE:

depression

SPECIFIC INDICATIONS:

CONSTITUTION, COMPLEXION, CHARACTERISTIC SYMPTOMS
- Gray, oxygen-poor complexion; smoker's complexion.

MIND, SENSES, NERVES, EMOTIONS, PERSONALITY
- Self-blame, guilt (Bach).
- *Calms the nerves*, increases introspection.
- Tired from doing nothing; needs exercise and inspiration.
- Tired after travel (a few drops of pine oil in a bath).

RESPIRATION
- Incipient colds and flus.
- Old sinus infections with viscid mucus, difficult to expel.
- Chronic bronchitis and lung infections, with viscid, green mucus, difficult to raise (extract, tincture, tea; oil as an inhalant).
- Strep throat, tonsillitis, laryngitis.
- Cough, spasmodic; croup, whooping cough, asthma.

DIGESTION
- Dyspepsia.
- Constipation (buds).
- Hemorrhoids (bark, external).

URINARY
- Edema; promotes urination.

MUSCULAR AND SKELETAL
- Chronic rheumatism and neuralgia; "a great deal applied" externally (turpentine; Christison, 1842, cited by Erichsen-Brown).
- Bones and joints; trophorestorative and protective (*Pinus montana*, gemmotherapy).

FEVER
- Smallpox.
- Dry skin; promotes perspiration and urine.

SKIN

- Sap or salve on a wound seals it up, keeps it antiseptic, and draws out impurities and objects (like bullets and splinters).
- Ulcers, fistula.
- Sores, burns (external poultice of the bark).
- Scurvy.

PREPARATION AND DOSAGE:

Pine is made into a wide variety of different preparations, including a decoction, tincture, pine tar, pine tar soap, and turpentine. I have not generally included the indications for pine tar and turpentine, which are used externally.

The inner bark from a young tree is collected in May or June and dried for use per decoction or soaked for use as a poultice. "The bark of the white pine . . . should be boiled and the soft part script out and beat in a poultice in a mortar, and then sufficiently moistened with the liquor and applied to burns or sores of any kind. Repeat the poultices and wash with the liquor until the sore is well. This will not terrify or smart in its application. A new skin will come on quickly without a scar. The same application is a cure for piles. A little tea of the bark should be drank while the external applications are continued" (Peter Smith, 1812). The young needles can be tinctured fresh, collected in July when they mature.

CONTRAINDICATIONS:

Strong tea and pitch should not be taken for kidney inflammation, as they stimulate the kidneys. Frequent use can irritate the kidneys (Michael Moore, 2003).

LITERATURE:

Traditional, Dietrich Gümbel (1), Edward Bach (2), Julia Graves (3), Matthew Wood (2-confirmed, 3, 5), Ben Charles Harris (7, 8), Peter Smith (14, 21), Dorothy Hall (4, 5), American Indian use (12–15, 18–22), Erichsen-Brown (10–15, 17–22), Max Tetau (16).

Polygala senega. Senega Snake Root.

This was an extremely important remedy for the American Indians, both medically and economically. It was still officinal in the standard pharmacopoeias of the United States and Europe as late as the 1950s, because of its great importance as a medicine in deep-seated bronchopneumonia. Its use here was replaced by the introduction of antibiotics.

Senega snake root was first introduced to the medical profession by Dr. John Tennant. While sojourning with the Seneca Indians, in Virginia, he noted that they had a very effective remedy for snake bite. For a fee, the plant was identified for him and he was allowed to watch its application in practice. He noted that it was most effective in cases where the toxemia produced symptoms like a deeply infected bronchopneumonia. He published his findings in 1745. They were read by Linnaeus, the father of botanical taxonomy, who used them for his own chronic bronchial problems with success.

Stamped with the personal approval of Linnaeus, Senega snake root became established in allopathic medicine as the standard of care for bronchopneumonia. It was also used in herbalism and homeopathy. During the two hundred years following its first appearance in print, Senega snake root was hunted almost to extinction. By the beginning of the twentieth century it was found only in the northwestern end of its range in any number. The 1900 federal census shows "snake root digger." to be the most common occupation on the Red Lake Indian Reservation, surrounded by northwestern Minnesota (Clara NiiSka). A farmer from central Manitoba tells me that Indians continued to pick snake root in his vicinity, north of Lake Winnipeg, until the 1960s.

"In croup this is a valuable medicine: and the discovery of it as such is due to Dr. Archer, of Harford county, Maryland," writes Dr. A. C. Gunn (1847, 623). He used bleeding, followed by a warm bath, then large doses of decoction of senega. Decoct 1 or 2 ounces of the root in a quart of boiling water in a closed vessel, until it is down to a pint; give a teaspoonful every hour or even 20 minutes. "It brings on a discharge of mucus or tough slime from the month and throat, which almost always relieves the person afflicted." I have needed to use senega snake root only twice for bronchopneumonia; it was both times quite helpful.

"The virtues of this root, in obstructions or stoppages of the menses or monthly discharges are absolutely incalculable; and every woman should return thanks to the Author of all good for giving such virtues to this root," continues Dr. Gunn. It is "possessed, perhaps, by no other, in relieving this diseased state of the female system which, of all others, is probably the most dangerous. When the menstrual discharge is looked for and does not appear, four ounces of the decoction above described ought to be taken in the course of a day." If it is too hard for the stomach to bear, cinnamon, ginger, or angelica can be given as a carminative to prevent vomiting. "The discovery of its virtues in female obstructions is due to Dr. Hartshorn, of Philadelphia, one of the best of men, and whose heart is devoted to suffering humanity."

SPECIFIC INDICATIONS:

- Hives (strong decoction).
- Violent colds.
- Croup (strong decoction).
- Bronchopneumonia.
- Edema.
- Menses obstructed.
- "Rheumatism of an inflammatory nature."
- Snake bite.

CAUTIONS:

Can cause emesis and purging.

LITERATURE:

John Tennant, A. C. Gunn (1–7).

Polygonatum spp. True Solomon's Seal.

Solomon's seal is a member of the lily family. Various species are native to Asia, Europe, and North America, where they have been used as food and medicine. The soft, sweet white/yellowish rhizomes look like bones and vertebrae, while the leaves wrapping around the stalk look like tendons and ligaments wrapping around bones, so Polygonatum has been used to strengthen the bones, marrow, and tendons. The "seals" on the rhizomes, where the stalk rises up, look like the sigils used by magicians (circles with marks inside them). Hence, the plant was named sigillum Salomanis *or Solomon's seal, after the wise king. It is one of the plants known in African American herbalism as "High John the Conqueror," in reference to magic or "conquering." It is worn as a mojo or chewed for "conquering."*

True Solomon's seal is used in Asia, Europe, and North America as a sweet nutritive for tendons and joints. The dried rhizomes look like bones, knuckles, and vertebrae, the leaves clasp around the stem, looking like a muscle attaching to a bone, and the flowers appear at the joints. It is of such widespread utility that it can help almost anyone with muscular and skeletal problems. It adjusts the tension on the tendons and ligaments; if they are too tight the tendon will not stretch as necessary or, if stretched, will not shrink back into place. It lubricates tendons, ligaments, muscles, and joints. If my knees are creaky, I take Solomon's seal tincture, a few drops externally, as needed. I have seen it remove bone spurs many times— it adjusts the tensions on the pelvis and legs that cause stress on bones and bone overgrowth resulting in bone spurs. This is not a disease of excessive calcification, except in a few cases, but of stress causing overgrowth. Bones are literally shaped by the pull on them.

The hydrated rhizomes of Solomon's seal, though they may still look like bones, also look like intestines and there is a long and persistent history of use of this medicine to curtail inflammation of the intestines. Leonard Thresher (1871, 328) reports this from Vermont. Phyllis Light reports it as a Southern folk usage. One American Indian practitioner reported that the mucilage in the rhizomes contains oligopolysaccharides that build up the flora of the colon. I have used Solomon's seal in several cases of severe intestinal inflammation. The demulcent nutritive constituents may soothe irritation of the mucosa of the lungs, gastrointestinal tract, and female system.

Solomon's seal also is considered to have a tonifying effect on the sexual system, both male and female. It definitely tightens the tendons holding up the uterus so that it is remedial in some cases of uterine prolapse. A friend of mine, acupuncturist Timothy Sartori, of Sun Prairie, Wisconsin, reported a case promptly cured. The woman, in her early forties, had just given birth to her first child; the womb was not in as good shape as that of a younger mother and was badly prolapsed. True Solomon's seal cured in five days.

Solomon's seal contains small amounts of cardiac glycosides, like its cousin *Convallaria majalis* (lily of the valley), but not enough to make it a toxic plant nor even a heart tonic. In my experience it will gently tone the pulse, making it more even, but I do not think of this as a cardiac usage so much as an indication that the mind is calmed. Notice its use in high blood pressure cited in the following paragraph.

Polygonatum spp. is used in Chinese herbalism, where it is known as "yellow essence." It is classified as a sweet, neutral yin tonic, or a moistening, lubricating, and nourishing tonic. It lubricates the heart and lungs, tones the middle region (abdomen), builds the marrow, and increases semen (essence). As a yin deficiency tonic it is used for dry throat and thirst, cough due to dry lungs, diabetes, and gray hair from kidney yin deficiency. Modern research shows that it can be used to bring down high blood pressure, protect the liver, treat fatty liver, and reduce blood sugar levels and blood fat (Lu, 1994, 203).

TASTE:

sweet, slightly acrid • cool, moist

TISSUE STATE:

atrophy

SPECIFIC INDICATIONS:

CONSTITUTION, COMPLEXION, CHARACTERISTIC SYMPTOMS
- Stretched, stiff, tight, or loose, weak tendons and ligaments.
- Nutritive food for weak and prostrated persons; tuberculosis.
- Irritation of the mucosa of the intestines, lungs, vagina.

RESPIRATION
- Pulmonary problems and hemorrhages.

CARDIOVASCULAR
- High blood pressure.

DIGESTION
- Intestinal upset; tension.
- Hemorrhoids.

FEMALE

- Profuse menstrual flow, vaginal irritation.
- Restores hormonal glow to the face, tonifies the ovaries, strengthens the estrogen side of the cycle.
- Ovarian pain.

MALE

- Premature ejaculation.

MUSCULAR AND SKELETAL

- Muscular and skeletal tensions, bone spurs resulting from such tensions.
- Repetitive use injury; carpal tunnel syndrome; arthritis associated with old injuries, calcifications, and muscular and skeletal tensions.

SKIN

- Bruises (external).
- Poison ivy (external).

PREPARATION AND DOSAGE:

The rhizomes are collected in the fall, dried for use by decoction or extracted fresh in alcohol. A high proof alcohol has to be used, since the sticky roots cause a sweet syrup if extracted in a low proof sweet alcohol like brandy. They can also be extracted in rubbing alcohol for external use only (add *Apios* for extra effect, Native American formula). Dose: external or internal use in small to large amount.

CONTRAINDICATIONS:

The seeds are toxic. It is considered to be environmentally challenged in some areas but it is one of the few native wildflowers that reestablishes itself in cities and yards, in flower beds and fence lines, throughout my area.

LITERATURE:

Traditional, John Gerard (1, 2, 12, 14), William Cook (3), Matthew Wood

(1, 3, 6, 12, 13), Henry Lu (5, 11), Julia Graves (9, 10), William Cullen (7), Chalid Ottway, Matthew Cameron (2, 4).

Populus candicans. Balm of Gilead.

The resinous buds of this northern tree are harvested and extracted in oil to make a "balm" used as a warming rub on the chest and joints, and as a disinfectant on wounds. These resins are also collected by bees to make propolis; hence this agent is similar to that one in properties (laryngitis, bronchitis). Balm of Gilead is used to promote dreaming (Anishinabe).

TASTE:

bitter • warm • stimulating

TISSUE STATE:

depression

SPECIFIC INDICATIONS:

- Laryngitis; restores the voice almost instantaneously.
- Hot, raw, dry bronchitis.
- Drying out of the membranes of the lungs, hence pleurisy.
- Hot, raw skin lesions (eczema, psoriasis).

LITERATURE:

Traditional, William Boericke (1), Matthew Wood (2), Beal P. Downing (3), traditional Anishinabe Ojibwe remedy (4).

Populus tremuloides. Trembling Aspen, Poplar.

The inner bark of the trembling aspen or poplar is used as a bitter tonic with nutritive effects. It contains phenolic glycosides (including salicin and populin), resins, tannins, and triterpenes.

Poplar is beneficial in conditions where there is fear, hyperadrenalism, hyperthyroidism, and overactivity of the sympathetic branch. William

LeSassier called poplar a remedy for "kidney nervousness." It has a similar mental state to the Bach flower essence poplar *(Populus tremula)*,
used for "fears of unknown origin." Because there is debility, weakness,
and poor digestion with sympathetic overactivity and exhaustion, poplar
bark "shows its influence best where there is general debility, very marked,
with impairment of the nutritive functions of the body" (Ellingwood,
1918, 317). It reduces fever and heat, and establishes groundedness and
strength, in people who are nervous (Matthew Wood).

Here is a case from my own practice. A middle-aged woman was suffering from hyperthyroid asthma (panting caused by a metabolic rate so
high the cells can't get enough oxygen). The asthma and the hyperthyroidism rapidly settled down with a tincture of *Populus tremuloides*,
dosage unrecorded. Recently I had another case of hyperthyroidism with
panting in hot weather. She tried a formula with melissa, lycopus, and
leonurus, which hadn't worked. Skullcap and poplar bark were, however, effective. The latter was more helpful with the asthma than the scutellaria.

The guts are not able to relax due to the high sympathetic activity.
"The stool becomes fluid when peristalsis (wave-like movements of the
bowel) is increased," writes Dr. J. V. Cerney (1976, 63). This can be caused
by mental stress, food allergies, or infection. In some of these cases aspen
will radically cure the complaint. Cerney cites a patient with chronic diarrhea stopped "within hours" of beginning poplar tincture, 10 drops in
sherry wine.

This weakness and debility can also manifest in the urinary sphere.
"Urinary organs are inherently weak and prone to recurring problems
such as *cystitis,"* writes Laurel Dewey (1999, 86). Since poplar bark is
so bitter, she sometimes uses a bath, especially for children.

Poplar is also beneficial for the alternating chills and fever of malaria
and influenza, which also represent a sympathetic excess (since that branch
of the autonomic is in charge of the shivering mechanism). Samuel
Thomson, Wooster Beach, and many of the early botanical physicians
utilized bitter poplar bark for intermittent fever, malaria, and hepatic
troubles where the autonomic innervations of the gallbladder are damaged by alternating chills and fever.

In American Indian medicine, poplar bark is used with rose thorns in
a formula for wounds that are healing slowly or for very serious wounds
that need immediate regrowth of tissue "if the part can be saved." It stops
the bleeding, dries and seals the wound, relieves pain, and stimulates

regrowth of the damaged tissue. I knew a woman whose badly infected foot was healed with this formula; the white doctors advised her that it might be necessary to amputate her foot. She went to a medicine man, who cured her. Interestingly, this woman was somewhat the opposite of the poplar type: almost apathetic and indolent. Indeed, she let her foot get very badly infected after wounding it with an ax.

TASTE:

bitter

TISSUE STATES:

constriction, atrophy, depression

SPECIFIC INDICATIONS:

CONSTITUTION, COMPLEXION, CHARACTERISTIC SYMPTOMS
- Persons who get a shaky feeling when nervous; shaky feeling in the stomach.
- General debility, impairment of the nutritive function, consumption or wasting.

MIND, SENSES, NERVES, EMOTIONS, PERSONALITY
- *Nervousness, fear, anxiety, sympathetic excess, hyperthyroidism.*
- Pain reducer.

RESPIRATION
- Panting asthma of hyperthyroidism (two cases).
- Catarrh; thick and intractable, in bronchitis and bronchorrhea.

DIGESTION
- Shaking; nervousness, intermittent fever (chills alternating with fever), with debility and weakness.
- Indigestion, accompanied by flatulence and acidity.
- *Atonic dyspepsia,* especially when there is debility, hepatic torpor, old age; poor digestion, assimilation, and anabolism leading to emaciation.
- *Chronic diarrhea.*
- Intestinal worms.

KIDNEYS AND BLADDER

- Cystitis; painful passage of urine, scalding, heat, burning in the urethra and meatus.
- Suppression and retention of urine; associated with weakness and debility.
- Tenesmus after urination.

MALE

- Enlarged prostate with neurasthenia (nerve wasting).

FEMALE

- Uterine congestion.

FEVER

- Chronic, relapsing, debilitating fevers, where there is an irregular element; night sweats, intermittent chills and fever.

MUSCULAR AND SKELETAL

- Tremor of Parkinson's and nervous debility.
- Arthritis, broken bones.

EXTERNAL

- Skin rashes, sore throat, minor burns, inflamed wounds (tea, external).
- Severe injury, the part may be lost, necrosis is feared (external application of rose thorns and poplar bark).

PREPARATION AND DOSAGE:

"When first I began to use this Samson among remedies of its class, I had to use decoctions of the bark—it was a nasty, bitter dose. How much better to use the specific medicine in from five to twenty drop doses" (John Fearn, MD, quoted in Ellingwood, 1918, 317). Michael Moore (2003) suggests using an infusion of the leaves to avoid the problem with bitterness in the bark. "The bark of the aspen tree may be made into powder form, decoctions, or tinctures. Start with a small amount. Determine the exact quantity you need by adding to each dose. This way you get to know what your own personal dosage may be" (J. V. Cerney, 1976, 63).

CONTRAINDICATIONS:

Poplar bark can be ineffective for people who have taken aspirin for many years or are currently taking it (Dewey, 1999, 89).

LITERATURE:

Traditional, American Indian specific formula (21), Michael Moore (6), Samuel Thomson (7, 8), Grover Coe (7, 8), Finley Ellingwood (2, 7, 8, 13–17), John William Fyfe (eclectic literature), R. Swinburne Clymer (2), Terry Willard, Dorothy Hall (1), Matthew Wood (5), William LeSassier (3, 4, 19), J. V. Cerney (10), Laurel Dewey (9, 10, 12, 13, 20).

Polytrichum juniperinum. Hairy Cap Moss.

This common little moss was incorporated into medicine during the American colonial era. Specific indications for its presentation were never developed, so that it sometimes worked spectacularly and sometimes failed miserably. It was generally dropped from practice by the early twentieth century. It is "a hydragogue diuretic; in some cases incredibly increasing the flow of urine," writes Rolla Thomas (1903). "It is most valuable in uric acid diathesis, lithemia, and suppression of urine from cold." Dose: "5 drops to 1 dram."

"According to the late Dr. A. M. Cushing, this remedy (hairycap moss or Robin's eye) will, in the tincture, or an infusion (*i.e.*, the moss steeped in water), have a powerfully good effect in the ills of old men suffering from a bad bladder or enlarged prostate—prostatitis. This he got from the old herbalists" (Anshutz, 1900, 145).

Prinos verticillatus. Black Alder, Winterberry.

This is the most northerly representative of the holly or Aquifoliaceae family in North America. It loses its leaves in the fall but retains the bright red berries. This is about the only time of the year when it is easily seen and is the season when the bark and fruits are harvested. Like other hollies, winterberry has a reputation in intermittent fever. It contains bitters, tannins (to 16%), resins, gum, sugar, and albumin, which suits it to use as an astringent bitter to purge and tone the gallbladder and digestive tract, while returning the autonomic nervous system to balance. It is suited to old, worn-out cases following lengthy fevers, and even to gangrene. Black alder grows on low ground, like its unrelated namesake, the true alder (Alnus).

"Black alder is common in thickets at the margins of pools and marshy places, from western Florida northward" to Canada (Millspaugh, 1892, 416). It is "another of the growing list of plants handed down to us by the aborigines, who used the bark both internally and externally as a tonic, astringent, and antiseptic, and is probably as well known to domestic practice as any indigenous shrub." The berries are also used. "It is so well known by its red berries, which the women in the country give their children for worms, that it needs no further description," wrote Dr. Samuel Henry (1814, 13). "The bark is good to boil in spring beer, which opens obstructions, purifies the blood, and keeps the body soluble."

To continue with Millspaugh: "In intermittent fever it has proved as generally applicable as Peruvian bark, and in such low typhoid forms associated with diarrhea, and in the later stages, where ulceration and hemorrhage are present, it is a very valuable agent. In general debilitated conditions of the system after long fevers, and where the body is depleted by exhausting discharges, it is also very useful, as well as in gangrenous affections and jaundice. Certain forms of chronic herpetic eruptions and ulcers are also benefited by its use as an external application. The berries are purgative and vermifuge, forming one of the pleasantest adjuvants in children's remedies, for the expulsion of lumbrici. Schoepf [1777] first noted the plant as having the above field of utility, and also mentioned its usefulness in anasarca."

Millspaugh and Shook mention a case in which twenty-five berries caused nausea, vomiting of bile without retching, passage of green diarrhea, with return to improved digestion and appetite. From the green discharges it is clear that black alder purges the gallbladder.

Alma Hutchins (1991, 4) is one of the few modern authors with extensive information on black alder. It is "very similar in action to Cascara when used for constipation," she writes. "Alder is an agent used for jaundice, diarrhea, gangrene, dropsy, and all diseases with symptoms of great weakness."

TASTE:

bitter • astringent

TISSUE STATES:

depression, relaxation, stagnation

SPECIFIC INDICATIONS:

CHARACTERISTIC SYMPTOMS

- Atonic conditions of the digestive tract with exhausting discharges and great exhaustion.

DIGESTION

- Gums infirm.
- Nausea and vomiting.
- Chronic dyspepsia, diarrhea, and dysentery.
- Typhoid with ulceration, hemorrhage, exhausting discharge, debility.
- Worms (berries).

LIVER

- Jaundice and dyspepsia.
- Anasarca, fluid in the abdomen due to liver disease.

KIDNEYS AND BLADDER

- Dropsy.

SKIN

- Chronic skin eruptions; old ulcers, sores; gangrene (external).
- Head lice (external).

PREPARATION AND DOSAGE:

Black alder is difficult to find until the leaves are off and the red berries are prominent. The fresh bark is gathered before the first autumnal frost (Shook).

Internal (bark): "Make sure you age the outer and inner bark, as the green bark will provoke strong vomiting, pain, and gripping in the stomach." One-half dram of the powdered bark to 1 dram of apple cider. Take 1 teaspoonful 3x/day, for three days in a row. Or make a decoction, let stand for two or three days, until the yellow color turns to black. "It will strengthen the stomach and procure an appetite" (Hutchins, 1991, 4).

Two ounces of the cut bark in 3 pints of water, boil down to 2 pints, strain, a wineglassful 3 or 4x/day (Shook). Fluid extract, 10–60 drops (John William Fyfe).

Internal (berries): combine with apple cider (1/2 dram to 1 dram), give a dose when the moon is full and the worms are most active, then fast the patient before bed, give a mild herbal laxative, fast again in the morning, and give alder again. Repeat again in four weeks to get rid of the eggs (Hutchins).

External: boil the inner bark in vinegar.

CAUTIONS:

Nauseating in large doses, when not dried.

LITERATURE:

Traditional (American Indian), Johann Schoepf, Samuel Henry (6), Charles Millspaugh (1, 3, 4, 5, 6, 7, 9), Edward Shook, Ben Charles Harris (8, 10), Alma Hutchins (1, 2, 11).

Prunella vulgaris. Self-Heal.

Long thought to be native to the Old World it has now been shown that Self-Heal was also indigenous to North America. This explains its many uses in Native American medicine. A full account is given with the medicinal plants of the Old World.

Prunus serotina. Wild Cherry.

Wild or black cherry is a member of the rose family native to eastern North America. In the nineteenth century it was considered an indispensable medicine by the Indian people and their students, the American pioneers. John Uri Lloyd declared it the most commonly used domestic remedy in the late nineteenth century. It was primarily used as a coolant in fever and irritative coughs. It did not receive a homeopathic proving, and is little used in homeopathy, but Dr. John Eberle (1834, 1:301) tested it on himself and produced symptoms of both excitation and depression. Wild cherry possesses flavonoids, bitter cyanogens, tannins, a bit of mucilage, resins, and volatile oils.

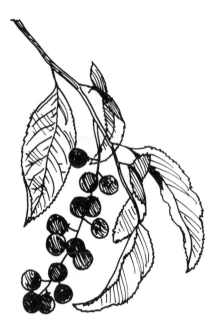

The Latin binomial Prunus virginiana *was originally applied to both wild cherry and chokecherry. Eventually the former was designated* Prunus serotina. *Mid-nineteenth-century literature often confuses the identity and uses of these two agents. Chokecherry is a powerful astringent, whereas wild cherry is a sedative. The former is thus used for diarrhea and dysentery.*

Dr. John Eberle (1834, 1:301) relates of the wild cherry: "When taken into the system, it produces a slight increase of the action of the heart and arteries, and induces, in some individuals, considerable drowsiness." It also tones the stomach and gives "vigour to the general system." However, in large doses, frequently repeated, it depresses the heart and circulation, weakens the digestion, and exhausts the system. "In my own person I have several times reduced my pulse from seventy-five to fifty strokes in a minute, by copious draughts of the cold infusion, taken several times during the day, and continued for twelve or fourteen days." Eberle pinpoints the action of wild cherry in (1) the heart and circulation, (2) stomach and digestion, and (3) lungs.

Flavonoids are cooling because they repair irritation in the capillaries that would otherwise slow down the blood flow, leading to capillary congestion and its side effects: heat, redness, swelling, tenderness, and rapid heartbeat. These are the classic symptoms of inflammation and fever, for which wild cherry has long been used. In addition, it contains cyanogens, which break down into hydrocyanic acid. This stops the Krebs cycle, which is the body's mechanism for producing energy. Thus, cyanogens cut down heat production at the cellular level. This is why too much cyanide can kill a person. Fortunately, the amount of cyanide in a small dose of wild cherry bark is only enough to cool. The cyanogens and flavonoids work together to sedate and cool the organism. They are most commonly found together in members of the rose family such as bitter almond, wild cherry, peach twig and leaf, apple seed, and pear seed.

From clinical observations we can, however, be somewhat more precise in our understanding of the action of wild cherry. It specifically reduces the amount of irritation due to histamine, the substance that the body uses to irritate the capillaries to increase local blood congestion and the inflammatory process. We see this in the fact that wild cherry is such a good remedy for irritative laryngeal cough. This type of cough can be produced as a side effect of the use of the ACE inhibitors, which increase bradykinins, a histamine analog.

The histaminic reaction can be observed on the surface by scoring the skin with a fingernail. After a period of blanching (whiteness), the area gets extra red as the cells produce histamine to bring in more blood and repair the slight damage caused by the scratch. Excess histamine is seen when there is an excessive, highly colored cherry red inflammation around a wound. This sort of aggravated histamine reaction is a specific indication for wild cherry bark. It will clear up both the redness (which is but a minor symptom) and other deeper problems in the system.

The ACE inhibitors were introduced into the market with the idea that they reduce blood pressure by inhibiting the angiotensin converting enzyme (ACE), which converts angiotensin I to II, increasing sodium retention in the kidneys and increasing blood pressure. However, they also increase bradykinin levels and this reduces blood pressure through another mechanism. The capillaries become irritated and open up to receive more blood. This reduces blood congestion in the internal organs, which produces high blood pressure. Thus, the increase in bradykinins increases peripheral circulation and reduces blood pressure. However, if peripheral irritation gets too intense, the tissues become inflamed and the pulse and blood pressure rise.

Wild cherry bark is probably a histamine normalizer. It acts on excessive heat and irritation, where the tissues are hot, red, and full, with a rapid pulse and high blood pressure. The skin easily turns red when it is irritated. This condition is more common in cherry redheads. They are more sensitive to the sun, their injuries tend to turn red easily, they heat up, they sometimes have food allergies (histamine is part of the immune response), and (as studies have shown) they bleed more at parturition (due to the irritated capillaries). However, wild cherry bark also acts on conditions where there is a lack of histamine. The extremities are cold, from poor circulation, the tissues are mottled red and blue, with a yellow tinge, and the blanching reaction is too long—when pressed, the skin stays white longer than normal. These people are usually thin, with cool skin and cold extremities. Wild cherry will warm them up, even though we think of it as a sedative. Wild cherry is often called for in cases where a combination of the above symptoms presents with, for example, cold skin but hot mucosa.

Wild cherry is suited to an irritable cough in the throat. By soothing the respiratory apparatus it increases expectoration. It is also good in old, exhausted coughs. William LeSassier noted that wild cherry is indicated for a hacking cough that weakens the sphincter of the colon, so it affects "the tubes at both ends," as he said in his unique fashion. It acts especially on the small intestine. It acts as a sedative in cases where there are food sensitivities and as a bitter where there is a lack of secretion. Finally, wild cherry is beneficial for the heart. It is useful when there are heart palpitations, arrhythmias, and "exalted action of the heart," as herbalist Darrell Martin of Biloxi says—and I quote this, not because it is original, but because it shows a contemporary herbalist still thinking along the same lines as Eberle and the nineteenth-century practitioners. Thus, it has been used for fever, nervousness, and rehabilitation after fever.

Here is something I have not seen anywhere else in the literature: "Cherry bark will dissolve stones but should be combined with other herbs and administered carefully and over a period of several months, as when taken too fast will expel the stones abruptly without being softened" (Alma Hutchins, 1991, 86). The type of stones is not designated; probably the reference is to gallstones. There must be some action on the gallbladder and liver, because I find that the skin is often yellow and red, with poor capillary reflux (blanching), when wild cherry is needed (cf. *Crataegus*).

Phyllis Light adds that wild cherry bark is an old Southern remedy for uterine fibroids.

Dr. Samuel Henry (1814, 178), of New York City, learned of a pulmonary formula from a man who had gotten it from a Dr. Kennedy, of Sussex County, New Jersey. This man had been in a "deep consumption"—that is, wasting with coughing, perhaps tuberculosis—when Dr. Kennedy gave him a "sirup chiefly composed of the lungwort taken from the north side of the white oak tree." This was used in lieu of Iceland moss. He "was perfectly restored to health in a few weeks: he also drank daily a tea made of the lungwort." The full formula is two handfuls lungwort moss from the north side of an oak tree, a handful each of white hoarhound, hyssop, sage, elecampane, fresh spikenard, inner bark of wild cherry, and button wood (probably sweet gum), boil in 2 gallons of water, down to 1, strain, and add molasses. Boil down to 4 quarts and store in an earthen pot. This represents an interesting combination of well-known British pulmonary herbs (white hoarhound, hyssop, elecampane) with native American medicinals (spikenard, wild cherry, button wood, and lungwort moss). This compound was probably the ancestor of "compound syrup of spikenard" or "pulmonary balsam," which was used in obstinate respiratory cases. It contained equal parts spikenard, comfrey, elecampane, bloodroot, white hoarhound, and wild cherry (Cook, 1869, 260).

Another variation on this formula is recorded by Vermont doctor Leonard Thresher (1871, 36). "At one time I was practicing medicine with a native Indian doctor in one of our New England cities, where a young lady about eighteen years of age came under our treatment for consumption of the lungs. She had been doctored, at different times, by four of the best Allopathic physicians in the city, and each of them pronounced her case incurable, with tubercles in the lungs. There was great excitation; profuse expectoration; pain in the chest, with other symptoms denoting the last stage of consumption of the lungs. The Indian made an examination of the case, and prepared a medicine in the form of a syrup, which, in the course of a few weeks, checked the progress of the disease and subsequently restored the girl to perfect health." If, as Thresher reports, there were tubercles present, this is an instance of remarkable doctoring. The formula was pleurisy root, elecampane, sumach bark, skunk cabbage, witch hazel bark and flowers, bayberry bark and flowers, white hoarhound leaves and flowers, gum arabic, liquorice, sugar, eggs, bloodroot, and lobelia.

TASTE:

bitter, sweet, sour • hot and cold, damp and dry • astringent

TISSUE STATE:

excitation

SPECIFIC INDICATIONS:

CONSTITUTION, COMPLEXION, CHARACTERISTIC SYMPTOMS
- *People with a tendency to red, irritable, histaminic reactions on the skin; little cuts develop a cherry red border; redheads.*

- Thin people with cold extremities and cool, damp skin.
- Fever with irritable tissue.

RESPIRATION

- *Irritated, histaminic, laryngeal cough.*
- *Old, tired coughs that linger after active infection has passed;* coughs with palpitations; debility of old, protracted, enfeebled congestion of phlegm.
- Accumulation of hardened mucus.
- Asthma, bronchitis, pleurisy, tuberculosis.

CARDIOVASCULAR AND CIRCULATION

- Irregular or intermittent action of the heart; cardiac irregularities in chronic bronchitis, anemia, and nervous palpitations.
- Convulsive action of the heart from overwork; heart palpitations, high blood pressure.

DIGESTION

- Nervous irritation of the stomach and intestines, dyspepsia, diarrhea.
- Exhausted, irritable, nervous conditions of the digestion after typhoid, low conditions.
- Hemorrhoids, irritable; weak rectal sphincter.
- *Celiac; food allergies; irritation of the small intestine.*
- Diarrhea of children (syrup).

LIVER

- Hepatitis, jaundice, cirrhosis of the liver, stones.

SKIN

- Skin cherry red, irritated, histaminic appearance; palms red and yellow.
- Herpes and shingles; when the eruption is on the tongue or in the mouth, not on the lips; when the eruption exhibits generalized redness rather than a vesicular appearance (cf. *Ranunculus bulbosus* when there are vesicles).

FEVER

- Fever, long continued, erratic, exhaustive.

- Lack of muscular tone in patients recovering from fevers and other exhausting diseases.
- Pulse weak and irregular.
- Reddish, slightly purple, and yellow skin that blanches under pressure and only slowly returns to its original color (cf. *Crataegus*).
- Fever; "irritable nervousness of hectic, and similar cases" (Cook).
- "Nervous irritability and arterial excitement" (Cook).

PREPARATION AND DOSAGE:

The bark of the branches is collected, but the bark of the root is the best (Darrell Martin). It is collected, not during the late winter, as is usual with most barks, but during the spring or fall when the sugar content is higher in the bark. It is more bitter with cyanogens in midwinter, when other barks are collected. William LeSassier gave the following advice about making wild cherry preparations. Check the bark from several trees to find one with the characteristic bitter almond taste and smell. There are two methods of preparation: (1) hydrolyze the fresh bark by soaking in lukewarm water in a covered vessel for 12–24 hours until the bitter almond smell comes off, then add alcohol. The longer the herb is left, the more astringent it becomes, so: (2) boil until the soothing and volatile parts are dissipated. Dosage of the tincture: 20–60 drops, up to 4x/day, and do not exceed this amount (Gagnon). I use 1–3 drops, 1–3x/day. Fluid extract, 10 drops in hot water every 4 hours in pleurisy (Ralph M. Russell).

CAUTIONS:

Wild cherry bark contains cyanide and should not be used in large or too frequent doses.

LITERATURE:

Traditional (3, 4, 5, 7, 10, 15), John Eberle (8, 20), Jack Ritchason (6), William LeSassier (12), J. I. Lighthall, John William Fyfe (8, 9, 15), Darrell Martin, Matthew Wood (1, 2, 13, 16, 17, 20, 21), Tommie Bass (12), Ralph M. Russell (7), Christopher Menzies-Trull (20), William Cook (11, 22, 23), Alma Hutchins (5, 7, 9, 10, 14, 22), Leonard Thresher (7), A. C. Gunn (15).

Ptelea trifoliata. Wafer Ash.

This little tree is found in low, moist ground in eastern North America. It was presumably an Indian remedy picked up by the settlers and doctors. The bark yields a good bitter; it was one of the innumerable bitters used in the nineteenth century to combat the digestive problems caused by malaria.

Ptelea unites the happy properties of a carminative: bitter, pungent, and astringent. Hence it is tonic to the stomach and digestion. Ellingwood (1918, 273) writes, "The agent is a mild tonic, exercising a direct influence upon the stomach and digestive apparatus, correcting certain faults of gastric secretion, overcoming dyspepsia and improving the appetite. It may be given to good advantage with other stomachic tonics and iron. It corrects atonic diarrhea and is of benefit in dysentery, its pungent properties and sufficient astringency render it of benefit in mild cases. In full doses it acts upon the skin as a diaphoretic. It has been given in lung troubles," especially asthma.

LITERATURE:

Traditional (American Indian), Johann Schoepf, Constantine Rafinesque, Horton Howard, Finley Ellingwood.

Quercus alba, Q. robur. White Oak, English Oak.

White oak (Quercus alba) is the officinal plant in North America, whereas English or European oak (Quercus robur) is used in the Old World. Since the constituent used in herbal medicine is the powerful astringency, which is found in all oaks, most members of the family can be used interchangeably with the officinal species. The inner bark of the oak contains tannins, saponins, and minerals.

Oak bark is a very powerful and relatively pure astringent. Michael Moore (2003, 177) calls it the "basic astringent." I would call it the "model astringent," against which others may be compared. Therefore, what we see in its symptom picture is a highly developed condition of tissue relaxation, with loss of tone, prolapse, outflow of fluids, and loss of minerals. The respiratory tract becomes atonic and there may be chronic loss of fluids through the sinuses or lungs. The stomach is damp and mucoid, either from its own hypersecretion, or because of fluids descending from the sinuses. The gums are weak, the teeth loose and easily cavitated, and there may be mouth sores. The intestines may be atonic, giving way to "relaxation of the bowels" or diarrhea. Digestion and assimilation are poor, and metabolism is low. The circulatory system is also affected, resulting in swollen, knobby blue-black veins in the legs and hemorrhoids. Undoubtedly there is going to be some kind of negative influence on the heart through such vascular deterioration. The lymphatics may be involved—oak bark has proved itself many times in my experience for chronic lymphedema from surgical excision of glands—and it is an old remedy for swollen spleen.

From the standpoint of traditional Chinese medicine, the above set of symptoms would be classified under deficient spleen yang. Actually oak is an old splenic medicine in the Western tradition. J. G. Rademacher introduced distilled tincture of acorn as a remedy for swollen spleen and bellyache emanating from the region of the spleen.

When the relaxed, atonic condition is well developed, the system will be somewhat cool from the air-conditioning-like effects of having a moist surface. There is a loss of potassium and electrolytes with the fluids, giving rise to weakness of the kidneys, with clear, copious urine, and a general demineralization of the hard structures. Thus, oak is indicated by a low body temperature, loss of fluids, clear, limpid urine, and demineralization of the teeth. Relaxation pushes so far that putrefaction sets in and there may be dead tissue and putrid discharges.

The above symptoms, long established by experience and tradition, have also been produced by oak, so that we may say that it is homeopathic to these symptoms as well. Dr. W. T. Fernie (1917, 15) noted that excessive consumption of acorns caused a disease in young cattle. "Its symptoms are progressive wasting, loss of appetite, diarrhea, sore places inside the mouth, discharge from the eyes and nostrils, excretion of much pale urine, and no fever, but a fall of temperature below the normal standard." Interestingly, Toronto herbalist Chalid Ottway (1933, 113) considered acorn to be "a wonderful medicine for fat people. It dries up the watery humor, aids sluggishness of the system and will reduce surplus flesh. It will bring high blood pressure down to normal."

My experience with oak led me to suppose that it must have a calcifying effect, since it is so beneficial for the teeth, improving both the hard parts and the tendons attaching the teeth to the jaw. It seems to put calcium into connective tissue, whether cartilage, tendon, or bone. There is little about this in the traditional literature, but Fernie (1917, 18) mentions some pertinent information. "Finely powdered oak bark, when inhaled pretty frequently, has proved very beneficial against consumption of the lungs in its early stages. Working tanners are well known to be particularly exempt from this disease, probably through their constantly inhaling the peculiar aroma given off from the tan pits." The body fights tuberculosis by enclosing the bacteria in a calcified cell, so resistance to tuberculosis is clearly related to calcium.

When the tissues are extremely relaxed they deteriorate or break down in a fashion analogous to the depressed tissue state. Thus, oak bark is remedial to putrefaction and necrosis, especially where an astringent rather than a stimulant is needed. This was brought out by none other than Samuel Hahnemann in his pre-homeopathic phase. In 1791 he contributed an article entitled "A Household Remedy for Gangrene" to a medical journal. He writes that the "surest and most certain household remedy for gangrene" is 6 ounces of powdered oak bark boiled down in a large quantity of water, compressed on the affected part, and changed every half hour. "Within a few hours the gangrene will stop spreading and will not smell when it is moist." After a while the gangrenous part becomes detached and the flesh forms an abscess. As the condition improves the compress is used hourly, then every few hours (Richard Haehl, 1927, 24). It is remarkable that in his homeopathic phase Hahnemann never advocated the use of oak bark.

The mental state for which oak is remedial is analogous to the physical condition. Oak is the great remedy when integrity of mind or body has been broken down by long, arduous suffering or usage. Dr. Bach introduced *Quercus robur* for those who fight on against adversity, who never give in but they never succeed. It helps a person choose the appropriate, winnable battles, instead of trying to "out-integrity" every obstacle. Doctors J. G. Rademacher, Compton Burnett, and Dorothy Shepherd developed the use of *Q. robur* in alcoholics to stop the desire for drink (cf. Wood, *The Book of Herbal Wisdom*).

TASTE:

astringent

TISSUE STATE:

relaxation

SPECIFIC INDICATIONS:

MIND, SENSES, NERVES, EMOTIONS, PERSONALITY
- *Persons who struggle against adversity; never give up but never succeed;* helps a person choose the battles they can win (flower essence, confirmed with the bark).
- *Alcoholism; persons who struggle with their addictions.*

HAIR, TEETH, GUMS
- Darkens and strengthens the hair.
- *Gum disease, dental caries, loose teeth, bad breath, canker sores, bleeding gums.*
- Whitens the teeth (bark).
- Thrush in children (bark tea).

RESPIRATION
- Swelling and puffiness under the eyes, yellow and blue discoloration.
- Sinus congestion, postnasal drip, mucus in the stomach, indigestion.
- Cough.
- Tuberculosis, early stages.

HEART AND CIRCULATION
- High blood pressure.
- Palpitation of the heart.
- *Blue-black, knobby varicose veins in the legs, surrounded by yellow infiltration.*

DIGESTION
- Lack of appetite, indigestion.
- Intestinal prolapse, diarrhea, dysentery, lack of tone.
- *Hemorrhoids.*
- Gastroenteritis (with raspberry; dried leaf tea).

KIDNEYS AND BLADDER
- Kidneys not concentrating the urine; clear, copious urine.
- Ulceration of the bladder, bloody urine, cystitis.

FEMALE
- Vaginitis.

MUSCULAR AND SKELETAL
- Osteoporosis.
- Hernia (poultice).

LYMPHATICS
- Strep throat, tonsillitis, swollen glands in throat.
- Lymphedema after surgical removal of glands.
- Swollen spleen; pain in the spleen.

ENDOCRINE
- Goiter.
- Fat people; dries up the watery humor, aids sluggishness of the system, reduces surplus flesh (acorn).

SKIN
- Bleeding, bruises.
- Excessive sweating on the feet or elsewhere.
- Erysipelas, eczema, irritation of the skin (ointment from the acorn).
- Ulcers, putrid, foul, gangrenous (external compress or wash).

OTHER
- Diabetes (powdered oak bark).

PREPARATION, CONTRAINDICATIONS, AND DOSAGE:

The inner bark is collected in late winter or spring and extracted fresh in alcohol or dried for use by decoction. Also used externally in sitz baths, poultices, salves, fomentations, etc. Large doses are too puckering and astringent. I use the bark of the twigs. Tommie Bass would use it in vinegar. The leaves and acorns can also be used.

CAUTIONS:

Do not spread oak wilt by using the same utensils to cut different trees.

COMPARISON:

Tommie Bass used red oak *(Quercus rubra)* differently than white oak. It was for cirrhosis of the liver.

LITERATURE:

Traditional, Edward Bach (1, 2), Johann Gottfried Rademacher (2, 25), Michael Moore (4, 15), Laurel Dewey (6, 17), John Scudder (16), Alma Hutchins (8, 18–20, 23, 26, 28), J. Compton Burnett (2, 7), Dorothy Shepherd (2), Finley Ellingwood, Matthew Wood (1, 2, 4, 13, 18, 21, 24), John Christopher (4), Tommie Bass (29), W. T. Fernie (10, 14, 15, 23), Chalid Ottway (3, 4, 5, 7, 9, 11, 12, 27, 30), Horton Howard (22), Daniel Cobb (31), Samuel Hahnemann (31), Juliette de Bairacli Levy (32), Deb Frances (21).

Rhus aromatica, R. coriaria, R. typhina. Sumach.

Sumach (R. coriaria) *has a long history of use in Greek and Arabic medicine. The name comes from the Greek* rhu *for "flux." It is one of the great remedies for fluid loss from any outlet. However, sumach is not native to Europe and was not much used in European medicine. It is widely used as a condiment in Middle Eastern cooking. It makes rice taste delicious, but it is primarily used (with basil) to increase the digestion of fats in meat.*

North America has many species of sumach and here either the Indian people taught the European settlers its use, or the settlers discovered it themselves. The various sumachs had important economic uses, especially in the dye industry, and country people were very familiar with them. Fragrant sumach (R. aromatica) *and smooth sumach* (R. glabra) *were officinal in nineteenth-century America. Staghorn sumach* (R. typhina) *was used in folk medicine. The indications seem to be relatively interchangeable.* Rhus glabra *received a homeopathic proving, so I have rendered a separate account of it based on this history. All of these species are nontoxic, unlike their unfriendly cousins, poison ivy* (R. toxicodendron) *and California poison oak* (R. diversiloba).

Sumach (*Rhus* spp.) is the superlative remedy for stopping excessive flux from any channel of elimination—skin, kidneys, colon, lungs, or menses. It is indicated when there are debilitating fluid losses. It especially strengthens the functions of the kidney, helping it to retain water in both diabetes mellitus type II and diabetes insipidus. It was for this that sumach was introduced into nineteenth-century American medicine by Dr. McClanahan (Fyfe, 1909). Subsequently it was used for dribbling and lack of retention of urine in the young and the old. And finally, as herbalist Phyllis Light informs us, it is indicated in "kidney anemia," when the kidneys do not signal the bone marrow to produce enough red blood cells.

Sumach not only helps the kidneys retain water in sugar diabetes, but helps the cells pick up blood sugar, reducing problems with eyesight and neuropathy and making blood sugar levels more manageable and less extreme. It evidently acts on vasopressin, the antidiuretic hormone secreted by the posterior pituitary, for it also has a profound influence on high blood pressure in some cases—evidently those that trace to insufficient action of vasopressin. I have seen some dramatic cases where it brought down high blood pressure and high sugar levels.

Moving into the respiratory sphere, sumach is indicated in runny secretion resulting in sneezy head colds, irritable coughing from excessive salivation overstimulating the cough reflexes, and watery discharges from the lungs. It is one of Phyllis Light's first selections in influenza and it is indicated when mucus is specked with blood, according to Australian herbalist Glenda Croft. The cough reflex needs a little bit of fluid to keep it happy; both lack and excess of fluids cause an irritable cough that sounds similar in either instance. Sumach is indicated when excessive saliva stimulates a "drippy cough" (cf. red clover, white hoarhound). This can cause choking/coughing episodes at night, when the saliva or nasal drip runs down, yet there is no ripened mucus.

In the gastrointestinal sphere sumach is indicated in excessive secretion, from the mouth (saliva) to the colon, resulting in diarrhea. The latter can be putrescent—this is particularly well documented in association with *Rhus glabra*, both in the nineteenth-century usage and in the homeopathic provings. I had a case where high blood pressure would accompany expansion of a rectal fissure. There was a history of heart disease in the family. *Rhus typhina* controlled both symptoms remarkably.

Sumach also acts on the menses. It is indicated when the menstrual blood is accompanied by a thin, watery discharge, according to Phyllis Light. She also recommended it when other fluids are not being retained, hence in nocturnal emissions, clear vaginal discharge, excessive blood loss from the kidneys, uterus, bowels, stomach, or lungs, and excessive expectoration. Yarrow, shepherd's purse, and sumach are Glenda Croft's basic threesome for the treatment of excessive menstrual discharge. She uses sumach in menopausal women with constant bleeding, the menses are profuse, thin (not clotted), constant, and dark, like the color of sumach berries. The burgundy red color of the berries is also a signature for blood building (cf. rehmannia root, beet root, yellow dock seeds).

The skin is also affected, and a capital indication is "excessive sweating and peeing." In other cases the skin or lungs or digestive tract is dried out, yet the kidneys or another channel are losing fluids. This led my friend Lise Wolff, an herbalist in Minneapolis, to describe sumach as the "leaky straw" remedy. It is indicated when there is a leak somewhere in the system that dries out the tissues elsewhere. The tongue is often dry in the center and wet on the edges, indicating that the core is drying out as fluids are being lost.

Glenda Croft uses *Rhus coriaria,* because it is available in Middle Eastern markets as a culinary spice. She lived in the Middle East at one time and noted that the Bedouin chew the stalks as a strengthening tonic. Later, as an herbalist in Australia, she took up its use. Both she and I noticed that sumach is indicated when there is a blue and gray complexion around the veins.

Sumach is considered to be a deer or elk medicine in American Indian woodlore. The branches of these small trees look like deer or elk antlers. Deer like to browse at the edges of fields, where this plant—a colonist from the forest—grows. That way they can eat the rich offerings of the field, but dash away into the forest. According to my friend Paul Red Elk, the Indian people noticed that the female deer would eat sumach then lick her vagina after giving birth, from which it was deduced that she was cleaning herself. Thus, sumach is used, not only to check the loss of fluids during menstruation, but to bring on a flow of fluids—many herbs have such dual actions. From an Iroquois woman I learned a related use: after menopause sumach is used to induce a watery discharge to cleanse the womb.

Sumach is sometimes indicated for nervousness, anxiety, fear, or even desperation. See the provings of *Rhus glabra* listed below. Herbalist Erica Fargione, of Minneapolis, had a case in which a woman had extreme anxiety and fear. Nothing really helped until it came out that she panicked after having profuse urination. *Rhus typhina* helped both the physical and the psychological symptoms become manageable. Glenda Croft made similar observations about the "very anxious" and "desperate" character of the emotions in other people needing sumach.

Sumach *(Rhus spp.)* is also beneficial in joint pain. Samuel Henry (1814, 109) gives the following case history. "For rheumatic complaints observe the following cure, discovered in a dream by a very pious baptist elderly lady whom I visited, labouring under violent rheumatic complaints, which caused her to use crutches: take four ounces of the fresh milky roots of upland sumach cut small, boil them in three pints of rum over the coals for one hour, then strain and apply flannels wet with this decoction over the hips, knees, or back, every hour until well. This proved effectual, according to the old lady's dream, in curing her in a few days. I applied a strengthening plaster warm over the part affected."

The dried inner bark contains a gummy emollient. "The inner bark powdered, or scraped, and stewed soft, forms an excellent emollient poultice. If there is matter [pus], it will bring it to a head; if not, it will allay the swelling" (Child, 1837, 124). A poultice of "white sumach" bark is "good for all kinds of swelling. Soothing, cooling" (Ralph Russell, 1911, 327).

TASTE:

(bark) astringent, gummy
    (berries) sour • cooling • astringent

TISSUE STATES:

(bark) relaxation
    (berries) relaxation, excitation

SPECIFIC INDICATIONS:

CONSTITUTION, COMPLEXION, CHARACTERISTIC SYMPTOMS
- *Excessive sweating and urinating.*
- Fatigued, pale, anemic, low immunity, weak bone marrow and kidneys, with fluid loss from the skin, lungs, bowels, kidneys; yet sometimes with local edema; lacking in will, whines, codependent.

MIND, SENSES, NERVES, EMOTIONS, PERSONALITY
- Anxiety, fear, panic, desperation.

HEAD
- Headache, occipital.
- Dark and/or pale under the eyes; puffy above the eyes; pale facial complexion, flushing during flu and fever alternating with gray pallor.
- Blackheads.
- Tongue dry in the center, wet on the edges.
- Spongy gums, canker sores, ulcerations in the mouth (rinse, *Rhus glabra, R. typhina, R. aromatica*).

RESPIRATION
- Colds and flus with copious secretion, postnasal drip, cough from secretion into lung; mucus stringy, adhesive (cf. homeopathic *Kali bichromicum*).
- Cold in nose causing stoppage.
- Sore throat with inflamed uvula and tonsils (but no pitting or pus).
- Bronchitis with copious, free secretion, weakness, lethargy, fragile capillaries, bleeding.
- Tuberculosis; bleeding, diarrhea, weakness, night sweats.

DIGESTION
- Stomach, gas.
- *Diarrhea, with profuse, painful discharges,* mucoid and hemorrhagic.
- *Diarrhea, dysentery;* with putrescent tendencies and tendencies to ulcerate; as in typhus and typhoid fever *(Rhus glabra).*

KIDNEYS
- Diabetes insipidus; large quantities of urine passed, no sugar, thirst.
- "Excessive activity of the urinary organs when there is no inflammation"; contraindicated in acute inflammation.
- Urine profuse, frequent, pale; with or without active inflammation; with exhaustion, weakness, anemia.
- "Profuse and painful discharges, mucus and hemorrhagic, from

the mucous surfaces of the kidneys, bladder, gastrointestinal canal, uterus, lungs and bronchi."
- Kidney stones, difficult passage of urine.
- *Diabetes mellitus with copious urine and perspiration;* urine pale, of high specific gravity, with sugar in it, with debility.
- "Chronic diabetes, when no sugar is found in the urine and a large quantity of urine is passed, and there is great thirst."
- *Incipient albuminuria.*
- Edema; with weakness, fatigue.

BLADDER
- *Chronic catarrh of the bladder and chronic cystitis.*
- *Bedwetting in the young and the old;* with weakness; frequent urination at night; unable to fill the bladder before needing relief; dribbling, lack of retention of urine.
- Constant dribbling.

MALE
- *Swollen prostate, with great pain on urination.*
- Impotence; with frequent urination at night.

FEMALE
- Leucorrhea.
- Profuse uterine bleeding.

MUSCULAR AND SKELETAL
- Stiffness, inflammation, and weakness of the lower back and knees (cf. homeopathic *Rhus toxicodendron*).

SKIN
- Skin fungus associated with dampness.
- "Clammy perspiration."

FEVER
- Fever with debility, fluid loss, night sweats, thirst; preceded by frequent urination.

OTHER
- Diabetic retinopathy; improves deteriorated eyesight *(Rhus typhina).*

- Cataract (reputed).
- "Antiseptic in infectious diseases."
- High blood pressure.
- "Chills, thirst, and constipation, with sugar in the urine" (Rolla Thomas).

PREPARATION AND DOSAGE:

The bark is collected in the spring, when the sap is running, and used per decoction or preserved in alcohol, glycerine, or sugar. The outer bark, though easily peeled, should be kept attached to the inner bark. The berries are collected as soon as they are ripe and are tinctured fresh to prevent the growth of worms. They are most potent if it has not rained for a week. Usual dose of the tincture, 5–30 drops (Fyfe).

LITERATURE:

Traditional, Phyllis Light (2, 5, 8, 9, 11, 12, 32), Erica Fargione (3), William Boericke (4, 7, 19, 27, 28), John William Fyfe (7, 13, 15, 18, 20, 22, 23, 24, 26, 27, 29, 37), Glenda Croft (3, 32), McClanahan (1, 17, 22, 25, 27, 28, 36), John King (30), Finley Ellingwood (31), Lise Wolff (7), Matthew Wood (1, 7, 22-confirmed, 33, 34-confirmed, 35, 37, 40-case history), Chalid Ottway (4, 6, 10, 14, 21, 25, 34, 39), Rolla Thomas (41).

Rhus glabra. Smooth Sumach.

A homeopathic proving of Rhus glabra *produced symptoms fairly similar to those associated with the other sumachs in botanical medicine. For the proving refer to Peter L. Tumminello (1997).*

The proving produces many of the same symptoms that characterize *Rhus aromatica* and *Rhus typhina*: anxiety, fluid excess, and deficiency. One is reminded of the enigmatic statement of Heraclitus the Dark, perhaps a commentary on the human condition: "too much, not enough." The connection with abuse is justified. Mental symptoms such as fear, timidity, anxiety, panic, and low self-confidence are associated with the kidneys. The hardhearted/softhearted dichotomy ought to suggest an association with the heart, but cardiac symptoms were not developed in the proving. One is reminded, instead, of the association to blood pressure maintained by the kidneys under influence from vasopressin and the posterior pituitary. Some of the mental symptoms are justified by the clinical experiences mentioned under the other sumachs—especially anxiety and lack of will. The desire to hurry may indicate a relationship to the bladder.

SPECIFIC INDICATIONS:

MIND, SENSES, NERVES, EMOTIONS, PERSONALITY
- Anxiety, panic, fears, wants to hurry.
- Cowardice, low self-confidence, timidity.
- Difficulty controlling thoughts.
- Mental debility, weakness of attention and memory.
- Feels hardhearted, haughty, abusive; alternately, softhearted, stabbed in the back, used, betrayed.

HEAD
- Headache.
- Nosebleed.
- Face, chin, nose, blemishes.
- Tongue furred white.

DIGESTION
- Mouth ulcers, small (cf. "aphthous stomatitis," from Boericke).
- Excessive salivation.
- Appetite excessive or deficient.
- Stomach upset by food or drink; acidity in stomach.
- Sharp cutting pains in the bowels.
- Diarrhea; brown and yellow (yellow indicates purging of the bile).
- Dry, hard stool.
- First part of stool hard and dry, succeeded by moist, loose stool.
- Sudden urging to stool, difficult expulsion, movement incomplete.

KIDNEYS AND BLADDER
- Urine scanty, dark.
- Profuse urination.

FEMALE

- Black, stringy discharge.
- Candida, vaginal, with discharge.
- Pale, brown blood of menses.
- Aching in lower back and legs, worse at start of menses.

MUSCULAR AND SKELETAL

- Pain in small of back; achy lumbar region.
- Wakes up stiff.

FEVER

- Skin hot and dry, followed by profuse sweat during sleep.
- "Profuse perspiration arising from debility" (Boericke).

PREPARATION AND DOSAGE:

Tincture, 1–30 drops (Boericke).

LITERATURE:

Peter L. Tumminello, William Boericke.

Rosa spp. Wild Rose.

Roses are used throughout the world in herbal medicine. I have already included them in the Old World volume of The Earthwise Herbal. *However, they were once very popular among the American Indians, and are in fact still used in Native medicine, so I have included some additional information germane to North America and Europe.*

There is a long history of usage in both the New and the Old World of rose for eye problems, though the lack of modern diagnostic terms makes the old literature difficult to interpret. The Indians used the bark of the root for the eyes. Moses Maimonides quotes his mentor on materia medica, Abu Merwan Ibn Zuhr, on the use of the petals in various eye problems. "A lotion made of the liquid of roses and sugar strengthens vision. The regular use thereof heals farsightedness." Ibn Zuhr adds, "This has been substantiated by experience and I do not veer from using it to strengthen vision" (Maimonides; Rosner, 1989, 3:347).

It is interesting that rose is also used to enhance nonmaterial vision. In the Scottish Lowlands the thoughtless picking of rose flowers and the breaking of small sticks used to be considered dangerous because it can call up the faeries from the Underworld. This method can also be used intentionally. In the ballad of *Tam Lin*, Janet wore her green tartan up above her knee, went to the hill of Carterhaugh, and boldly plucked roses and broke sticks to call up a virile young knight caught by the faeries on the hilltop. "How dare you pull those flowers! / How dare you break those wands! / How dare you come to Carterhaugh / Withouten my command?" he exclaims. Through a series of bold actions—including pregnancy and threatened abortion—she manages to drag him out of the Underworld. The Faery Queen cries out in disgust that if she'd known Tam Lin was going to get away she'd have torn out his heart—because love saved him from captivity—and his eyes—because now he can see in both worlds.

The tradition is very precise in associating the rose with the heart *and the eyes*. By comparison, hawthorn, the tree of the faeries, is associated with the heart *and the tongue*. As reward for his service to the Queen of Elfland, Thomas the Rhymer is given "the tongue that cannot lie." They met under a hawthorn.

Rubus idaeus var. canadensis, R. strigosus. Red Raspberry.

Species of raspberry are found around the world, even in Australia. It grows wild from the Canadian Arctic to Southern California. The berries have long been used as food and the leaves as medicine. Although known in the medicine of Europe, India, and China, much of our modern knowledge comes from the American Indians. Raspberry contains tannins, flavonoids, mucilage, carbohydrates, pectin, volatile oils, and minerals.

Red raspberry leaf is a milder astringent than its cousin blackberry leaf or root bark. The taste is sweet, indicating nutritive capacity, and astringent, making it an excellent tonic for relaxed tissue. It especially acts on the intestines and uterus. The Indian people introduced it as a female tonic for pregnancy. It nourishes the mother and child, tones the uterus, and makes it conducive to quick and efficient labor. Herbalist midwife Willa Shaffer (1986, 1) writes that it prevents morning sickness, strengthens the uterus, prevents miscarriage "in most cases," makes the delivery more rapid, and prevents tearing of the cervix. Juliette de Bairacli Levy (1973, 56) adds a further observation: "The action of the herb on the organs of reproduction is mainly tonic: hence its further use for sluggish stud dogs." This agrees with the Chinese pharmacopoeia, which considers raspberry leaf to be a male tonic. Indeed, a considerable number of astringents fit this classification by restraining the loss of fluids and resultant exhaustion. In her work on herbs for humans, our gypsy herbalist (Juliette de Bairacli Levy, 1974, 119) cites raspberry as "an acclaimed remedy for sterility in male and female." Upon her suggestion it has been widely used to help deliver pug dogs, whose huge heads make natural parturition difficult.

After delivery, raspberry leaf serves as a medicine for postpartum pains. It is used during lactation to enrich the milk and to reduce breast discomfort. It is considered to be a general breast remedy, according to a friend of mine from an Anishinabe Ojibwe reservation.

Raspberry leaf is used to check diarrhea of recent origin. It is indicated in "relaxation in infants and adults" (Neil, 1998, 31)—that is, diarrhea. It is probably not as effective in intestinal disorders as blackberry. It is widely used as a mild astringent tonic for the eyes. It is my remedy of choice for allergies or influenza with copious free discharge of clear mucus from the upper respiratory tract. Raspberry is also used in flu with GI involvement. Surprisingly, it is also used in chronic constipation. The leaves are "one of the best remedies for constipation of the bowels," writes Derby herbalist George Slack (1919, 116). He recommends a formula of equal parts flaxseed, raspberry leaf, and poplar bark as "one of the best opening medicines that can be used. Make a strong decoction of them, and give a wineglassful every hour till they operate (Slack, 1919, 111)."

The fruit is said to nourish the blood (cf. blueberries, elderberries, blackberries).

TASTE:

(leaf) sweet, slightly sour • astringent

TISSUE STATES:

relaxation, excitation, atrophy

SPECIFIC INDICATIONS:

MIND, SENSES, NERVES, EMOTIONS, PERSONALITY
- Nervousness.

HEAD AND EYES
- Cataract.
- Canker sores.
- Teething.

RESPIRATION
- Colds, flus, copious nasal discharge, postnasal drip, coughs.
- Sore throat; with postnasal drip; relaxed tissue (raspberry fruit vinegar).
- Strep throat.

DIGESTION
- Stomach; "weak and queasy."
- Diarrhea, colic.
- Relaxed small intestine or colon, benign diarrhea (internal, or external; enema).
- Constipation.

FEMALE
- Menstruation: irregular flow, pain.
- Vaginitis, uterine weakness, uterine prolapse.
- *Partus preparator: to prevent miscarriage, to nourish mother and child, to reduce morning sickness.*
- *Delivery: to eliminate pain and bleeding at birth, to expel the afterbirth.*
- Postpartum: afterbirth pains.
- Lactation: discomfort, enriches milk.
- Breast health.

MALE
- Prostate.
- Sexual sluggishness, exhaustion.
- Sterility, barrenness, frigidity, in male (and female).

SKIN

- Scars (cf. ginseng, comfrey, turmeric, lentil, teasel).
- Proud flesh (with or without slippery elm).

FEVER

- Fever, influenza (leaves, berries).
- Distemper in dogs.

PREPARATION, TOXICITY, AND DOSAGE:

The leaves are used fresh or dry but not in between because they are somewhat toxic during the drying stage. Infusion, tincture.

LITERATURE:

Traditional, W. T. Fernie (6, 22), John Gerard (8), V. G. Rocine (8), Julia Graves (10), George Slack (11), Edward Shook (14), John Christopher (2, 14), Matthew Wood (5-confirmed), Clara NiiSka (18), Juliette de Bairacli Levy (7, 13, 14, 15, 17, 20, 21, 24), William LeSassier (22), J. V. Cerney (23), Ben Charles Harris (3).

Rubus villosus, R. fruticosus. Blackberry.

Blackberry is native to both the Old World (Rubus fruticosus) *and the New* (R. villosus). *It is used in both places as an astringent for the stomach and intestines. In Europe the leaves are used, whereas in North America—following Indian practice—the bark of the root is preferred. The properties are very similar. Today the leaves are available in herbal commerce. Blackberry contains tannins, plant acids, and flavonoids.*

Galen wrote that blackberry leaf was one of the agents most beneficial to the stomach (*De Victu Attenuante;* Maimonides; Rosner, 1989, 3:318). It is used as an astringent to tone the stomach and intestines. It was particularly used in children with a damp stomach (spitting up of mucus and food) and intestines (diarrhea). Because of its commonness, it fell from professional into domestic practice.

British herbalist John Hill (1740, 88) writes, "The most neglected things have their use. The buds of the bramble-leaves boiled in spring-water, and the decoction sweetened with honey, are excellent for a sore throat. A syrup made from the juice of the unripe fruit, with very fine sugar, is cooling and astringent. It is good in immoderate fluxes of the menses, and even in purgings. The berries are to be gathered for this purpose, when they are red."

Dr. Wooster Beach describes an instance when the Oneida Indians saved themselves from a contagious intestinal flux, while hundreds of their white neighbors died from the use of mercury. Blackberry root bark entered into American folk medicine. At one time "blackberry cordial" was a staple of American home medicine. Blackberry root "is especially indicated when there is evidence of relaxation and enfeeblement of the mucous coats of the stomach and bowels, and the discharges are large, watery and clay-colored. It is also useful in some cases of cholera infantum and dysentery" (John William Fyfe, 1909). Today the leaves are used for the same purposes.

Blackberry leaves are one of the staple simples used by Juliette de Bairacli Levy (1973) in her wide-ranging treatment of animals and humans. She used a hot lotion of blackberry on abscesses, to ripen and open them, internally as a blood tonic in anemia, to settle a cough, and for eczema.

Donald Law (1973, 33) writes, "Some legends say that witches feared the brambles but the reason for this is not clear." I don't know what to make of this. I still remember a dream I had at about age five, in which I was terrified to go into the blackberry brambles. This is one of the few dream feelings I have never managed to "process," so I still have a deep fear when I approach a blackberry bramble.

TASTE:

sweet, sour • cool, dry • astringent

TISSUE STATES:

irritation, relaxation

SPECIFIC INDICATIONS:

MIND, SENSES, NERVES, EMOTIONS, PERSONALITY

- People who are too intellectual; too much energy accumulated in the head; moves energy downward so that they can act on their thoughts (flower essence).

MOUTH
- Mouth ulcers.
- Loose teeth (the young shoots eaten as a salad).
- Sore throat.

RESPIRATION
- Milk allergies.
- Cough.
- "Whooping cough in its spasmodic stage."

CARDIOVASCULAR
- "Dropsy from feeble, ineffectual circulation."
- Anemia.

DIGESTION
- Digestive complaints associated with headaches and sluggish feelings.
- Atonic conditions of the gastrointestinal tract, accompanied by excessive discharges; large, watery, clay colored.
- Passive hemorrhage from the stomach, bowels, or uterus.
- Diarrhea; from lack of tone of the intestines; acute and chronic.

EXTERNAL
- Eczema.
- Hemorrhoids.
- Varicose veins.
- Ulcers; inflamed, foul (external wash).
- Abscess (hot lotion).

PREPARATION AND DOSAGE:

The root is used by decoction or tincture, the leaf by infusion or tincture. The root is more effective than any other part (tradition, confirmed by Rosemary Gladstar). The berry, green or ripe, is also used. Usual dosage of the tincture, 5–60 drops, every 2–4 hours in acute cases (Fyfe).

LITERATURE:

Traditional (13), Flower Essence Society (1), William T. Fernie (3, 7, 8,

12, 15), John William Fyfe (11, 12, 13), Juliette de Bairacli Levy (6, 9, 14, 17), Tommie Bass (2, 4, 5, 16), Daniel Cobb (17), J. V. Cerney (10), Matthew Wood (13-confirmed), Alma Hutchins (15).

Sabatia angularis. American Centaury.

This is an American representative of the gentian family used early by the pioneers, and probably the Indians before. It is not used much today. One of the last authors to write of it in familiarity is Alma Hutchins (1991).

"There are many species and colors: the English distinguish between them by using the red centaury in disease of the blood, the yellow in choleric diseases, and the white in those of phlegm and water."

"Excellent, old American remedy, bitter tonic, preventive in all periodic febrile diseases, dyspepsia, and convalescence from fevers; it strengthens the stomach and promotes digestion. An aid to rheumatic and all joint pains. The following in a warm infusion is a domestic remedy for expelling worms and to restore the menstrual secretions: Of the powder, ½ to 1 dram, of the extract, 2–6 grains.

"The loose dried herb, 1 teaspoonful to 1 cup of boiling water. Although bitter, this effective herb is a good accompaniment to all herbal teas and preparations. For taste, combine with other herbs such as anise, cardamom, peppermint, ginger, fennel, etc." (Alma Hutchins, 1991, 76).

TASTE:

bitter

TISSUE STATE:

stagnation

SPECIFIC INDICATIONS:

- Homesickness.
- Head cold.
- Vanishing of sight.
- Inflammation of the eyes.

- Diarrhea.
- Fever.
- Intermittent fever.

PREPARATION AND DOSAGE:

The whole herb is used, yielding itself to alcohol or water.

LITERATURE:

Traditional, William Cook, Alma Hutchins.

Salix nigra. Black Willow.

The American black willow had a distinctive application in nineteenth-century medicine that bears little similarity to the use of white willow as a source of natural aspirin. It was a sexual tonic, the specific indications including nocturnal emissions, impotence, ovarian pain before and after menses, nervous disorders, and leucorrhea. The willows contain hormones; they were once used (particularly the black willow) to stimulate rooting by nurserymen because they contain growth hormones.

Black willow possesses salicin, like the European willow, and can also be used as a pain reliever. It acts like aspirin but is soothing to the stomach instead of irritating. "Willow is valued as a nerve sedative because it leaves no depressing after-effects" (Tenney, 1983, 132).

TASTE:

bitter • dry • astringent

SPECIFIC INDICATIONS:

CONSTITUTION, COMPLEXION, CHARACTERISTIC SYMPTOMS
- Nervousness, inflammation, infection, pain.

HEAD
- Headache.
- Dandruff.
- Earache.

RESPIRATION
- Hay fever.
- Tonsillitis.

DIGESTION
- Heartburn.
- Diarrhea and dysentery.
- Worms.

SEX
- Impotence, nocturnal emissions, nymphomania, sexual excitability; when due to irritation of the parts more than mental preoccupation.
- Ovarian congestion.
- Ovarian pain, before and after the periods.
- Leucorrhea.
- Night sweats.

MUSCULAR AND SKELETAL
- Muscles sore.
- Neuralgia.
- Rheumatism, gout.

FEVER
- Fever and chills.
- Flu.

SKIN
- Corns.
- Eczema.
- Bleeding and ulceration.

PREPARATION AND DOSAGE:

Appalachian herbalist Tommie Bass felt that the power of willow bark was increased when it was burned to an ash before use. Dose of the tincture: 10 drops, 3x/day (Yadubir Sinha).

LITERATURE:

Traditional, Finley Ellingwood (10, 12, 13), Frederick Petersen (10, 11), Louise Tenney (1–10, 12, 14–21).

Sassafras albidum. Sassafras.

This beautiful little tree or shrub is native to eastern North America, from Canada to Mexico. "The Indians use a strong decoction to purge and clean the body in the spring," wrote Constantine Rafinesque in 1830. "We use instead the tea of the blossoms for a vernal purification of the blood." The early settlers made much from the export of sassafras, but after a fad career as an antisyphilitic it was dropped by polite people and remained a favored drink among the rural population.

The leaves are famous in Cajun cooking, the mucilage of the pith and twig is used as a lubricant in herbal medicine, and the root and root bark are a warm, sweet, spicy medicinal. The root bark is picked in the spring to thin the blood, the mucilage in the fall, to thicken it. The root bark contains volatile oils (including up to 80% safrole), lignans, alkaloids (in the bark), and tannins. Safrole is a neurotoxin and carcinogenic in isolation, but tests have shown that people who drink the tea for years actually have a reduced rate of cancer. Still, the unaltered sassafras root and root bark remain suspect.

The root bark is sweet, pungent, astringent, and warming. Sassafras tea is used to thin the blood (increase the cooling watery proportion), hence to further circulation in acute fever as well as in the chronic thickening of the blood typical of old age. This is one of the most important Indian remedies for fever, along with wild cherry bark, mountain mint, and sycamore heartwood. It is a stimulating diaphoretic, whereas wild cherry bark is a sedative diaphoretic. Like yarrow and elder, sassafras stirs up the blood and brings deep, stagnant, hot blood to the surface. It opens the pores of the skin and releases perspiration.

Sassafras root bark is traditionally taken in the spring because it thins the blood, increasing the watery proportion. Indeed, taken on a hot summer day it is cooling. One would think it would work the other way around, as a warming remedy, because it is so spicy and warm. However, its action on the blood makes it cooling. Since it thins the blood, sassafras root bark is also used to prevent stroke and heart attack caused by thick, coagulated blood, to promote clear thinking in old age from good circulation to the brain, to improve peripheral circulation to rid the joints of arthritic depositions, and to promote diuresis.

Sassafras root bark is also used like a carminative to improve digestion and assimilation. It contains volatile oils that stimulate the lungs and remove wind from the stomach. Passing through the kidneys, these oils stimulate renal function. It was thus used to remove stones and arthritic deposits and was thought to protect against cancer. It is contraindicated in winter, when thin blood makes a person cold. However, the mucilage can be used to help thicken the blood.

Because of concerns about cancer and neurotoxicity, sassafras should be used only as a specific medicine, on specific indications, and therefore in smaller doses. I use 1–3 drops, 1–3x/day. Sassafras is specifically indicated, in my experience, where there is thick, adhesive, coagulated, dark, blackish blood. Look for a dark, sooty complexion around the veins or eyes or a blue/black appearance in association with a bruise. Also look for a thick, oatmeal-like consistency to the blood passing under the finger when the pulse is taken. Of course, in some persons, only a trace of the discoloration will appear. Sassafras is indicated when the "black bile" is present—that is to say, blood that is easily congealed, heavy, thick, requiring thinning and purification.

Sassafras is a premier bruise remedy. This usage, adopted from the Native people, achieved a level of prominence among white lay and professional practitioners in the nineteenth century. The oil was often used as a direct application, or a poultice of the root bark. Dr. William Cook (1869) thought this to be the most promising use for sassafras. "The powdered bark will be found of much value in bruises and congested swellings; and combined with mullein, makes a superior appliance in swollen face, chronic abscesses, and similar cases," he writes. "Under such circumstances, it both relieves the suffering and promotes the absorption of effused materials."

"Always treat a bruise, because a bruise can turn to bad blood, and bad blood can turn to cancer." Thus spoke Tis Mal Crow when he lectured to some of his "herblings" on Sassafras. This is, indeed, virtually a motto in Indian communities. "Yes," agreed a Kickapoo Indian woman in one of my classes. "We were always taught that from childhood up." She looked around for agreement. Much to her surprise, the white people in the class had a blank look.

TASTE:

sweet, spicy • cool/warm • stimulating, mucilaginous

TISSUE STATES:

depression, atrophy

SPECIFIC INDICATIONS:

CONSTITUTION, COMPLEXION, CHARACTERISTIC SYMPTOMS
- *Sooty, dark, blackish complexion, especially around the eyes.*

MIND, SENSES, NERVES, EMOTIONS, PERSONALITY
- Depression, melancholy.

RESPIRATION
- Colds, bronchitis, with dry skin.

CARDIOVASCULAR AND BLOOD
- Used to thin the blood in the spring to cool the system.
- Thick, viscid blood; thins the blood to prevent stroke, ischemia.

DIGESTION
- Lack of appetite, indigestion, flatulence.
- Constipation, diarrhea, cramps, colic.

KIDNEYS AND BLADDER
- Kidney stones, edema, cystitis.

FEMALE
- Postpartum; afterbirth pains.

MUSCULAR AND SKELETAL
- Stiff muscles and joints.
- Deposits in muscles and joints that cause arthritis and rheumatism.

SKIN
- *Pimples* and boils, angry, red, purulent; on the legs; ingrown hairs.

- *Skin diseases*, eczema, *psoriasis*, poison ivy; increases perspiration and thins the blood to lessen the heavy, oily content.

FEVER
- Fever with cold extremities, lack of perspiration.
- Influenza.

WOUNDS
- Bruises *with a blackish blue complexion.*
- Insect bites with putrefaction.

PREPARATION AND DOSAGE:

The soft inner bark of the root is used for its mucilaginous properties. It is prepared by infusion with hot water, or cold maceration overnight, rather than by decoction, since it is "rendered almost worthless by boiling" (Cook). The root and root bark are used for the spicy, warming, blood-thinning, astringent properties. Traditionally, tea is made from the root and root bark. The tincture should be prepared without the use of heat. Only a small or external dosage should be used. The oil is used as an external stimulant for blood stagnation or cold rheumatism.

CONTRAINDICATIONS:

"Sassafras should not be used by thin-blooded persons" (J. H. Greer)—that is, cold extremities, easy bleeding and bruising (damp/relaxation tissue state). Also, it should be used only in the summer as a blood thinner and it should not be used in combination with a prescribed blood thinner because it is very effective.

TOXICITY:

Possibly carcinogenic. In large and prolonged doses safrole is a nerve toxin producing lowered body temperature, exhaustion, tachycardia, and collapse (Bisset and Wichtl, 1994, 456).

LITERATURE:

Traditional (2–11, 13–16), Constantine Rafinesque, William LeSassier (12), Matthew Wood (1, 5, 15), Louise Tenney (3, 6, 7, 9–13).

Scrophularia nodosa, S. marilandica. Figwort, Pilewort.

The European and American species are almost identical in appearance and properties. They have long been used interchangeably for the treatment of scrofula or king's evil (nodes in the neck, with sores, pimples, and even fistulous burrowings, associated with stagnant lymphatics). The nodular roots gave rise to the common names figwort and pilewort. They resemble swollen nodular hemorrhoids, scrofulous nodes or fistulous burrowings and swellings, and this is what they have been used for.

Scrophularia is indicated in conditions where the lymphatic system is "tainted," hence where there are swollen glands, often associated with acne and facial redness, sometimes with a cheesy discharge from the glands typical of scrofula. What is distinct about scrophularia is that the symptoms of "toxic blood" and lymphatic stagnation are associated with symptoms of blood stagnation, so that acne and skin lesions are not only swollen, red, and inflamed, but sometimes exhibit a blue cast (see indications by Culpeper below; confirmed, Matthew Wood).

Scrophularia has an organ affinity to the throat, hence the association with scrofula (swelling and disease of the glands in the neck). It is also a very important remedy (internal or external) in many kinds of eczema. The Chinese species, which is probably interchangeable with the European and American, is used for epidemic fever that causes swelling and soreness in the throat. It is traditionally combined with *Isatis* (woad), which is a remedy for low-grade fever analogous to baptisia. This is a sensible and useful association. The other remedy that should be associated with this group is scrofulawort *(Helianthemum canadense).*

Culpeper summarizes the traditional authors. "The decoction of the herb taken inwardly, and the bruised herb applied outwardly, dissolves clotted and congealed blood within the body, coming by any wounds, bruise, or fall; and is no less effectual for the king's evil, or any other knobs, kernels, bunches, or wens, growing in the flesh wheresoever; and for the hemorrhoids, or piles." He also recommends that it be used to dry up "the superfluous virulent moisture of hollow and corroding ulcers," redness, spots, freckles, scurf, leprosy and foul deformities of the skin.

"The leaves are most medicinal, though the roots also are employed," writes Cook (1869). "They are used in irritable forms of scrofula, and in scaly and irritable forms of skin affections; for which purposes they are best combined with such articles as rumex and stillingia. By limiting their alterative use to cases of the above class, the happiest results will be obtained. They exert an unusually excellent influence on the kidneys, moderately promoting the flow of urine, relieving torpor, and imparting a soothed and toned impression to these organs. In weakness of the female generative organs, with painfulness and irregularity in menstruation, they deserve especial notice; and I would respectfully, but confidently, commend them to the profession as among the most desirable soothing tonics for these cases. An ointment on lard is of much service in soothing burns, inflammation, sore nipples, ringworm, eczema, and piles. A decoction is made by digesting two ounces of the herb in a pint of hot water, and straining with strong pressure; of which two fluid ounces may be given three or four times a day."

Eli Jones, one of the few old-time authors capable of writing competently on the subject of cancer treatment by botanical medicines, says that *Scrophularia marilandica* is "one of the most valuable remedies we have in the treatment of cancer in its advanced stages, when there are lumps in the neck and in the axilla. It has been handed down to us by the fathers of the Eclectic School of Medicine. This is one of the remedies that helped them to make their splendid reputation in the successful treatment of cancer" *(Cancer: Its Causes, Symptoms & Treatment).*

Michael Moore (2003, 118) discusses the "doctrine of signatures" under his treatment of *Scrophularia*. Partisans of the doctrine "considered the plant useful for skin eruptions because of the glandular nodes found on the roots and leaves of the main European species. Even though this happens to be the case, it does not reflect the validity of that old doctrine so much as the ability of old physicians to find something in the plant's appearance that related to its previous empirical use. By that doctrine, Figwort could just as easily have been used for the following: mouth problems (flower shape), heart disease (shape of some leaves), cuts and abrasions (leaf serrations), or ligament problems (stem form), not to mention clotting blood (color of the flower)," putrefaction (smell of the flowers), swollen glands and hemorrhoids (nodular seed capsules), and fistulous discharges of pus (shape of roots). In fact, *Scrophularia* is used for all of these complaints. What is necessary for the appropriate use of the doctrine of signatures is a sense of the underlying pattern in the plant that emerges out through its signatures. Scrophularia is traditionally used for taints to the system, manifesting in chronic swollen glands about the neck especially, hardening of the tendons in and about the neck (this is brought out in the homeopathic provings), putrid discharges, including sanies from the glands in the neck, all of this set against a background of dark, easily congealed blood.

TASTE:

bitter, earthen, pungent • warm • putrid smelling

TISSUE STATES:

torpor, depression

SPECIFIC INDICATIONS:

CONSTITUTION
- *The great remedy for scrofula* (swollen glands, purulent, discharging glands, discharging cracks behind the ears, sanies or yellow discharge from *glands in the neck*, skin diseases).

MIND, SENSES, NERVES, EMOTIONS, PERSONALITY
- Miserable, despondent state.
- Mentally sluggish, sleepy, yet restless.

HEAD
- *Cradle cap.*
- Headache associated with swollen glands and tight neck tendons and muscles.
- Acne; reddish inflammation with blue from blood stagnation.
- Skin cracking open behind ears, discharges yellow sanies.
- Swollen glands in the throat; stiffness in the neck.

RESPIRATION
- Asthma in scrofulous persons.

DIGESTION
- Constipation, hemorrhoids, pain in abdomen.

LIVER
- Pain in liver.

CARDIOVASCULAR
- Varicose veins.
- High blood pressure.
- Inflammation and blood stagnation.

LYMPH/IMMUNE
- *Eczema of the ear; around the back, inside.*
- *Hard, nodular glands, fistulous burrowings and purulent discharges, in the throat and elsewhere; associated with chronic swelling of the lymphatics.*
- Hodgkin's disease.

KIDNEYS AND BLADDER
- Edema.

FEMALE
- Nodosities in the breasts.
- "Specific affinity to the breasts; very useful in the dissipation of breast tumors" (Boericke; cf. Eli Jones).
- Amenorrhea.

SKIN
- *Eczema.*
- Scruffy skin conditions; scabies, impetigo, athlete's foot, ringworm.
- Skin tumors, rashes, scratches, bruises, wounds.
- Keratonosis (drying out, thickening, callousing of palms).

PREPARATION AND DOSAGE:

"The juice of the fresh-gathered root is an excellent sweetener of the blood taken in small doses, and for a long time together" (Hill, 1740, 174). The root, fluid extract, 3–10 drops.

LITERATURE:

Traditional, Nicholas Culpeper (1-case history), William Boericke (1, 3, 4, 5, 8, 9, 10, 11, 15, 16, 17, 19, 20, 22), Eli Jones, Matthew Wood (1, 2, 3, 5, 6, 7, 8, 9, 14, 15, 16, 17, 20, 21, 22-all confirmed).

Scutellaria lateriflora, S. galericulata. Skullcap.

Skullcap was originally introduced into American folk medicine as a simple for rabies. It was a secret remedy used by several generations of the Lane family of central Westchester County, New York, for the bite of the mad dog. One of their neighbors planted the seeds given in the tea and so learned the identity of the remedy. It was introduced to the burghers of New York City by Robert Bowne, of the old Bowne house in Flushing (brother of my great-great-great-grandmother). After this it was used (supposedly successfully) in the treatment of "thousands" of cases of rabies in New York City by a Dr. Vanderveer and others. However, subsequent authors scorned this intelligence. One who used it, Dr. Henry Taylor (1860, 234), writes, "It is, however, but the part of candor to say that but small hope may be cherished when the virus has once entered the system." Nevertheless, this introduction led to the use of skullcap, which was eventually classified (like so many of its mint relatives) as a nervine. Skullcap is a bitter mint with sedative properties like Leonurus *and* Lycopus. *It is only partly analogous to the great Chinese medicinal,* Scutellaria baicalensis.

Skullcap is "a sure treatment for almost any nervous system malfunction of a mild or chronic nature, from insomnia to fear to nervous or sick headaches, and as a basic palliative-restorative when pasturing out from stress," writes Michael Moore (2003, 235).

Dr. Grover Coe (1858, 345) gives a good description of the properties of skullcap. It "soothes and quiets the irritability of the nervous system, giving tone and regularity of action, lessens cerebral excitement, abates delirium, diminishes febrile excitement, excites diaphoresis and diuresis, and accomplishes its work without any subsequent unpleasant reactions." Scutellaria is "of great service in fevers and other acute diseases in which there is a tendency to delirium. It seems to have the power of lessening cerebral excitement, and at the same time proves febrifuge. It is equally useful in the treatment of acute dysmenorrhea, menorrhagia, and other female disorders in which the head is liable to be unpleasantly affected. It would seem to have an especial influence in equalizing the flow of the nervous currents, and so lessening the tendency to congestions." This is a creative picture from which to work.

As the irritation of the nerves increases, there are tendencies to spasm and convulsion. Scutellaria therefore "is an excellent remedy in the treatment of convulsions, chorea, hysteria, etc., more as a radical remedy during the remissions, however, than as a means of overcoming the immediate spasm." It is given either between or during the spasms. It is indicated in "threatened trismus, tetanic cramps, and other spasmodic disorders." We begin to see how skullcap could in fact live up to its reputation as a remedy for hydrophobia, or bite of a mad dog. "In all cases of nervous irritability, debility, hysteria, dysmenorrhea, etc., indications will be found for its employment. . . . In the management of the disorders of children. For nervous irritability, wakefulness, slight febrile disturbances, flatulence, colicky pains, etc."

"Its diuretic powers are considerable, but not uniformly displayed. In many cases we have found it to induce a copious flow of urine, while in others no appreciable diuretic effects were observable. When taken in warm solution it proves gently diaphoretic, and is useful in breaking up a recent cold."

Skullcap has an affinity for the peripheral nervous system, according to herbalist Daniel Gagnon, of Santa Fe. For that reason, colors are too bright, lights are too intense, and things are felt too intensely in general and they feel nervous inside. Muscles are often twitchy; twitching during sleep. "Wants to crawl out of their skin."

Skullcap "is the perfect nervine," comments William LeSassier. "It doesn't drag on the rest of the system, good for all formulas. Sedates fire in the small intestine that would otherwise burn off energy too quickly. Good for skinny people. . . . Holds energy in the body. Good for overthinkers."

TASTE:

bitter

TISSUE STATES:

excitation, constriction, atrophy

SPECIFIC INDICATIONS:

CONSTITUTION, COMPLEXION, CHARACTERISTIC SYMPTOMS
- Lack of resistance to stimulation, headaches after stimulating meetings and events (take beforehand as a preventative).
- Oversensitivity; too bright, too colorful, too intense.

MIND, SENSES, NERVES, EMOTIONS, PERSONALITY
- *Nervous fear, anticipation.*
- *Restlessness, irritability, nervousness, wakefulness.*
- Children; nervousness, restlessness, wakefulness, fever, digestive constriction.

DIGESTION
- Colic, flatulence, pains in the gastrointestinal tract.

FEMALE
- Menstrual pain, irritation, spasm.

RESPIRATION
- Recent colds, mild fever with nervousness and irritation, lack of perspiration.

FEVER
- High fever affecting the mental and nervous processes, delirium.
- Restorative after fever and influenza have left the nervous system and circulation out of order.

OTHER
- Sunstroke; chronic side effects, never entirely recovered from its effects; the sun's rays produce dizziness, headache, nervous tremblings, wakefulness, indigestion.
- *Gestational diabetes*; fetus agitated, mother's skin somewhat irritated (cf. *Scutellaria baicalensis*).

MUSCULAR AND SKELETAL
- *Twitchy muscles, twitching during sleep.*
- *Hysteria, with inability to control the voluntary muscles; nervousness manifesting itself in muscular action.*
- Chorea, convulsions, tetanus, tremors, delirium tremens, hysteria, monomania.

PREPARATION AND DOSAGE:

Often adulterated and mislabeled in herb commerce. Best identified and picked by a knowledgable person in the field. Dose: "5 drops to 1 dram in 4 ounces of water. Sometimes quite large doses will be required" (Rolla Thomas).

LITERATURE:

Traditional (9, 10), George Royal (homeopathic provings: 1, 3, 4), William Boericke (3, 4, 10, 15), Grover Coe (5, 6, 7, 8, 9, 11, 15), John King (12), Daniel Gagnon (2, 13), Matthew Wood (3, 9, 12-all confirmed), Rolla Thomas (14).

Selenicereus grandiflorus. Night Blooming Cereus.

See the listing under the old name, *Cactus grandiflorus.*

Senecio aureus. Life Root.

In the British Isles, Senecio vulgaris or groundsel (a member of the aster family) has long been used as a menstrual remedy, hence the common name ragwort. The American species, Senecio aureus was used after the colonization of America. It had a similar reputation among the Indian people, as the names unkum, waw weed, and squaw weed testify. The names life root and female regulator are not without interest. "The American species was used by the English colonists of New England from the earliest settlements," relates William Cook (1869, 691), although Samuel Henry (1814, 176) presents it as a recent discovery. Senecio contains pyrrolizidine alkaloids, which are quite toxic. Cattle have been killed feeding on the plants in pastures. For this reason it has fallen out of fashion in modern practice. Small doses, however, effectively represent the plant without danger. Senecio contains bitter alkaloids, flavonoids, fatty acids, volatile oils, and resins.

"Its special action is on the reproductive organs of both sexes, but especially the female. A tonic to the nervous and muscular structure of the reproductive organs of the female, with a tendency to bring about normal action and therefore applicable alike to amenorrhea, metrorrhagia, menorrhagia, or dysmenorrhea. We think of it in a relaxed condition of the uterus and its appendages, relaxed condition of the support of the uterus resulting in displacements" (Petersen, 1905, 140). It also seems to have some action on the blood or blood vessels. "Of value in capillary hemorrhage, haematuria in large doses, albuminuria, especially during pregnancy, leucorrhea, chlorosis."

Samuel Henry (1814) writes, "I have found it a sure cure for all complaints of the gravel and pains in the breast, is a febrifuge, a powerful diuretic, relieves melancholy and causes cheerfulness." These, strangely, are not the symptoms for which it became famous in the nineteenth century.

TASTE:

bitter, pungent (Cook) • astringent (Menzies-Trull)

TISSUE STATE:

relaxation

SPECIFIC INDICATIONS:

CONSTITUTION, COMPLEXION, CHARACTERISTIC SYMPTOMS
- Relaxed, atonic conditions in women; chlorosis (kidney anemia), pallor, blood loss, excess secretion (mucoid, purulent), uterine prolapse, leucorrhea, watery blood, infertility, diarrhea, feeble appetite, backache.

MIND, SENSES, NERVES, EMOTIONS, PERSONALITY
- Melancholy, low spirits; causes cheerfulness.

RESPIRATION
- Old and debilitated coughs.

DIGESTION
- Feeble appetite and backache common in women.
- Dyspepsia attended with flatulence after meals.
- Excessive secretion of gastric juice, with acidity and heartburn.
- Subacute and chronic dysentery.

KIDNEYS AND BLADDER
- Kidney problems associated with menstrual complaints.

FEMALE

- *Pelvic congestion, irritation, or atonicity.*
- *Uterus: relaxation of the supportive ligaments and the muscles.*
- Menstrual irregularity with pain and weakness in the pelvic region, headache in top or back of head.
- Pain worse at menstrual period.
- *Sensation of weight, fullness, and dragging in the pelvis.*
- *Leucorrhea:* uterine or cervical; purulent.
- Chlorosis (watery blood); pale, moist skin, anemic.
- Uterine prolapsus, subinvolution.
- *Menorrhagia, passive; due to relaxation and atonicity of the uterus.*
- *Amenorrhea, atonic and languid cases.*
- Closure of the fallopian tubes, underactive ovaries, fallopian congestion.
- Pregnancy: albuminuria, with occasional attacks of hematuria.
- Parturition: uterine and nervous fatigue (warm infusion).
- Menopause: hot flashes, vasomotor disorder.

MALE

- Engorged, *relaxed conditions* of the sexual organs.
- Fullness and weight in the perineum, with dragging sensation in the testicles.
- Urination difficult and tardy.
- Urinary irritation from engorgement; pain and straining.
- Gonorrhea, gleety discharge, prostatorrhea.
- Hematuria.

PREPARATION AND DOSAGE:

"It is of moderately slow and rather persistent action" (William Cook, 1869, 691). "The remedy acts slowly, and sufficient time must be given" (Scudder, quoted by Fyfe, 1909, 211). "Its action is slow and it must be continued for some time for good results" (Frederick Petersen, 1905, 141). Well, so much for impatient herbalists. Unfortunately, pyrrolizidine alkaloids should not be taken long term. Thus, the dose needs to be very small. Dose of the tincture is 1–15 drops (John William Fyfe, 1909). However, some people may feel most comfortable using it in low homeopathic doses (3x, 6x) or very low material doses (1/10 drop to 1 drop).

TOXICITY:

Senecio contains pyrrolizidine alkaloids, which are mutagenic, hepato-toxic, and carcinogenic. In pastures it has killed cattle.

LITERATURE:

Traditional, William Cook (1, 3, 4, 7, 8, 10, 14, 16, 17, 18, 20), Frederick Petersen (1, 9, 10, 11, 12, 14, 15, 17, 18, 21, 23, 26, 28), Samuel Henry (2), Darrell Martin (8-confirmed), John Scudder (1, 24, 25), John William Fyfe (1, 5, 6, 13, 14, 15, 16, 28), Finley Ellingwood (14, 16, 20, 27, 28), Christopher Menzies-Trull (19, 22), Mary Bove (9, 19).

Serenoa repens. Saw Palmetto.

Saw palmetto is a small palm native to the underbrush of Florida. Many of the old books list it under the name Sabal serrulata. It first came to the attention of the medical faculty in the nineteenth century when the berries were utilized as a starvation food by the survivors of a shipwreck. The naturalized wild swine of Florida fatten up in the spring on the berries. The berries are high in saponins, which build up the steroidal tone of the adrenal cortex and gonads. Saw palmetto is often thought of as a male remedy for swollen prostate. It is very good here, but it has many other uses. It is also a female tonic. One of the women who participated in the homeopathic provings in the late nineteenth century experienced breast growth—she was thin and undernourished. Saw palmetto is best classi-fied as a nutritive tonic; hence it is suited to thin persons and it should be used when there is such a background with prostate problems (David Winston).

Saw palmetto contains steroidal saponins, which give it an obnox-ious, soapy taste; flavonoids; fixed acids up to 26%; fatty acids includ-ing capric, caprylic, palmitic, and oleic; volatile oils; polysaccharides; and resin. These properties explain its usefulness as a nutritive tonic, sexual tonic, and sedative for heat/excitation.

"Saw palmetto relieves irritability of the entire nervous system, stimu-lates digestion, improves the appetite and aids assimilation," writes John William Fyfe (1909, 700). It improves nutrition and assimilation and rebuilds the adrenocortical base, which calms down nervousness and hyperadrenalism. By decreasing atrophy and dryness it also decreases heat and irritation. "In diseases characterized by irritation of the nose, throat, and larynx, it has been extensively employed with marked advantage, and in various catarrhal affections it has often proved serviceable. It exerts a sedative influence in irritable conditions of the reproductive organs, and at the same time acts as a nutritive tonic to them. It undoubtedly favors normal functional activity of the reproductive system through its power to reinvigorate and balance the entire nervous system." It has been known to increase the size of the breasts, testicles, and reproductive organs generally, when there was malnutrition. However, its effect on the prostate is to reduce swelling and irritation.

"The saw palmetto, on account of its tonic effects, together with its special diuretic action, becomes an efficient remedy in many urinary troubles. In this respect it is said to be the friend of the old man—the most positive remedy we possess for the relief of some of the difficulties that beset the declining years of about four-fifths of our old men" (William Bloyer, quoted by John William Fyfe, 1909).

TASTE:

sweet, soapy • moist

TISSUE STATES:

atrophy, excitation

SPECIFIC INDICATIONS:

- Acute and chronic catarrh; asthma, pertussis.
- Chronic laryngitis, chronic pharyngitis, and chronic bronchitis.
- Functional inactivity of the reproductive system of both male and female.
- Atrophy of the prostate, mammae, uterus, or testes.
- Feebleness of the urinary organs.
- Enuresis, incontinence, cystitis, urethritis.
- Prostatic enlargement.
- Orchitis, ovaritis.
- Polycystic ovarian disease, hirsutism, hyperandrogenism.

- Lactation; inhibits prolactin.
- Infertility, decreased sperm, testicular atrophy, reduced libido.
- Malnutrition, muscular wasting.

PREPARATION AND DOSAGE:

Fluid extract, 10 drops to 2 drams; usual dose, 10–30 drops, in water, 3x/day (Fyfe).

LITERATURE:

Edwin Hale, John William Fyfe, David Winston, Christopher Menzies-Trull.

Sisyrinchium spp. Blue Eyed Grass, Spiderwort.

Blue eyed grass resembles a small iris with leaves like grass, but it is a member of the lily family. It is native to American prairies, but unlike many wildflowers, it is widespread around human habitations, growing out of cracks and gaps in the sidewalks, in alleys, and by mailboxes.

Sisyrinchium was used by a number of Native American tribes as a menstrual regulator, and considered to be a preventative for conception when taken over long periods of time. The root was used to break fevers, malaria, and scarlet fever, and as a physic (Robert Dale Rogers).

Smilacina racemosa. False Solomon's Seal.

False Solomon's seal is related to Polygonatum *(true Solomon's seal) in botany and in properties. Both are useful for dehydrated, inflexible tendons and ligaments so it is often hard to determine when one is needed rather than the other. One will not always substitute for the other. In addition,* Smilacina *possesses its own unique characteristics. It appears to be more active on the nervous system.*

False Solomon's seal, like true Solomon's seal, is an important remedy for the tendons and ligaments, which it moistens, strengthens, and loosens or tightens to gain the healthy tension on joints and the muscular and skeletal system. It is useful to relax the symphysis pubis before birth, if that joint is not loosening up (Lise Wolff).

In addition to its use with tendons, Brent Davis, DC, points out that smilacina is beneficial for the liver. It is restorative to the cells or tissues and functions. He recommends it in women who are experiencing hormonal irregularities (cf. *Taraxacum, Smilax, Artemisia vulgaris*) and suffer from a history of mental and emotional stress. Since estrogen and progesterone readily break down in the bloodstream this indicates that it is useful for androgen excesses, which are burdensome to the liver. Imbalance is frequently associated with anger, frustration, and stress. The smudge is an old Indian remedy for severe premenstrual syndrome, crying babies, and hysteria (Foster and Duke).

William LeSassier said that constipation will always be present in a case requiring false Solomon's seal. This may indicate that smilacina improves bile secretion, hence lubrication of the stool.

TASTE:

(rhizome) sweet • moist • mucilaginous

TISSUE STATE:

atrophy

SPECIFIC INDICATIONS:

MIND, SENSES, NERVES, EMOTIONS, PERSONALITY
• Crying baby (smudge, burn the root).

HEAD
• Headache, frontal; caused by indigestion.

RESPIRATION
• Throat; sore, inflamed.
• Lung infections.

DIGESTION
• "Always some constipation."
• "Clears and relaxes the lower burner"—that is, pelvic region.

LIVER

- Restorative to the parenchyma of the liver.
- Increases liver function, hence elimination by the bowel.

FEMALE

- PMS, hysteria, pain (smudge, burn the root).
- Hormonal irregularities in women with a history of mental and emotional stress.
- Loosens the symphysis pubis before birth.

MUSCULAR AND SKELETAL

- Tendinous problems, with pain.

PREPARATION AND DOSAGE:

Roots and rhizomes tinctured in alcohol. Small to moderate dosage, 1–15 drops per dose.

LITERATURE:

Traditional American Indian (1, 9, 10), Tis Mal Crow (1, 9, 10), Michael Moore (2, 3, 4), William LeSassier (5, 6, 10), Brent Davis (7, 8, 10), Lise Wolff (11, 12), Matthew Wood (12).

Smilax officinalis, S. ornata, S. spp. Sarsaparilla.

Sarsaparilla is a member of the lily family native to Central America. The root was very important in nineteenth-century herbalism and is still in use today. It has a North American cousin, variously known as green briar, cat briar, or blasphemy vine, which is found in forests.

Sarsaparilla is mildly pungent, sweet, nutritive, and stimulating. Like many plants that contain saponins (cf. yucca, saw palmetto), it is an adrenal and sexual system tonic, improving nutrition and strength. In addition, it brings the function of the liver into relationship with steroid hormones. The liver processes lipids into cholesterols, which the adrenal cortex and sex glands need to make steroidal hormones—cortisone, aldosterone, and sex hormones. Although many of these break down easily, some, such as the androgens, are difficult for the liver to catabolize, so that they stress the liver and favor the creation of what we call "dirty blood." By detoxifying the blood, the liver clears the bloodstream so that the hypothalamus can get a better reading on the contents and regulate the endocrine system. Sarsaparilla is therefore an adaptogen that can normalize steroid activity.

Dorothy Hall paints a precise picture calling for sarsaparilla. It is suited to periods in life when there are sex hormone imbalances—puberty, periods, pregnancy, menopause—and the need for it can be more obvious in women. Sarsaparilla balances estrogen, progesterone, and testosterone. Indications include wild fluctuations in hormones involving the pituitary, thyroid, adrenals, sex glands, and pancreas. Hyperadrenalism, nervousness, worry, sensitivity, and overreactiveness are characteristic. Fatigue alternates with excessive enthusiasm.

TASTE:

pungent, sweet • balancing

TISSUE STATES:

stagnation, atrophy, depression

SPECIFIC INDICATIONS:

- "Despondent, sensitive, easily offended, ill humored and taciturn."
- Worry, anxiety, nervousness, hyperadrenalism.
- *Fatigue with pimples, boils, dark rings under the eyes.*
- Hot, flustered, and tired.
- Overenthusiastic, alternating or giving way to underactivity.
- Weakness, emaciation, and dryness, with aggravation from stimulation, weather changes, foods, hormonal shifts.
- Colds, catarrh, flu.
- Poor digestion, heartburn, flatulence, colic, with backache.
- Diabetes.
- Exhaustion and pain after urination.
- Puberty: hormonal imbalances with acne and boils.
- Uterus: difficulty getting pregnant or easy conception.
- Menopause: hot flashes.

- Lack of interest in sex; from exhaustion, hyperadrenalism.
- Men: low sperm count, premature ejaculation, difficulty getting an erection, low interest in sex, low libido, worry, anxiety, nervousness, sensitivity.
- Multiple sclerosis.
- Rheumatism, gout, joint aches, poor peripheral circulation.
- Spine out of joint all the time.
- Skin emaciated, withered, hard, indurated, dry, itching, faulty perspiration.
- Eczema, psoriasis, rashes, boils, pimples, age spots, ringworm.
- Heavy metal toxicity.

PREPARATION AND DOSAGE:

Decoction or tincture. Traditionally combined with burdock root in alterative formulas; combine with raspberry leaf for fertility.

COMPARISON:

Herbalist Tommie Bass said that the native species of *Smilax*, of which there are plenty, could be used in place of the imported species. There is, however, wide variation in quality among members of this genus.

LITERATURE:

Traditional, William Boericke (1), William LeSassier (3), Dorothy Hall (2, 4, 5, 9, 11, 12, 14, 16), Jack Ritchason (17, 21).

Spilanthes acmella, S. oleracea. Toothache Plant.

Spilanthes stimulates secretions from the mucous membranes. It stimulates the immune system. Specific indications are ear infections, colds, influenza, respiratory tract infections, fungal and viral infections, candida, herpes simplex, and malaria.

Stillingia sylvatica. Queen's Root.

Stillingia is native to the sandy coasts of the South, from North Carolina to the Gulf of Mexico. These once useless and isolated soils came into high demand for coastal housing developments, leading to an unfortunate loss of habitat, endangerment, and scarcity in the availability of the plant. In the nineteenth century it was widely used as a deep-acting alterative and blood cleanser for the "syphilitic taint"—that is, deterioration of the fluid, cartilaginous, and bony structures of the body. It is much less commonly used today. Dr. Brent Davis confirms that it works at the "inherited level" and is bactericidal and antineoplastic.

Scudder writes that Stillingia "increases waste and excretion, but its principal action probably is upon the lymphatic system, favoring the formation of good lymph, hence good blood and nutrition." Also "in cases of chronic disease where the tissues are feeble and not readily removed and renewed."

TASTE:

sweet, earthen

TISSUE STATES:

atrophy, torpor

SPECIFIC INDICATIONS:

- Tumid, red, glistening mucosa, with scanty secretion.
- Chronic sore throat; irritation of the superior pharynx and just behind the fauces, causing cough.
- Paroxysmal cough accompanied by laryngeal irritation.
- Irritation of the mucosa of the nasal cavities, throat, larynx, and bronchial tubes; hoarse, croupy cough, without secretion.
- Irritative coughing; croup (in combination with Lobelia); tuberculosis.
- Ulcers of the stomach.
- One of the most important anti-cancer remedies; bone cancer.
- Skin diseases with irritation, moist, thin, acrid discharge.
- Chronic furunculosis (combine with Arctium).

PREPARATION AND DOSAGE:

Must use the fresh root, or within a year of picking (traditional, confirmed by John Uri Lloyd, Brent Davis).

LITERATURE:

Traditional, John Scudder (1, 2), Finley Ellingwood (2–5), Brent Davis (7, 9).

Thuja occidentalis. Cedar.

Ripened, brown cedar cones were the remedy of choice to induce healthy labor in American Indian communities. The recipe I have says to simmer the tea of the cones for at least an hour. Use in a bath or on a warm towel on the womb. "No woman ever drank cedarberry tea without being 'talked about,'" reported an old Ozark woman (Randolph, 1947, 194).

This North American remedy was picked up by Samuel Hahnemann and given a homeopathic proving which brought out many details of interest, including skin growths, warts, moles, skin tags, and skin cancers (Boericke, 1927). Many antitumor remedies are abortifacient. Dermal uses came over into eclectic medicine (see Finley Ellingwood, 1918). The latter is reprinted by David Hoffmann (2003). I have seen Thuja remove warts.

Trillium cernuum, T. erectum, T. spp. Beth Root, Birth Root.

Trillium is a beautiful spring wildflower native to mature woods in North America. It was used by the American Indians as a female medicine and was adopted by the pioneers and professional doctors. The root contains saponins, steroidal glycosides, resins, and tannins, giving it a very bad taste.

Trillium erectum has an erect, red flower, while *T. cernuum* has a white flower bent toward the ground. The American Indian people viewed them as a single, sexed species called "reds and whites"—a name recorded by Rafinesque (1830). The red ones were considered male, the white ones female. (This "signature" could be thought to justify the association of

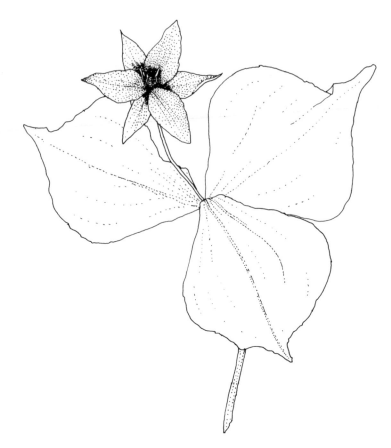

trillium flower essence as a remedy for women undergoing difficulties in relationships.)

Trillium was particularly associated with gynecology and obstetrics in Eastern Woodland Indian society. Tis Mal Crow informed a class that the trillium floral design was worn by the Indian midwife as a symbol of her vocation. In Indian society a plant or animal could be used by a vocation, represent the vocation, and appear in the dreams of people called to that vocation. The three leaves signature the torso and the legs spread to give birth.

Trillium root is used to "bring down the baby." It increases the downward expulsive power of the uterus. It is also used after pregnancy to tighten up and tone the uterus and stop postpartum bleeding. The homeopathic proving, on one woman, produced symptoms of pelvic collapse and profuse bleeding. Herbalist Julia Graves notes that trillium improves the tone in the tendons and muscles in the legs and thighs and lessens cramping. This effect can even be helpful in men. (Nettles acts on the muscles of the inner thighs to improve their tonus for childbirth.)

Trillium passed over into pioneer society as "birth root" or "beth root." "It is considered a specific for female weakness and leucorrhea, or the whites" (Hutchins, 1991, 22). By "weakness" she must mean the lack of tonus, or relaxation, for which birth root is remedial. The relaxed tissue state is associated with watery discharges such as leucorrhea. Trillium is suited to "cases that are characterized by a *relaxation* of the *tissues* accompanied by mucous discharges, and active and passive *hemorrhages* that are complicated by fainting." So writes Dr. Alexander Blackwood (1922, 85), a homeopath who used material or herbal doses. Relaxation, profuse bleeding, leucorrhea, and fainting would all be associated with "thin blood" and "low blood" in Southern folk medicine.

Trillium, in my experience, is a specific in endometriosis, an otherwise hard-to-treat condition. It is suited to this problem because it stimulates downward, expulsive movement in the uterus, and also because it controls heat, irritation, and overgrowth in the endometrium.

Birth root not only checks the bleeding but reduces inflammation and putrefaction connected with hemorrhage. In the mid-nineteenth century it was one of the standbys for hemorrhage of all kinds and was widely used for the bleeding associated with tuberculosis. The bleeding and mucus of the latter disease were associated by the Indians with the red and white flowers (Rafinesque, 1830). Trillium was often used in combination with lycopus to stop bleeding (see Grover Coe and other mid-nineteenth-century authors).

Samuel Henry (1814, 40) introduced beth root and bloodroot for the treatment of gangrene. "This poultice is also a certain cure for old putrid ulcers, obviates the gangrene or mortification, and will prevent the cutting off of many limbs in our hospitals, and on board ships of war." Henry had served with the U.S. Army in the War of 1812 and had been a prisoner among the Creek Indians. So much for Rafinesque's (1830) claim to have introduced trillium into medicine. Trillium was classified as an antiseptic. It prevented or treated sepsis associated with wounds or bleeding.

TASTE:

acrid, pungent • astringent

TISSUE STATES:

relaxation, depression

SPECIFIC INDICATIONS:

CONSTITUTION, COMPLEXION, CHARACTERISTIC SYMPTOMS
- *Women* with gynecological problems starting with or associated with inequalities in sexual and romantic relationships.

BLOOD
- Rush of blood to the head, with dizziness, faintness, and unsteadiness.
- Bleeding from the nose, lungs, stomach, bladder; with heat and excitation; tuberculosis.

DIGESTION
- Dysentery.

FEMALE
- *Relaxation of the uterus, prolapse, with weak expulsive power downward, with profuse bleeding, exhaustion, dizziness, and faintness.*
- *Uterine hemorrhage* with falling-apart sensation in the pelvis and hips.
- *Menstruation;* with heat, irritation, pain, intensity, and engorgement, with local relaxation and atonicity of tissues.
- *Endometriosis;* endometrioma.
- Profuse menstrual hemorrhages and postpartum bleeding.
- Prolapsus uteri; from muscular relaxation; frontal prolapse; frequent urging with scanty urine from pressure on bladder.
- Engorgement of the cervix uteri.
- Vaginal and uterine leucorrhea; chronic vaginitis; atonic mucosa with viscid, acrid, irritating discharges.

SKIN
- Gangrene.
- Erysipelatous irritations and ulcers.
- Diabetes.

PREPARATION AND DOSAGE:

"The roots are medicinal," writes William Cook (1869, 717). "The properties all [species] seem to be the same. When fresh, they have an acrid and bitterish taste; when dry, they are bitterish and slightly astringent. Water and diluted alcohol extract their virtues." Due to environmental concerns, trillium should be used only in small doses. A fifty-year-old plant can yield a root the size of a thimble. Fortunately, small doses are efficacious. Large ones can disturb the circulation, as with bloodroot. My dosage is 1 dropperful of the tincture diluted in an ounce of alcohol taken in 3 drops, 1–3x/day.

CAUTIONS:

Trillium has been generally regarded as safe, but the extremely bad taste may have prevented poisonings. The glycosides may have an effect on the heart. Some derangement of the circulation and blood distribution is often felt on taking a modest quantity of the root.

LITERATURE:

Traditional (American Indian), Samuel Henry (13), Constantine Rafinesque, Grover Coe, William Cook, Edwin Hale, Henry Minton (homeopathic proving, 5–8, 10–13), Matthew Wood (1, 5, 6, 9), Flower Essence Society (1), Tis Mal Crow.

Tsuga canadensis. Hemlock Tree.

The hemlock is a noble conifer native to eastern North America—not to be confused with poisonous hemlock (Conium maculatum). *It likes to grow along creeks in ravines in the mountains in the Appalachian Mountains and northward throughout New England and eastern Canada. Where it grows the temperature will be significantly cooler. It will also grow in other places but this is its preferred habitat. Unfortunately, it is being attacked by an insect that is endangering it through much of its range.*

Hemlock is a warming astringent. It is an important American Indian remedy. Putnam Flint, the father of herbalist Margi Flint, of Marblehead,

Massachusetts, gifted us with a story illustrating its use by a Native practitioner. In the late 1920s his father was in rural Maine representing a Boston chocolate company when the weather turned bad and he got caught in the back country. Worse followed when he came down with dysentery and his life was in danger. An Indian came out of the woods on snowshoes; he said he had heard about the case. The traveling doctor studied the sick man, went back into the woods for several hours, and came back with a tea. Through the use of this tea the chocolatier from the city was completely restored to health. The only ingredient he remembered was hemlock. This warming astringent would indeed be perfectly suited to a septic fever with bleeding and diarrhea.

Samuel Thomson, who grew up in New Hampshire, tried hemlock in his "composition powder," a spicy mix, but found it too astringent for general use. It is so warming that Dr. Beal P. Downing, after fifty years wandering on the American frontier, recommended that if one was caught outside in the winter, one could sleep on the boughs to stay warm. Oil of hemlock found a place in American medicine in the nineteenth century as a strengthening application to the lower back and kidney region. The warmth and astringence strengthen the kidneys, tendons, and ligaments. (This would be a remedy for "kidney yang deficiency" in traditional Chinese medicine—for fluid loss and weakness of the lower back due to lack of fire in the kidneys.) The use of a warming or even burning poultice over the kidneys as a stimulant goes back to Hippocrates.

Mrs. Lydia Child (1837, 112) recommended hemlock as a decoction in the bath for "spotted fever or other malignant fever"—that is, smallpox or other fever that is having a hard time erupting. As a stimulant it brings the rash to the surface. "For rheumatic pain in the bones, it is good to soak the feet in very warm water, with hemlock branches steeped in it. Keep covered with blankets and get into a hot bed."

Ulmus rubra, U. fulva. Slippery Elm.

Slippery elm is a member of the elm clan native to ravines and valleys where water is abundant in the Eastern Woodland region of North America. Samuel Henry (1814, 110) reports it being particularly abundant "in the Indian Nation, and West Florida"—that is, in Georgia, Alabama, and Mississippi. The thick, mucilaginous bark yields a gruel that the Indian people used for the malnourished, sick, and convalescent, when the strength of the system needed to be rebuilt. It was also used as

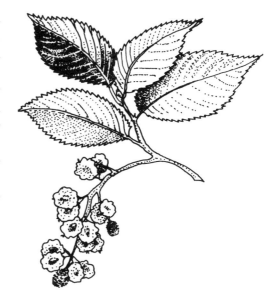

a lubricant for the throat, for the bowels, and for the passage of the baby during labor. It was adopted by the pioneers and botanical doctors and today occupies an important niche in the Western herbal materia medica. In addition to mucilage it contains sugars and minerals, especially calcium, magnesium, phosphorus, and potassium.

Slippery elm bark not only is a fine mucilage but is moderately sweet and slightly earthen in flavor, showing that it possesses nutritious sugars and minerals. It is a tonic food/medicine used to rebuild patients run-down by fever, disease, and malnutrition and also exerts a specific influence on the mucosa of the respiratory, digestive, and sexual-urinary tract, to promote lubrication, cleansing, cooling, nutrition, and healing.

In the digestive tract slippery elm neutralizes excess acidity with its alkaline salts, thus reducing stomach acidity and ulceration. It combines with and emulsifies fats and oils, thus assisting digestion in the small intestine. It contains fruit sugars, which are attractive to the healthful bacteria that live in the large intestine, hence it stimulates their growth and reproduction. As a lubricating substance, it helps normal or hard, scybalous stool pass an irritated, constricted part of the intestine or an irritated, fissured, torn rectal sphincter. Chronic diarrhea and colitis will often cause constriction in the intestinal tract; slippery elm soothes the tissue and softens the stool so that it can pass by better. The tea is taken for its direct influence on inflammation of the mouth and throat. The tea or capsules are used for acute gastric and duodenal ulcer, gastritis, gastric catarrh, weakness of the stomach, enteritis, diarrhea, dysentery, and mucus colitis. A dose lasts thirty hours in the digestive tract, so it need not be given frequently.

Dr. John Eberle (1834, 2:452–4) writes that it exerts a specific action in dysentery or chronic diarrhea, which is not explained by its mucilaginous content alone. "I have very frequently used it in this disease, from the very commencement through its whole course," by itself or in conjunction with other medicines. "It does not seem probable to me, that its efficacy in dysentery depends entirely upon its demulcent quality; for other vegetable demulcents, such as flaxseed tea, solution of gum arabic, &c. are not equal to it in this respect." He quotes physicians who used it in severe and hopeless cases of dysentery in children, with "excruciating tormina in the umbilical region," where the effect was "so immediate that it appeared like a charm."

Slippery elm bark also influences the respiratory tract. It gives a feeling of expanded capacity in the lungs. "It is of great value in bronchitis, bleeding from the lungs and consumption," says Dr. Edward Shook. "It is most healing to the lungs, soothing and checking cough, building up the tissues and preventing or checking the wasting of tissue." Because it is high in calcium it helps the body wall off tubercular infection. High levels of calcium are needed in this disease.

Samuel Henry (1814, 111) recommends it as a partus preparator. "Its constant use is very proper for pregnant women during the seventh month [until the end of the pregnancy], as it facilitates the birth and causes a speedy and easy delivery." Rafinesque (1828–30) reported that slippery elm was "a specific to procure easy labor to pregnant women by using the tea for 2 months previous." This was "well known to Indian women, whose easy parturition has often been noticed; now becoming in general use." It moistens and lubricates the passages and relaxes slightly.

A douche is used for vaginitis, suppositories for hemorrhoids and fissures. Poultices are applied externally for burns, scalds, abrasions, rashes, sores, ulcers, boils, carbuncles, inflamed wounds, and poison ivy. Eberle recommends the internal decoction for skin diseases as a general remedy, saying that it must sometimes be used for several months. If it stimulates increased diuresis and aggravates the eruption on the skin, then it is most likely to bring about a cure. He also recommends it externally for "ulcers, eruptions, gun-shot wounds, chilblains, etc." After recounting many skin conditions that slippery elm cures, Samuel Henry notes that it "is the best poultice I know of for fresh wounds, burns, and ulcers."

William LeSassier felt that slippery elm had a very profound nerve-relaxant capacity, also beneficial for related emotional imbalances. He learned this from an older practitioner when he was young. From some old notes I repeat his comments. Slippery elm is "for instability of emotions. Manic/depressives. Has lots of calcium and trace elements. A muscle relaxer, good in combination with chamomille. Good for hyperkinetic kids. Emotional seesaw formula: skullcap, slippery elm, a little angelica seed."

TASTE:

sweet, earthen • moist • mucilaginous

TISSUE STATE:

atrophy

SPECIFIC INDICATIONS:

CONSTITUTION, COMPLEXION, CHARACTERISTIC SYMPTOMS
- *Weak, debilitated, from poor nutrition; convalescence after long sickness; nourishing to the body during cancer and cachexias.*
- Adrenocortical deficiency.

RESPIRATION
- Irritable sore throat; tonsillitis.
- Irritable lungs; cough, influenza, bronchitis, asthma, pneumonia, tuberculosis; deepens respiration.
- Independent of the mucilaginous effect, slippery elm deepens respiration.

DIGESTION
- *Stomach acidity, ulceration, flatulence.*
- Facilitates digestion of milk products.
- Diabetes mellitus.
- Jaundice.
- *Hard stool, difficult and painful to pass; constipation, rectal fissure.*
- *Diarrhea, colitis, appendicitis, diverticulitis, hemorrhoids, dysentery.*
- *Dysentery with severe tormina (cramping pain) in the umbilical region.*

KIDNEYS AND BLADDER
- Irritated kidneys; increases diuresis.
- Irritable bladder; cystitis.

MUSCULAR AND SKELETAL
- Fractures (external, internal).

SKIN
- *Abscesses, boils, ulcers, herpes, wounds, burns, eczema, diaper rash, warts, skin diseases (external and internal).*
- *Inflamed, irritated, dried, or ulcerated surfaces (external).*

PREPARATION AND DOSAGE:

Easily distinguished in the spring, when the large seeds are present. Confirm by a touch to the bark on the twigs; it gives slightly under pressure, indicating the presence of mucilage.

The powder, as it comes to market, is often adulterated. It should have a slightly grayish/fawn color. It will not work if dark or reddish. It may be necessary to purchase whole pieces of the bark to avoid adulteration. It is powdered coarse for making poultices, fine for internal use. The powder absorbs a large amount of water and swells up, but it tends to clump up in lumps so it has to be carefully mixed. It is best to stir in a little cold water, to make a paste, then stir in boiling water. About one heaping teaspoonful of the powder makes 1 pint. Herbalist Dorothy Hall recommends that it simply be stirred in with yogurt or mashed banana, since it combines more readily with fats and oils. Dr. Edward Shook recommends that a teaspoonful be beaten up with an egg, then add boiling milk and some sweetening or flavor.

CAUTIONS:

Environmental concerns. Slippery elm is slightly less susceptible to Dutch elm disease because of the thick, mucilaginous bark. However, the population of large trees is being decimated by this disease. Small trees are often weedy.

CONTRAINDICATIONS:

Excessive dosing can cause it to absorb too much of the intestinal secretion, resulting in a dried-out condition. (Here we see the homeopathic principle: slippery elm causes what it cures.) Long-term overuse is also detrimental; folk herbalist Eva Graf recommended a twenty-one-day course.

LITERATURE:

Traditional, Samuel Henry, Constantine Rafinesque, Edward Shook, Dorothy Hall, Eva Graf, John Eberle (12, 13).

Usnea barbata. Old Man's Beard.

This unusual agent is a lichen growing on trees in moist climates. It contains mucilage, vitamin C, sterols, and lichenic (or usnic) acid, an antimicrobial. Thus it is used against viruses, bacteria, and fungus infections involving the mucosa of the respiratory, digestive, and sexual-urinary tract. It is indicated for gum diseases, sore throat, sinusitis, respiratory infections, bronchitis, pleurisy, pneumonia, and even tuberculosis (lung or skin). In addition, it acts on intestinal infection, dysentery, and cholera, urinary tract infections, vaginitis, cervical dysplasia, mastitis, impetigo, and boils.

LITERATURE:

Stephen Buhner, Laurel Dewey.

Uva Ursi. Bearberry.

See *Arctostaphylos uva-ursi.*

Vaccinium macrocarpon. Cranberry.

Native to acid peat bogs in the northern hemisphere, the North American representative has the larger berry, bred for food and used as a medicine. They are members of the heath family, closely related to the blueberry and bilberry. High levels of vitamin C made cranberry an excellent food to prevent scurvy and, more recently, the juice is used as a urinary antiseptic. The fruits contain flavonoids, fruit acids, sugars, pectin, tannins, carotene, vitamins (vitamin A, vitamin C, and the B-complex vitamins riboflavin and niacin), and minerals (sodium, potassium, calcium, magnesium, phosphorus, copper, sulfur, iron, and iodine).

Cranberry is largely used as a urinary antiseptic, to prevent or cure bacterial infections in the urethra. This usage depends on the tannins, which coat the mucosa. It is also used as an "antioxidant" based on the high content of flavonoids. These uses are, of course, based on a mechanical way of looking at the plant. From an energetic standpoint we would call cranberry cooling and drying. This reflects the markedly sour and astringent properties of the plant—the flavonoids, fruit acids, vitamin C, and tannins. However, cranberry has not generally been used "energetically."

Because it is acidic, cranberry has been used as an escharotic, to burn away the skin, cancer, and warts. This usage is preserved by Mrs. Lydia Child (1837, 127). "Cranberries, stewed, applied as a poultice frequently and perseveringly, are recommended by Indian doctors as a cure for cancer." The root is used for diabetes by some Native Americans.

TASTE:

sour

TISSUE STATE:

excitation

SPECIFIC INDICATIONS:

- Common cold (juice, tincture, fresh or dried berries, syrup, decoction).
- Influenza (juice, tincture).
- Diarrhea (juice, tincture, syrup, decoction).
- Constipation (dried berries, tincture for adults, syrup for children).
- Cystitis (juice, decoction, douche).
- Bedwetting (tincture).
- Candida, vaginitis (juice, tincture).
- Rheumatism (decoction, tea, juice).
- Gout (decoction, tea).
- Skin; inflamed spots, pustules, acne (juice, tincture, poultice, wash).
- Psoriasis (tincture, decoction, poultice).
- Shingles (tincture, juice, poultice).
- Chicken pox (decoction, external wash).
- Wounds, burns, sunburn (juice, poultice).

LITERATURE:

Traditional, Jill Rosemary Davies.

Vaccinium spp. Blueberry.

Blueberry is the North American analog of the Old World bilberry. It has similar constituents, food properties, and medicinal uses. However, there are so many different kinds of blueberry that we cannot always speak of a specific species in association with the common name.

Blueberry was one of the most important foods and medicines for the Indian people in the old days. The Anishinabe herbalist Keewaydinoquay wrote a book about the blueberry. She points out that it was considered the most important food for the Anishinabe or Ojibwe people. If fire or an enemy threatened a village, dried blueberry was the first food to be taken. The name for the blueberry in Anishinabe is *min,* which not only means "berry, fruit, or grain" but even infers what we would mean by the word "essence" or primal procreative material. Blueberry is known simply as *min,* and thus it is the essential or primordial berry from which all others derive, so to speak. It also means "all things that grow, that are God-made, not manmade."

Women born in the moon when the blueberries ripened were thought to be the most juicy or desirable. However, like the alchemists of the Old World, the Indian medicine men and women knew that the essence was the doorway through the personal, sexual, genetic, racial world to the realm of the spirit.

In addition, the blueberry is the choice food of the bear, who is the totem of the herbalist or food preparer in American Indian lore. The berries are one of two major types of "bear medicine," the other being the brown, furry, oily roots, which provide nutrition in spring, after a long winter hibernation (*Ligusticum porteri, Lomatium dissectum, Balsamorhiza sagittata,* etc.). Bill Mitchell, ND, pointed out the connection of these two types of food sources: the oily plants build up the fat and food reserves of the bear while the berries contain flavonoid antioxidants that preserve these fats and oils. Thus, they are cooling, sedating plants that are welcome by both bear and human in the middle of the summer.

The blueberry fruit is high in fructose, fruit acids, tannins, and flavonoids. Although it is high in sugar it does not cause a high glycemic reaction but actually helps to temper or moderate the effect of carbohydrates on the body. The fruit acids trap oxygen to prevent oxidation, and the flavonoids prevent oxidation and wear and tear in the capillaries. Thus, blueberry concentrate is used to stabilize blood sugar levels and reduce heat. It is excellent for thin hypoglycemics as a source of immediately ready blood sugar that will not cause a sudden sugar spike and drop, while it is also beneficial for diabetics and people with hyperinsulinism, who need to keep their blood sugar levels regular. Blueberry leaves are not sweet, but highly astringent and antiseptic, like other members of the heath family. They are beneficial for loss of fluids through the kidneys, as commonly occurs in diabetes.

Diabetes is a disease of the essence or *min*, in the sense that one is too stuck on the level of the fruit *(min)*, the juicy outer world, and needs a visit to the world of the spirit to develop greater personal identity and resistance to the sugary appeal of the world, with its food, pleasures, and consumer opportunities. This is almost the disease of the modern era.

Huckleberry (*Vaccinium* spp.) is the second choice for swollen prostate after red root (Tommie Bass—confirmed, Matthew Wood).

Verbena hastata. Blue Vervain.

Blue vervain is a member of the vervain family common in open ground in eastern North America. It is an intense, nauseant bitter, hard to hold down in medium to large doses. Such emetics were once fashionable for fever, especially malaria. It was utilized in the Revolutionary War, when quinine was unavailable, for intermittent chill and fever. It was found to be suited to cases where it was very hard to induce sweating. The deeper properties of the plant were brought out by Dr. O. Phelps Brown, of Jersey City, New Jersey, shortly before the Civil War. He tested many members of the Verbena *species and felt that the* hastata *was the most powerful. It is used in a fashion similar to European vervain (Verbena officinalis). The deeper properties of blue vervain are brought out in the moderate to low doses, which are not emetic. It contains bitters, saponins, tannins, volatile oils, and iridoid glycosides.*

Blue vervain is an intense bitter that deeply influences the nervous system, sending a profound shiver through the body that awakens the shivering mechanism, which is under sympathetic control. Hence, it is useful in cases where the sympathetic, governor of the surface, is unable to correctly regulate the skin. It is suitable to fever where the skin is tightly closed, or to hot flashes and night sweats where the sweat comes on uncontrollably and there is persistent fluid loss. These symptoms originate in what would be cited, in traditional Chinese medicine, as exhaustion of the yin, so that the yang cannot be restrained. The yin is being burned out by the too excessive flushing, heat, or yang, resulting in either profuse perspiration or no sweating at all.

These physical properties are analogous to the personality and physical conditions for which blue vervain is remedial. It is suited to people who are very intense, even fanatical, laying impossible standards on themselves or others. They strain to live up to these impossible standards, or to impose them on others. Yet, they have not the strength to sustain this activity, so that they are too intense mentally and emotionally, but suffer from physical weakness. I always say, "Strong above, weak below," meaning that they are strong in the head but weak in the digestion and sexual centers.

Blue vervain is useful in the same kind of cases where Dr. Bach used

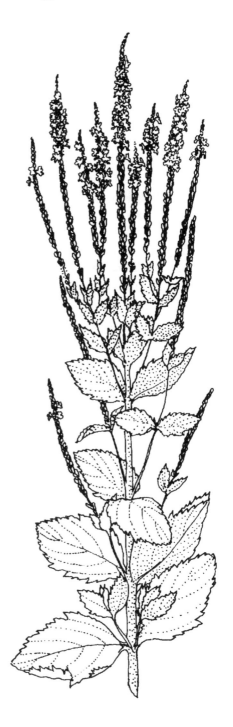

the European vervain as a flower essence: intense, fanatical people who have high standards for themselves or others. Dorothy Hall (1988) says that they make lists. I remember one teenage girl with heart palpitations. I asked her if she made lists and she replied that she made lists of other people's faults! That fits blue vervain to a tee. The remedy relaxed the heart and within several months she had her first boyfriend. She moved from unreasonably high standards to attainable ones.

This extreme intensity can have a hormonal origin and is sometimes associated with food craving and binging in women during their menstrual cycle. It is probably related to excess progesterone or intolerance to progesterone, as this hormone makes one want to eat more. In thin women who are not accustomed to eating a great deal this can be very unpleasant, especially in the second half of the cycle, when progesterone is high. William LeSassier cured a woman who exclaimed that one week a month she felt like "a school of piranhas on a feeding frenzy." The rest of the month she ate hardly anything. Blue vervain/vervain people can have unpleasant, too intense sexual desires. These can be complicated and built up by inappropriate self-imposed sexual morals. O. Phelps Brown noted that blue vervain "establishes a brisk circulation" to the genitals; it brings the energy down from the head into the body and genitals and is grounding.

The vervain person has "too much energy up above and too little energy below" (cf. *Capsella*). They are mentally intense and demanding but physically weak or thin and not powerful. Great tensions build up and show up as tension in the neck, which sometimes goes off in explosive seizures—this was Dr. Brown's famous remedy for epileptic seizures that began in the neck. Sometimes the neck is stiff, but the head hangs down a little—a picture of the plant with its stiff, rigid neck and hanging flower tops. Tension extends through the digestive tract—Dr. Brown cited blue vervain for harassing dyspepsia. It causes and cures nausea and vomiting. Dr. F. Wheeler, a friend of Dr. Bach, used European vervain to help remove a kidney stone—the strong-willed patient was back at work later in the day.

There is probably no better remedy than blue vervain for menopausal night sweats and hot flashes, especially in women who are intense and driven. The specific indication to look for in all cases is stiffness in the nape of the neck. It is suited to the "stiff-necked" people who mean the best and strive for perfection, but whom the Lord found so irksome in the Hebrew Bible.

Michael Moore (2003, 255) writes, "I have also observed vervain tea to have a particular affinity for recovering alcoholics with frequent blood sugar imbalances, emotionally induced peripheral vasodilation, and an easily excited, flushed face, a genial, happy external disposition with private episodes of depression that bring the word *vapors* to mind." He also cites it as a remedy for "metabolic brittleness." The expression is not further defined, but this so perfectly fits my experience of blue vervain as a remedy for overly intense, but brittle, easily undermined persons.

TASTE:

bitter, acrid

TISSUE STATES:

constriction, atrophy

SPECIFIC INDICATIONS:

CONSTITUTION, COMPLEXION, CHARACTERISTIC SYMPTOMS
- Thin, strong-willed, but lacking stamina to sustain effort; overexertion.

MIND, SENSES, NERVES, EMOTIONS, PERSONALITY
- *High-minded, idealistic, driven, intolerant of shortcomings in self and others; sexual neurosis.*
- Mental overactivity, excessive thinking, excessive talking, loud voice.

HEAD AND NECK
- Headache; earache.
- Eyes; weak, sore, inflamed.
- Mouth ulcers; soft, spongy gums (mouthwash); adenoids.
- *Stiffness of the nape of the neck.*

RESPIRATION
- Colds, catarrh, irritable, spasmodic cough, whooping cough, croup, asthma, pneumonia.
- Wheezing, irritation, congestion.

DIGESTION
- Dyspepsia; harassing pain, sluggish digestion; constipation.

LIVER
- Malaria ague, hepatitis; liver congested, swollen, cirrhotic; biliousness, indigestion, jaundice, gallstone colic.

CARDIOVASCULAR
- Atrial fibrillation; poor peripheral circulation.

KIDNEYS AND BLADDER
- Kidney stone colic.
- Incontinence; bladder spasm.

FEMALE
- Menstruation; painful and irregular.
- *PMS; anger before the period; tension and cramping.*
- Food craving before the period; driven to eat.
- *Menopause; hot flashes,* hormonal drives, nymphomania.
- Labor.
- Mastitis; lack of lactation.

MALE
- Impotence.

MUSCULAR AND SKELETAL
- Epileptic seizures and spasms beginning in the neck.
- Sprains and strains, especially hyperextension.
- Deep bruises.

FEVER
- Fevers with profuse sweating, loss of fluids, stiffness in the neck, headache.
- Stubborn fevers with complete lack of sweating; where it is difficult to get a sweat going.
- Convulsions following fevers that have depleted the fluids.

OTHER
- Eczema, dry skin.

- Liver congestion, cirrhosis.
- Children; especially useful in children who get fidgety and cranky at the commencement of illness.
- For immediate use after burn to remove heat (leaf poultice).

PREPARATION AND DOSAGE:

The roots, leaves, and mature seeds are used by the Indians; alternatively, the flower tops are gathered at the height of flowering and extracted fresh in alcohol or dried for use as an infusion. Dose: 1–3 drops, 1–3x/day.

CAUTIONS:

None. Too bitter to produce side effects from large doses.

LITERATURE:

Traditional, O. Phelps Brown (7, 8, 10, 11, 21, 22), Edward Bach (2), Matthew Wood (1, 2, 3, 7, 12, 14, 18, 23), Jack Ritchason (4, 5, 6, 8, 9, 10, 11, 12, 14, 15, 20, 23, 25, 26, 28, 29), F. Wheeler (13), William LeSassier (7, 16, 17, 26), Michael Moore (8, 10, 24, 30), E. P. Anshutz (27), Anishinabe traditional use (31).

Viburnum opulus, V. trilobum. Cramp Bark.

Dr. John King was informed by some of his patients about the use of cramp bark for menstrual cramping; they learned about it from a "neighboring Indian tribe." He introduced it under the name Viburnum opulus, but this is the name of the European species (guelder rose), whereas the Indians were undoubtedly using the native species, Viburnum trilobum. Since that time these two articles have been used interchangeably and come to market in herbal commerce mixed together. (I know this from talking to wildcrafters.) Guelder rose is an ornamental naturalized on uplands in North America, whereas the trilobum is native to low ground. There are also some physical differences: the American species is more sour, the European more acrid. They are members of the Caprifoliaceae (honeysuckle) family, which has many cooling remedies. V. opulus contains hydroquinones, coumarins, and tannins.

Cramp bark is sour and acrid. It contains valerianic acid, a parasympathetic relaxant. As a consequence, it is suited to smooth muscle cramping with irritation and heat. The European species *(V. opulus)* is more acrid, while the American *(V. trilobum)* is more sour, so one is a little better for cramping, the other for heat. Some members of the honeysuckle family are used for heat (elder, honeysuckle), so this usage should not be forgotten. There are not too many plants that unite the sour and acrid flavors to fight heat and tension, so this is an important point of differentiation between viburnum and other plants.

"The specific influence of the agent is exercised in relieving irregular spasmodic pains of the womb and ovaries. It is antispasmodic in its action upon the entire pelvic viscera, influencing spasmodic contractions of the muscular structure of the bladder, and spasmodic stricture to a limited extent" (Ellingwood).

Cramp bark is used for cramps, for irritation and vomiting of pregnancy, and to prevent abortion from nervous irritation, like its cousin, black haw *(Viburnum prunifolium)*. Ellingwood continues, "Given prior to labor it is a partus preparator of much value, but its action is limited largely to its antispasmodic influence upon erratic pains. It is given with much benefit in severe after-pains, in hysterical conditions, with convulsive phenomena, and in spasmodic dysmenorrhea." He notes that it will prevent miscarriage, "but to an extent greatly inferior to *Viburnum prunifolium,* which agent, in fact, fully covers the field of operation of this agent, except in its antispasmodic influence." Black haw is more nutritive.

William LeSassier noted that cramp bark has a strong affinity to the kidneys. It is indicated when there is pain, weakness, stiffness, and soreness in the lower back. It strengthens weak kidneys, improving poor pumping action with insufficient removal of waste products and retention of minerals. It is beneficial for chronic debility associated with chronic, low-grade pain beginning in the back. By comparison, he says, *Viburnum prunifolium* has more of an affinity to the ovaries. With cramp bark, the pain tends to center in the ovaries. This agrees with Ellingwood's account of cramp bark: "pain from the pelvic organs which begin[s] in the back, extending through to the loins and down the thighs."

In Russia the berries are the part used; fresh or dried they are applied for high blood pressure and heart disease.

TASTE:

sour, acrid • cool

TISSUE STATES:

irritation, constriction

SPECIFIC INDICATIONS:

CHARACTERISTIC SYMPTOMS
- *"Cramp-like pains, pain recurring at intervals"* (Rolla Thomas).

MIND, SENSES, NERVES, EMOTIONS, PERSONALITY
- Nervous tension.

RESPIRATION
- Acute spasms of bronchitis, whooping cough, and asthma.

CARDIOVASCULAR
- Heart palpitations; irregular pulse; high blood pressure.

DIGESTION
- Nervous indigestion, flatulent stomach, vomiting of pregnancy.
- Painful intestinal cramping.
- Sudden abdominal cramps and colic.
- Catarrhal conditions of the gastrointestinal tract and related structures associated with spasmodic tension.
- Enteritis, colitis, dysentery.

LIVER
- Congestion and hardening of the liver.

KIDNEYS AND BLADDER
- Spasmodic stricture in urinary tract infections.
- Enuresis, cystitis.

FEMALE
- *Uterine relaxant;* irritation from IUD excess reaction and hyper-contraction.

- *Menses: bearing down pains precede the period; period late, scanty, with cramps; heaviness, aching in ovaries, pubes, sacrum, down the back of the thighs.*
- *Menstruation: cramping with "expulsive" pains* (Rolla Thomas).
- Menstrual cramping in younger women (*V. prunifolium* in older women).
- Pregnancy: cramping during.
- Pregnancy: repeated, early miscarriage.
- Labor: "pain assumes the form of spasmodic contraction, the muscular tissues of the perineum being also involved" (Rolla Thomas).
- Postpartum: afterpains.

FEVER
- Brings blood to the skin, balances pH.

OTHER
- Back pains and cramps; stiff, sore nape of neck, sacrum.
- Upper and lower back; "old whiplash stuff."
- Epilepsy, fits, convulsions, fainting.
- Cramping and fever.
- Neuralgia.
- Lockjaw.
- Poison oak.
- Kidneys (twigs and berries).

PREPARATION AND DOSAGE:

The bark tinctured fresh yields the best preparation. Dosage can be small or large. Dose: "10 drops to 1/2 dram in 4 ounces water" (Rolla Thomas).

LITERATURE:

Traditional, Rolla Thomas (1, 15, 19), William Boericke, William LeSassier (13, 23, 28), Matthew Alfs (16), Lise Wolff (20), Jack Ritchason (2, 3, 4, 7, 9, 12, 17, 20, 24, 25, 26, 27), Anishinabe traditional use (29).

Viburnum prunifolium. Black Haw.

Black haw is a member of the viburnum clan native to the lower Midwest and upper South. The bark was used from an early time to prevent miscarriages. It is a cousin of cramp bark, but possesses more depth, especially in its tonic properties. It contains coumarins, phenolic acids (including salicin), flavonoids, and triterpenes. Finley Ellingwood (1918) was one of the most knowledgeable of the eclectic physicians on obstetric and gynecological remedies. He gives an extensive account of black haw. I have rearranged some of the text in order to facilitate the flow of his ideas.

Margi Flint tells us how to look at this plant. "It is not just the alternative to crampbark, but is more versatile, powerful, and well rounded, with more medicinal qualities." In addition to the relaxant properties it is a nutritive tonic, improving the powers of digestion and nutrition in the body. "The bark is thick and rich, with a red, chestnuty color, denoting the blood building properties. The branches reach out in the forest in a protective manner, yet the flowers on the tips are delicate, like baby's breath, showing a purity and delicateness. It is indicated in delicate, sensitive women with weak digestion, lack of nervous tone, and weak circulation." Now let us turn to Ellingwood.

First, black haw operates on the nervous system. "The agent exercises its influence through the nervous centers, soothing nerve irritation and possessing marked antispasmodic properties. [In large, poisonous doses] it influences the motor side of the cord, producing progressive muscular weakness, loss of reflex action and ultimate paralysis. It apparently directly influences the action of the heart, as it lowers arterial pressure to a marked degree.

"Its sedative influence upon the nervous system is conveyed to the uterus and appendages and there becomes apparent. It overcomes all forms of nervous irritation, and irregular functional action in these organs. It is the direct remedy for nervous conditions of the pregnant state."

Second, it is tonic. "Viburnum is well classed among the tonics, as there is usually a general improvement in all the body functions while it is taken. It has a very satisfactory effect upon derangements of the stomach and intestinal tract, especially in females when the whole system is out of tone. It restores the nerve influence, improves the circulation, supplies nutrition to the womb and ovaries. It is valuable in dysmenor-rhea which is due to debility.

"It is the remedy for sympathetic disturbances of the heart, stomach and nervous system, common to sensitive ladies with irritable nervous systems, preceding or during the menstrual epoch, depending on vaso-motor derangement. It must be given in advance and continued through the period."

Third, it acts specifically on the female system. "It is the remedy for dysmenorrhea, especially that characterized by cramp-like pains of spas-modic character. It promotes normal uterine contractions and antago-nizes those of an irregular character. It is valuable in menorrhagia and metrorrhagia, either of an acute or a passive character. In all of these cases its use should be begun a few days in advance of the anticipated disor-der and continued through and beyond the menstrual period.

"It must not be overlooked in the treatment of irregular, sudden, men-strual flow, occurring during eruptive and low continued or violent inflam-matory fevers, especially in young ladies. This occurrence is not uncommon in smallpox, scarlet fever, diphtheria, measles, pneumonitis, pleuritis, phthisis and typhoid fever. It is sometimes of serious import, and masked sepsis undoubtedly occurs in the cases, with severe peritonitis or metri-tis, to which the patient may succumb.

"In a number of cases, when given for menstrual irregularities, or for the distress induced by uterine displacement, in previously sterile females, pregnancy has promptly occurred, proving the influence of the agent in restoring normal functional ovarian activity."

"Viburnum prunifolium is especially a uterine sedative in threatened miscarriage. It is particularly indicated in habitual abortion, preventing an anticipated occurrence and permanently overcoming the habit. I have had practical experience extending over thirty years, and have perfect confidence in the agent based on repeated success.

"In habitual cases it is necessary to give the agent in occasional doses for one, two or more weeks preceding the time of the miscarriage, which usually occurs each time at the same month of the fetal life. As the time approaches the patient is kept quiet and free from excitement, and the agent is given three or four times daily. The interval is shortened to one or two hours with the first suspicious indications at the usual time. If no symptoms appear the agent is continued beyond the period, and then per-haps in daily doses only for a week or two longer. The physicians should advise the patient to remain constantly on the watch for indications suggesting the necessity of an increase in the doses. The agent will stop induced miscarriage, as well as other forms, if no injury has been done to the membranes.

"In small doses, it is an excellent partus preparator, materially improving the conditions when irregular and distressing symptoms are present and greatly facilitating a speedy and uncomplicated normal labor. It controls after pains and prevents postpartum hemorrhage. It insures normal involution and assists in retaining a normal position of the womb subsequently, where malposition had previously existed.

"In its influence in overcoming reflex nervous disturbances, it is often most efficient in controlling the morning sickness of pregnancy and the entire train of distressing symptoms present at this time. It changes the mental condition of the patient from that of depression and despondency, to one of cheerfulness and hopefulness."

Fourth, it has an antiseptic quality, as described above.

Fifth, it acts on high blood pressure. Ellingwood wrote before the era when blood pressure was monitored. It is especially useful for the high blood pressure of pregnancy. It is almost "always successful" in this complaint, according to Margi Flint, and is also useful in high blood pressure "at other times."

TASTE:

sweet, slightly acrid • astringent

TISSUE STATES:

atrophy, constriction

SPECIFIC INDICATIONS:

CONSTITUTION, COMPLEXION, CHARACTERISTIC SYMPTOMS
- Delicate, sensitive women; nervous, excitable.

MIND, SENSES, NERVES, EMOTIONS, PERSONALITY
- Nervous excitement, nervousness with moderate pain, restlessness, and suffering.
- Depression, despondency.

FEMALE
- Painful menses, pain in the ovaries, down the legs, whether the flow is scanty or profuse, especially in middle-aged women.
- Membranous discharge.
- Amenorrhea and menorrhagia.
- High blood pressure; during pregnancy or not.
- Habitual abortion, sterility.

MUSCULAR AND SKELETAL
- Cramps in the legs.
- Arthritis.

PREPARATION AND DOSAGE:

The inner bark is the usual part to be used. Dose: "10–20 drops in 4 ounces water" (Rolla Thomas).

CAUTIONS:

The berries have caused nausea in some people.

LITERATURE:

Traditional, Constantine Rafinesque, Finley Ellingwood (1, 2, 4, 6, 8), Tommie Bass (9), Margi Flint (1, 7), Matthew Alfs (4).

Viburnum trilobum. Cramp Bark.

Refer to *Viburnum opulus*.

Xanthorhiza apiifolia. Yellow Root.

This small relative of goldenseal is native to stream banks in southern Appalachia. It is considered to be milder than its cousin and is better suited to use as a "tonic" than a "natural antibiotic." Yellow root enjoys local popularity.

Xanthoxylum americanum. Northern Prickly Ash.

Prickly ash is the most northerly member of the citrus family native to North America. It is found in old fields that are abandoned and returning to forest. The sharp thorns keep out intruders and allow nature to reassert her dominion. It has the stimulating properties associated with the citrus family. The thorns can cause a lot of pain—they remind one of the flagellum *or whips used by the Romans to scourge Jesus and other prisoners. This may be taken as a signature—prickly ash is a very powerful remedy for torturous pain. A taste of the bark or berry produces an electric-like current through the nerves. Although it is best known in nineteenth-century literature as a remedy for the mucosa, it is an important nervine for damaged, numb, tingling, or horribly painful nerves. It is also a powerful stimulant to the capillaries and is used as an "accelerator" or catalyst in combination with other plants in a formula.*

Prickly ash bark is as powerful a remedy as it looks and feels. The young branches have sharp thorns that rip the clothing and the skin. Any remedy that can inflict pain should be able to cure it. The bark and berry cause an intense tingling on the tongue and throat that can quickly become torturous. This stimulating impression moves down the throat and through the body, awakening the nervous system, left and right. Samuel Thomson included it among his handful of "diffusives"—remedies that cause a diffusing sensation through the nerves and act as stimulating catalysts in a formula.

According to Jonathan Carver, an eighteenth-century explorer of the interior of North America, the Indian people used the bark of the root as a specific for gonorrhea. From this usage it came into popularity as a remedy for debility of the mucosa, but this application does not bring out the full genius of the remedy. Albert Isaiah Coffin, who introduced Thomsonian herbalism to Britain, testified that it was used by an old Indian woman to cure him as a lad; it brought on a life-saving sweat in combination with other plants. It improves capillary circulation, bringing the blood to the skin and mucosa.

Xanthoxylum was given a homeopathic proving. It produced such symptoms as a sensation as if the ovaries were being ripped out by wires—torture. It also produced symptoms of numbness, tingling, and pain in the nerves—all of which probably represent overstimulation and understimulation. One of the conditions for which it is considered remedial in homeopathic literature (Boericke, 1927) is hemiplegia, or one-sided paralysis (Bell's palsy). One side of the body becomes intensely painful. Usually, the only relief comes over months, as the nerves slowly become debilitated and weak, and a semi-paralysis sets in. This condition perfectly corresponds to the essence of prickly ash, which is a remedy for imbalance in the charge on the nerves. It will rectify conditions where the nerves have been injured, torn, or overstimulated, are numb, tingling, or torturously painful, and it will do it with a power that is hard to believe.

Experience has taught me that prickly ash is a remedy for people "writhing in agony." They suffer so much pain that they cannot sit still or find solace. One woman begged her doctor to "cut the nerve," but of course they couldn't cut the sciatic. She writhed in agony until I gave her a dose of prickly ash. Months later she reported that the pain was now quite bearable, though not completely gone. Another woman writhed back and forth in the chair from a torn disk in her neck. The pain was completely removed within a month. And another, after spending more than twenty years on welfare, overcame her chronic menstrual pain (feeling like her ovaries were being ripped out by wires) to find a new job, boyfriend, and life. In other cases it has restored sensation where there was numbness or tingling.

TASTE:

(bark) pungent • slightly warm • highly stimulating and diffusive
(fruit) pungent • warm • moderately stimulating and diffusive

TISSUE STATE:

depression

SPECIFIC INDICATIONS:

CONSTITUTION, COMPLEXION, CHARACTERISTIC SYMPTOMS
- Spare, withered women in late middle age, afflicted with chronic wasting diseases; or robust, full persons with nerve injuries causing intense torment.
- Writhing in agony, can't sit still from the pain; torment of the most intense kind, bringing the patient to their knees.
- *Nerve damage; numb, tingling, painful.*
- *Hemiplegia (Bell's palsy); one-sided pain, numbness, paralysis.*

- *Nerve debility, withered, weakness.*

HEAD
- Paralysis of the tongue and mouth.
- *Mouth sores.*

RESPIRATION
- Sore throat and respiratory tension and discomfort.
- Deep respiratory infection, with debility and chronic illness.
- Asthma.

DIGESTION
- Weak digestion.
- Colic, cramps, gas.
- Diarrhea.
- Cholera (cf. *Ballota*).

KIDNEYS AND BLADDER
- Edema.

MUSCULAR AND SKELETAL
- Cold extremities and joints.
- Arthritis, rheumatism.
- Raynaud's disease (cf. *Carthamus*).

WOUNDS
- Wounds slow to heal.
- Ulcers.

FEVER
- Intermittent chill/fever.

PREPARATION AND DOSAGE:

The bark is collected in the late winter (or anytime; this is a pernicious weed in old pastures). Extracted fresh in alcohol, dosage very small, 1–3 drops, 1–3x/day. Dried for use by decoction, or roll a small piece on the tongue until the sensation becomes too intense. The berries are also used but have a slightly different flavor.

LITERATURE:

Traditional, homeopathic provings and clinical experience, Matthew Wood (1–5, 7, 8), William Boericke (1, 3, 4, 5), Louise Tenney (6, 7, 10–17, 19–20), William LeSassier (9), Phyllis Light (18).

Yucca glauca. Soap Plant.

This member of the lily family is native to temperate North America and is cultivated as an ornamental throughout the world. It has long been used by the Indians as a medicine and soap. It contains high levels of saponins, which are released when it is chopped up in water. These have a steroid-like property. Yet, the amount of these substances that can get into the body appears to be very limited, so yucca does not have much of a modern pharmacological reputation. However, the fiber and saponins in yucca act on the bowel, improving gut flora. It has been suggested that this is the source of the healing powers of the plant. Refer to Michael Moore (2003) for the chemistry and pharmacology.

Specific indications have not been well developed, but yucca's properties are fairly predictable from its prominent constituents. From a Native American perspective it would be considered a "bear medicine"—that is to say, a brown, furry root or stem with fixed oils that nourish the adrenal cortex.

TASTE:

soapy, bitter • moist, cool

TISSUE STATES:

atrophy, stagnation

SPECIFIC INDICATIONS:

HEAD
- Strengthens and straightens the neck and spine; removes blockages.
- Headache.

- Dandruff.
- Allergies.
- Cataracts.

DIGESTION
- Aphthous ulcers (canker sores).
- Indigestion.

CARDIOVASCULAR
- Hypertension, high cholesterol, triglycerides.

KIDNEYS AND BLADDER
- Urethritis.

LIVER AND GALLBLADDER
- Bilious problems.

MALE
- Prostatitis.

MUSCULAR AND SKELETAL
- *Arthritis,* gout, bursitis.
- Rheumatoid arthritis, osteoarthritis.

SKIN
- Skin and scalp problems.

ENDOCRINE
- Adrenocortical deficiency; Addison's disease.

OTHER
- Cancer.

PREPARATION AND DOSAGE:

The outer bark is too strong, so the inner pith is used.

CAUTIONS:

Large doses can be purgative and cause intestinal cramping.

LITERATURE:

Traditional, Jack Ritchason (3, 4, 5, 7–16), Julia Graves (1), Christopher Menzies-Trull (2, 6), Michael Moore (12, 13).

Zea mays. Corn Silk.

A member of the grass family, corn was developed into a major source of food by ancestors of the American Indians. The difference between the wild ancestor and the domesticated crop plant represents a genetic jump that is impossible to bridge from modern knowledge. The silk has long been used as a demulcent in bladder inflammation. The high nitrogen content of corn and the urinous smell of growing corn are "signatures" pointing to this use.

Corn silk is an old American Indian remedy that was passed to the pioneers. It is a simple domestic remedy for bladder infection. It is a mild demulcent, healing and soothing to the mucosa of the urinary tract. It is also beneficial in irritated mucosa of the colon and strengthens uterine muscle tone.

Cornmeal is a lesser known folk remedy for fungus growing under the nails of the toes, a common problem. White or yellow cornmeal is poured into an inch of warm water and the feet are soaked in this concoction once a day, or even just a few times a week. This has reportedly cured thousands according to popular accounts in the media. Another folk remedy for nail fungus is to paint the nail with henna (Jim McDonald).

TASTE:

sweet, slightly bitter • moist

TISSUE STATES:

irritation, constriction, atrophy

SPECIFIC INDICATIONS:

KIDNEYS AND *BLADDER*
- *Acute and chronic inflammation of the bladder.*
- *Painful urination, irritation of the bladder.*
- *Catarrhal cystitis; purulent urine indicating the presence of bacterial infection.*
- Bedwetting.
- *Excessive alkalinity of the urine.*
- Gravel; increases the quantity of urine and decreases the excessive proportions of urates.
- Urinary problems of the aged, and dropsies connected with heart disease (cf. rosemary).

OTHER
- Irritation of the intestinal mucosa.
- *Toenail fungus* (cornmeal infusion externally).

PREPARATION AND DOSAGE:

Infusion of corn silk to make a tea. It also works as a tincture made in alcohol or vinegar.

TOXICITY:

Corn can cause allergies and anaphylaxis. I have seen anaphylactic shock occur from exposure to dried corn silk (antidote: gentian).

LITERATURE:

Traditional (1–7), Tommie Bass (4), Matthew Wood (8).

We consider the bear as chief of all animals in regard to herb medicine, and therefore it is understood that if a man dreams of a bear he will be expert in the use of herbs for curing illness. The bear is regarded as an animal well acquainted with herbs because no other animal has such good claws for digging roots.

—SIYAKA, DAKOTA MEDICINE MAN (DENSMORE, 1926, 324)

REFERENCES

INTRODUCTION AND PART I: SPECIFICITY IN HERBAL MEDICINE

Arroyo, Stephen. *Astrology, Psychology, and the Four Elements: An Energy Approach to Astrology & Its Use in the Counseling Arts.* Sebastopol, CA: CRCS Publications, 1975.

Barnes, Broda. *Hypothyroidism.* New York: HarperCollins, 1976.

Beach, Wooster. *The American Practice of Medicine.* New York: Privately published, 1833.

Boericke, William. *Pocket Manual of Homoeopathic Materia Medica.* 9th ed., revised and enlarged. Philadelphia: Boericke & Runyon, 1927.

Cavender, Alexander. *Folk Medicine in Southern Appalachia.* Chapel Hill: University of North Carolina Press, 2003.

Cech, Richo. *Making Plant Medicine.* Williams, OR: Horizon Herbs Publishing, 2000.

Clymer, R. Swinburne, MD. *Nature's Healing Agents: The Medicine of Nature, (or the Natura System).* Revised ed. Quakertown, PA: The Humanitarian Society, 1973.

Cornford, Francis. *Plato's Cosmology: The Timaeus, Translated with a Running Commentary.* 1st ed., 1935. New York: Liberal Arts Press, 1957.

Culpeper, Nicholas. "A Key to Galen's Method of Physick." In *Culpeper's Complete Herbal, & English Physician.* Glenwood, IL: Meyerbooks, 1990.

Fernie, William T. *Old Fashioned Herbal Remedies.* Originally published 1917 as *Herbal Simples.* Reprint. Toronto: Coles, 1980.

Fyfe, John William, MD. *Specific Diagnosis and Specific Medication.* Cincinnati: The Scudder Brothers, 1909.

Hall, Dorothy. *Creating Your Herbal Profile.* New Canaan, CT: Keats Publishing Co., 1988.

Hoffmann, David. *Medical Herbalism: The Science and Practice of Herbal Medicine.* Rochester, VT: Healing Arts Press, 2003.

Moss, Kay K. *Southern Folk Medicine, 1750–1820.* Columbia: University of South Carolina Press, 1999.

Payne-Jackson, Arvilla. *Folk Wisdom and Mother Wit: John Lee—An African American Herbal Healer.* Westport, CT: Greenwood Publishing Group, 1993.

Pelikan, Wilhelm. *Healing Plants: Insights through Spiritual Science.* Vol. 1. German ed., 1988. Translated by A. R. Meuss. Spring Valley, NY: Mercury Press, 1997.

Phatak, S. R. *Materia Medica of Homeopathic Medicines.* New Delhi: Indian Books & Periodicals Syndicate, 1977.

Priest, A. W., and L. R. Priest. *Herbal Medication: A Clinical and Dispensary Handbook.* London: L. N. Fowler & Co., Ltd., 1982.

Quelch, Mary Thorne. *Herbs for Daily Use.* London: Faber and Faber, 1945.

Rafinesque, Constantine M. *Medical Flora, or Manual of the Medical Botany of the United States.* 2 vols. Philadelphia: Atkinson & Alexander, 1828–30.

Russell, Ralph, MD. *Home Medicine Book.* Birmingham, AL: Published by the author, 1911. [This book has an unusual section on Southern folk herbal materia medica.]

Scudder, John M. *Specific Diagnosis: A Study of Disease.* Reprint of the 1st ed., 1874. Cincinnati: John M. Scudder and Sons, Medical Publishers, 1893.

_____. *Specific Medication and Specific Medicines.* 4th revision. 1st ed., 1870. 10th ed. Cincinnati: Wilstach, Baldwin & Co., Printers, 1881.

Shaffer, Willa. *Midwifery and Herbs.* Provo, UT: Woodland Books, 1986.

Thurston, Joseph M. *The Philosophy of Physiomedicalism.* Richmond, IN: Privately published, 1900.

Winston, David. "Definite Medication: Specific Herbs for Specific Symptoms," in *Official Proceedings of the Gaia Symposium on Naturopathic Herbal Wisdom.* Harvard: Gaia Herbal Research Institute, 1995.

_____. "Definite Medication: Specific Medication for Specific

Symptom Pictures," pp. 198–99 in *American Herbalists Guild, 8th Annual Symposium, "Integrating Herbal Medicine into American Health Care."* Cincinnati: October 17–19, 1997.

_____. *"The 10 Tastes": The Energetics of Herbs.* Broadway, NJ: Published by the author, 1999.

Wood, Matthew. *The Earthwise Herbal: A Complete Guide to Medicinal Plants of the Old World.* Berkeley, CA: North Atlantic Books, 2008.

_____. *The Practice of Traditional Western Herbalism.* Berkeley, CA: North Atlantic Books, 2004.

_____. *Vitalism.* Berkeley, CA: North Atlantic Books, 1992.

BOTANY

Britton, Nathaniel Lord, and Addison Brown. *An Illustrated Flora of the Northern United States and Canada.* 3 vols. Originally published 1913. Reprint ed. New York: Dover Publications, 1970.

Foster, Steven, and James Duke. *A Field Guide to Medicinal Plants: Eastern and Central North America.* Peterson Field Guides. Boston: Houghton Mifflin Co., 1990.

HERBAL MATERIA MEDICA, ANCIENT GREEK AND ROMAN

Dioscorides. *The Materia Medica of Dioscorides, Englished by John Goodyear, 1655.* Edited by Robert T. Gunther. London and New York: Hafner Publishing Co., 1933.

Maimonides, Moses. *Maimonides' Medical Writings: The Medical Aphorisms of Moses Maimonides.* Translated and annotated by Fred Rosner, MD. Vol. 3. Haifa: The Maimonides Research Institute, 1989.

Plinius Secundus. *The History of the World commonly called The Natural History of C. Plinius Secundus, or Pliny.* Selected from the translation by Philemon Holland, 1601, and introduced by Paul Turner. New York: McGraw-Hill Book Company, 1962.

HERBAL MATERIA MEDICA, MEDIEVAL LATIN

von Bingen, Hildegard. *Hildegard von Bingen's Physica: The Complete English Translation of Her Classic Work on Health and*

Healing. Translated from the Latin by Priscilla Throop. Rochester, VT: Healing Arts Press, 1998.

_____. *Holistic Healing.* Original title: *Causae et Curae.* Manfred Pawlik, translator of the Latin text; Patrick Madigan, SJ, translator of the German text; John Kulas, OSB, translator of the foreword; Mary Palmquist and John Kulas, OSB, editors of the English text. Collegeville, MN: The Liturgical Press, 1994.

Macer, Aemilius. *Virtue of Herbs.* Translated by Daniel Patrick O'Hanlon. New Delhi: Hemkunt Press, 1981.

Strehlow, Wighard, Dr., and Gottfried Hertzka, MD. *Hildegard of Bingen's Medicine.* Translated from the German by Karin Anderson Strehlow. Santa Fe, NM: Bear & Co., 1988.

HERBAL MATERIA MEDICA, MEDIEVAL AND MODERN ARABIC

Avicenna (Abu Ali al-Husayn ibn Abd Allah ibn Sina). *The Canon of Medicine (al-Qanun fil-tibb).* Adapted by Laleh Bakhtiar. Series editor, Seyyed Hossein Nasr. Chicago: Great Books of the Islamic World, Inc., 1999.

Chishti, G. M. Hakim, ND. *The Traditional Healer: A Comprehensive Guide to the Principles and Practice of Unani Herbal Medicine.* Rochester, VT: Healing Arts Press, 1988.

Niazi, H. M. *The Egyptian Prescription.* Cairo: Elias Modern Press, 1988.

Ottway, Chalid. *Your Health, Planet and Herbs.* [Toronto: Privately published,] 1933.

HERBAL MATERIA MEDICA, RENAISSANCE ENGLISH

Banckes, Rycharde. *An Herbal [1525]; Edited and Transcribed into Modern English with an Introduction by Sanford V. Larkey, MD, and Thomas Pyles, PhD.* New York: Scholars' Facsimiles and Reprints, 1941.

Blochwitz, Martin. *The Anatomie of Elder.* English translation from the Latin ed. of 1629. London: 1664. [For some extracts see Matthew Wood, *The Book of Herbal Wisdom.*]

Buchan, William. *Domestic Medicine.* Edinburgh: 1779.

Coles, William. *Adam in Eden: or, Nature's Paradise.* London: Printed by J. Streater, for Nathaniel Brooke, 1657. [One of the few books organized upon the doctrine of signatures.]

Culpeper, Nicholas. *Culpeper's Complete Herbal, & English Physician, Enlarged*. First published 1653. Reprint of the 1814 London ed. Glenwood, IL: Meyerbooks, Publisher, 1944.

Gerard, John. *The Great Herbal or General History of Plants*. The Complete 1633 Edition Revised and Enlarged by Thomas Johnson. New York: Dover Publications, Inc., 1975.

Hill, John, MD. *The Usefull Family-Herbal*. 1st ed., 1740. A New Edition, Corrected. London: Wilson and French, 1789.

Palmer, Thomas. *The Admirable Secrets of Physick & Chirurgery*. Modern imprint of an original unpublished ms. of 1696. New Haven, CT: Yale, 1986. [It is unfortunate that the author's book of Indian remedies, bound in deer hide, has not survived.]

Quincy, John, MD. *Pharmacopoeia Officinalis &c. Extemporanea; Or, A Complete English Dispensatory, In Four Parts*. London: Thomas Longman, 1736.

Salmon, William, MD. *Botanologia, or The English Herbal*. London: 1710. [Salmon had some firsthand knowledge of North American flora and fauna, having participated in the settlement of South Carolina, which he calls the "West Indies."]

_____. *Medicina Practica, or Practical Physick*. London: printed by W. Bonny, for T. Hawkins in George Yard, in Lombard-street, and J. Harris at the Harrow in the Pultrey, 1692.

Turner, William. *A New Herball*. Parts I, II, and III, in 2 vols. Facsimile of the original ed. of 1551. Edited by George T. L. Chapman and Marilyn N. Tweddle. Cambridge, NY, Melbourne: Cambridge University Press, 1995.

HERBAL MATERIA MEDICA, AMERICAN INDIAN

Densmore, Francis. *How Indians Use Wild Plants for Food, Medicine and Crafts*. Formerly titled "Uses of Plants by the Chippewa Indians." 1st ed., 1926. New York: Dover Publications, Inc., 1974.

Erichsen-Brown, Charlotte. *Medicinal and Other Uses of North American Plants: A Historical Survey with Special Reference to the Eastern Indian Tribes*. New York: Dover, 1989. [An excellent general survey.]

Garrett, J. T. *The Cherokee Herbal: Native Plant Medicine from the Four Directions*. Santa Fe, NM: Bear & Co., 2003. [An outstanding work on American Indian medicine.]

Gates, William. *An Aztec Herbal: The Classic Codex of 1552*. 1st ed. Baltimore: The Maya Society, 1939. Mineola, NY: Dover Publications, 2000.

Lake, Medicine Grizzlybear. *Native Healer: Initiation into an Ancient Art*. Wheaton, IL; Madras, India: Quest Books, Theosophical Publishing House, 1991. [The author, otherwise known as Bobby Lake-Thom, is one of the few authors whose works on Indian medicine are really deep and authentic.]

Mooney, James. *Myths of the Cherokee and Sacred Formulas of the Cherokees*. Reproduction of the 19th and 7th Annual Reports of the Bureau of American Ethnology. Nashville: Charles and Randy Elder–Booksellers, 1982.

Smith, Huron H. *Ethnobotany of the Menomini Indians*. Bulletin of the Public Museum of the City of Milwaukee. Vol. 4, no. 1. Milwaukee: Published by Order of the Board of Trustees, 1923. [The author used herbs and was familiar with the eclectic materia medica.]

_____. *Ethnobotany of the Meskwaki Indians*. Bulletin of the Public Museum of the City of Milwaukee. Vol. 4, no. 2. Milwaukee: Published by Order of the Board of Trustees, 1923.

_____. *Ethnobotany of the Ojibwe Indians*. Bulletin of the Public Museum of the City of Milwaukee. Vol. 4, no. 3. Milwaukee: Published by Order of the Board of Trustees, 1923.

_____. *Ethnobotany of the Forest Potawatomi Indians*. Bulletin of the Public Museum of the City of Milwaukee. Vol. 7, no. 1. Milwaukee: Published by Order of the Board of Trustees, 1933.

HERBAL MATERIA MEDICA, AMERICAN FOLK MEDICINE

Crellin, John K., and Jane Philpott. *Herbal Medicine, Past and Present: Volume II, A Reference Guide to Medicinal Plants*. Durham, NC, and London: Duke University Press, 1990. [An excellent example of the "historical" method of verifying the actions and uses of an herb. The authors trace the use of medicinal plants from early America to their own time, then compare with information received from a contemporary herbalist, Tommie Bass.]

Janos, Elisabeth. *Country Folk Medicine: Tales of Skunk Oil, Sassafras Tea, and Other Old-Time Remedies.* New York: Galahad Books, 1990. [Old-time New England and New York area remedies collected from elderly people in rest homes.]

Leighton, Ann. *Early American Gardens: "For Meate or Medicine."* Boston: Houghton Mifflin Co., 1970.

Matteson, Antonette. *The Occult Family Physician and Botanic Guide to Health.* 1st ed., 1894. Glenwood, IL: Meyerbooks, 1993.

Moss, Kay K. *Southern Folk Medicine, 1750–1820.* Columbia: University of South Carolina Press, 1999.

Patton, Darryl. *Mountain Medicine: The Herbal Remedies of Tommie Bass.* [Birmingham, AL]: Natural Reader Press, 2004. [An excellent account of Tommie Bass by his devoted student and friend. Not too different from Crellin and Philpott, but where there are differences Patton reflects Bass more faithfully.]

Payne-Jackson, Arvilla. *Folk Wisdom and Mother Wit: John Lee—An African American Herbal Healer.* Westport, CT: Greenwood Publishing Group, 1993. [A sympathetic view of a traditional African American herbalist; including diagnosis by the blood.]

Richel, Jonas. *The Indian Physician.* New Berlin, PA: Joseph Miller, 1828. Reprint.

Smith, Peter. *The Indian Doctor's Dispensatory Being Father Smith's Advice Respecting Diseases and Their Cure.* Originally published in Cincinnati, 1812. Reprint with Biography by John Uri Lloyd. Cincinnati: Lloyd Library, Bulletin of the Lloyd Library of Botany, Pharmacy and Materia Medica, 1901.

HERBAL MATERIA MEDICA, EARLY AMERICAN

Bigelow, Jacob. *American Medical Botany.* Vol. 3. Boston: Cummings and Hilliard, 1817–20.

Brown, O. Phelps, MD. *The Complete Herbal, or, The People Their Own Doctor.* Jersey City, NJ: Published by the author, 1863.

Child, Mrs. [Lydia]. *The Family Nurse; or Companion of the American Frugal Housewife*. Revised by a member of the Massachusetts Medical Society. 1st ed. Boston: Charles J. Hendee, 1837. Reprint. Bedford, MA: Applewood Books, 1997.

Cobb, Daniel J. *The Medical Botanist, and Expositor of Diseases and Remedies*. 2 vols. Castile, NY: Published by the author, 1846.

Downing, Beal P., MD. *Doctor Downing's Reformed Practice and Family Physician*. Utica, NY: Roberts & Sherman, 1851. [An *extremely unique* herbal by a frontier physician who "practiced without a book" for twenty years, so decided to write one.]

Eberle, John, MD. *A Treatise of the Materia Medica and Therapeutics*. 2 vols. 4th ed. Philadelphia: Grigg & Elliot, 1834.

Gunn, A. C., MD. *Gunn's Domestic Medicine, or Poor Man's Friend*. Revised ed. Louisville, KY: Alston Mygatt, Publisher, 1847.

Henry, Samuel, MD. *New and Complete American Medical Family Herbal*. New York: Published by the author, 1814. [This is the second popular herbal written and published in the United States, and the first to have significant readership. Henry's herbal is based on considerable therapeutic experience and gives many interesting case histories and details of medical practice of the time. Unfortunately, the botanical nomenclature is often faulty.]

Howard, Horton, MD. *Howard's Domestic Medicine*. Cincinnati and Philadelphia: H. M. Rulison and D. Rulison, 1859.

_____. *An Improved System of Botanic Medicine*. 3 vols. Columbus, OH: Published by the author, 1836.

Monroe, John. *The American Botanist and Family Physician*. Compiled by Silas Gaskill. Danville, VT: Eben'r Eaton, Printer, 1824.

Porcher, Francis P. *Resources of the Southern Fields and Forests, Medical, Economical, and Agricultural*. 1st ed., Richmond, VA, 1863. Reprint. San Francisco: Jeremy Norman Co., 1991.

Rafinesque, Constantine M. *Medical Flora, or Manual of the Medical Botany of the United States*. Vol. 1. Philadelphia: Atkinson & Alexander, 1828.

_____. *Medical Flora, or Manual of the Medical Botany of the United States*. Vol. 2. Philadelphia: Atkinson & Alexander, 1830.

Taylor, Henry S., MD. *The Family Doctor: A Counsellor in Sickness, Pain, and Distress.* Philadelphia: John E. Potter, 1860.

Thresher, Leonard, MD. *The Family Physician, Nurse's Guide, and Farmer's Horse and Cattle Doctor.* Montpelier, VT: Argus and Patriot Job Printing House, 1871.

Wood, Geo. P., and E. H. Ruddock. *Vitalogy, or Encyclopedia of Health and Home Adapted for Home and Family Use.* Chicago: Vitalogy Association, 1916.

HERBAL MATERIA MEDICA, THOMSONIAN AND PHYSIOMEDICAL

Clymer, R. Swinburne, MD. *Nature's Healing Agents: The Medicine of Nature, (or the Natura System).* Revised ed. Quakertown, PA: The Humanitarian Society, 1973.

Coffin, A. I., MD. *Botanic Guide to Health.* 49th ed. London: Haynes, Coffin & Co., c. 1900. [The author and book that brought physiomedicalism to Britain.]

Colby, Benjamin. *A Guide to Health, Being an Exposition of the Principles of the Thomsonian System of Practice.* 4th ed. Milford, NH: John Burns, 1848. Reprint ed. Orem, UT: BiWorld Publishers, c. 1987.

Cook, William H., MD. *The Physio-Medical Dispensatory: A Treatise on Therapeutics, Materia Medica, and Pharmacy.* Original ed. Cincinnati: Published by the author, 1869. Reprint. Portland, OR: Eclectic Medical Publications, 1985. [The most important and comprehensive physiomedical materia medica.]

_____. *A Compend of the New Materia Medica.* Chicago: Published by the author, 1898.

Fox, William, MD. *The Working-Man's Model Family Botanic Guide.* Sheffield: William Fox and Sons, Medical Botanists, 1916.

Greer, J. H. *A Physician in the House.* 1st ed., 1915. n.p.: Stein Publishing House, 1963.

Hool, Richard Lawrence, FNAMH. *Common Plants and Their Uses in Medicine.* Lancashire: Lancashire Branch of the NAMH, 1922. [A unique and gifted herbalist.]

Menzies-Trull, Christopher. *Herbal Medicine: Keys to Physiomedicalism, including Pharmacopoeia.* Newcastle: Faculty of Physiomedical Herbal Medicine, 2003.

Priest, A. W., and L. R. Priest. *Herbal Medication: A Clinical and Dispensary Handbook*. London: L. N. Fowler & Co., Ltd., 1982.

Shook, Edward, ND. *Advanced Treatise in Herbology*. New and Enlarged Edition. Lecture notes first published 1946. Beaumont, CA: Trinity Center Press, 1978.

_____. *Elementary Treatise*. Lecture notes first published 1946. Banning, CA: Enos Press, 1978.

Skelton, John. *Family Medical Advisor*. 11th ed. Leeds: Published by the author, 1878.

Slack, George. *Slack's Herbal: A Treatise on the Pathology of Disease, Designed for the Use of Families*. London: Potter & Clarke, 1919.

Thomson, Samuel. *The Thomsonian Materia Medica, or Botanic Family Physician*. "Thirteenth edition." Albany, NY: J. Munsell, 1841. [Actually the work of John Thomson, with some editing by his father, Samuel.]

_____. *New Guide to Health; or Botanic Family Physician.... To Which Is Prefixed a Narrative of the Life and Medical Discoveries of the Author*. 2nd ed. Boston: Printed for the author, 1825.

Webb, William Henry. *Standard Guide to Non-Poisonous Herbal Medicine*. Southport, UK: Visitor Printing Works, 1916.

HERBAL MATERIA MEDICA, ECLECTIC

Beach, Wooster, MD. *The American Practice Condensed, or the Family Physician*. New York: James M'Alister, 1849.

Brinker, Francis, ND, ed. *The Eclectic Medical Journals: A Re-Printing of Selected Articles from the Eclectic Medical Journals*. Vol. 1, nos. 1–6. 1995.

_____. *The Eclectic Medical Journals: A Re-Printing of Selected Articles from the Eclectic Medical Journals—1864*. Vol. 2, nos. 1–2. 1995–96.

Coe, Grover, MD. *Concentrated Organic Medicines*. 1st ed., 1858. 2nd ed. New York: R. Keith & Co., 1860. [Excellent description of plant uses.]

Ellingwood, Finley, MD. *American Materia Medica, Therapeutics and Pharmacognosy*. Originally published 1918. Reprint ed. Portland, OR: Eclectic Medical Publications, 1989.

Felter, Harvey, MD, and John Uri Lloyd, MD. *King's American Dispensatory.* 11th ed., 3rd revision. Entirely Rewritten and Enlarged, 1898. 2 vols. Reprint. Portland, OR: Eclectic Medical Publications, 1983.

Fyfe, John William, MD. *Specific Diagnosis and Specific Medication.* Cincinnati: The Scudder Brothers, 1909.

Jones, Eli, MD. *Cancer: Its Causes, Symptoms & Treatment.* Reprint. New Delhi: B. Jain Publishers, Ltd., c. 1990.

_____. *Definite Medication.* 1st ed., 1910. Reprint. New Delhi: B. Jain Publishers, Ltd., 1988.

Lighthall, J. I., and W. O. Davis, MD. *The Indian Household Medicine Guide.* Originally published in Peoria, IL: by the author, 1882. Paperback reprint retitled *The Indian Folk Medicine Guide,* New York: Popular Library, 1973.

Lloyd, J. U., and C. G. Lloyd. *Drugs and Medicines of North America.* Vol. 2. Bulletin of the Lloyd Library of Botany, Pharmacy, and Materia Medica. Bulletin No. 31. Reproduction Series, Vol. 2, no. 9. Originally published 1886–7. Cincinnati: Lloyd Library, 1931.

Locke, Frederick J., MD. *Syllabus of Eclectic Materia Medica and Therapeutics.* Edited by Harvey W. Felter, MD, with notes by John Uri Lloyd. Cincinnati: John M. Scudder's Sons, 1895.

Petersen, Frederick J., MD. *Materia Medica and Clinical Therapeutics.* Los Olivos, CA: Published by the author, 1905.

Scudder, John M., MD. *Specific Diagnosis: A Study of Disease.* 1st ed., 1874. 9th ed. Cincinnati: John M. Scudder and Sons, Medical Publishers, 1893.

_____. *Specific Medication and Specific Medicines.* 4th revision. 1st ed., 1870. 10th ed. Cincinnati: Wilstach, Baldwin & Co., Printers, 1881.

Thomas, Rolla. *Eclectic Practice of Medicine.* Cincinnati: Scudder Brothers, 1903.

Watkins, Lyman. *A Compendium of the Practice of Medicine.* 2nd ed. Cincinnati: The Scudder Brothers Company, 1901.

HERBAL MATERIA MEDICA, MODERN AMERICAN, ENGLISH, CANADIAN, AUSTRALIAN, ETC.

de Bairacli Levy, Juliette. *The Complete Herbal Book for the Dog.* American ed. New York: Arco Publishing, 1973.

_____. *Common Herbs for Natural Health.* American ed. New York: Schocken Books, 1974.

Cameron, Matthew K. *Herbal Remedies from Nature's Pharmacy.* Toronto: Canadian Free Press, 1989.

Cerney, J. V., DPM. *Handbook of Unusual and Unorthodox Healing Methods.* West Nyack, NY: Parker Publishing Co., Inc., 1976.

Christopher, John R., ND. *The School of Natural Healing.* Original ed., 1976. Revised and Expanded 20th Anniversary Edition. Springville, UT: Christopher Publications, 1996. [The compendium from the most important American herbalist of the mid-twentieth century. Christopher was a physiomedicalist.]

Dewey, Laurel. *Plant Power: The Humorous Herbalist's Guide to Finding, Growing, Gathering & Using 30 Great Medicinal Herbs.* East Canaan, CT: ATN/Safe Goods, 1999.

Elliot, Rose, and de Paoli, Carlo. *Kitchen Pharmacy.* London: Tiger Books International, 1991.

Fernie, William T., MD. *Old Fashioned Herbal Remedies.* Originally published 1917 as *Herbal Simples.* Reprint. Toronto: Coles, 1980.

Gagnon, Daniel. *Liquid Herbal Drops in Everyday Use.* 4th ed. Santa Fe, NM: Botanical Research and Education Institute, Inc., 2000.

Gosling, Nalda. *Herbs for Colds and Flu.* Boulder, CO: Shambhala, 1981.

Grieve, M[aude], FRHS. *A Modern Herbal.* Edited and introduction by Mrs. C. F. Leyel. 1st ed., 1931. Reprint. London: Tiger Books International, 1994.

Hall, Dorothy. *Creating Your Herbal Profile.* New Canaan, CT: Keats Publishing Co., 1988.

Harris, Ben Charles. *The Compleat Herbal.* Barre, MA: Barre Publishers, 1972.

Hemmes, Hilde. *Herbs with Hilde Hemmes.* Edited by Andrew Tobin. 1st ed., 1992. 4th ed. Ridgehaven: South Australian School of Herbal Medicine, 1995.

Holmes, Peter. *The Energetics of Western Herbs.* Vol. 1. 3rd ed. Boulder, CO: Snow Lotus Press, 1997.

Kloss, Jethro. *Back to Eden: A Human Interest Story of Health and Restoration to Be Found in Herb, Root and Bark.* 1st ed., 1939. Coalmont, TN: Longview Publishing House, 1962.

Kuts-Cheraux, A. W., MD, ND. *Naturae Medicina and Naturopathic Dispensatory.* Des Moines, IA: American Naturopathic Physicians and Surgeons Association, 1953.

Law, Donald. *The Concise Herbal Encyclopedia.* New York: St. Martin's Press, 1973.

Lucas, Richard. *Magic Herbs for Arthritis, Rheumatism, and Related Ailments.* West Nyack, NY: Parker Publishing Co., 1981.

_____. *The Magic of Herbs in Daily Living.* West Nyack, NY: Parker Publishing Co., 1972.

Mitchell, William A., ND. *Plant Medicine: Using the Teachings of Dr. John Bastyr.* Edinburgh: Churchill Livingstone, 2003.

Moore, Michael. *Medicinal Plants of the Mountain West.* Revised and expanded ed. Santa Fe: Museum of New Mexico Press, 2003.

Neil, James. *The New Zealand Family Herb Doctor: A Guide to Recipes and Herbal Remedies.* First published 1891 by Mills, Dick & Company, Dunedin, New Zealand. Reprint. Twickenham, UK: Senate, an Imprint of Tiger Books International, 1998.

Ritchason, Jack, ND. *The Little Herb Encyclopedia.* 3rd ed. Pleasant Grove, UT: Woodland Health Books, 1995.

Rogers, Robert Dale. *Rogers' Herbal Manual.* Edmonton, Alberta: Karamat Wilderness Ways, 2000.

Smith, Keith Vincent. *The Illustrated Earth Garden Herbal: A Herbal Companion.* Victoria, Australia: Lothian, 1978.

Tenney, Louise. *Today's Herbal Health.* 2nd ed. Provo, UT: Woodland Books, 1983.

Thomas, Lalitha. *10 Essential Herbs.* Originally published 1992. 2nd ed. Prescott, AZ: Hohm Press, 1996.

Tierra, Michael, CA, OMD. *Planetary Herbology: An Integration of Western Herbs into the Traditional Chinese and Ayurvedic Systems.* Edited and supplement by David Frawley, OMD, and Christopher Hobbs, CA. Santa Fe, NM: Lotus Press, 1988.

Tietze, Harald W. *Herbal Teaology.* Bermagui South, AU: Published by the author, 1996.

Willard, Terry, PhD. *Textbook of Modern Herbology.* Calgary: Progressive Publishing Inc., 1988.

Wood, Matthew. *The Book of Herbal Wisdom.* Berkeley: North Atlantic Books, 1997.

HERBAL MATERIA MEDICA, NUTRITIONAL APPROACH

Adams, Rex. *Miracle Medicine Foods.* Paramus, NJ: Prentice Hall, 1977. [Provides case histories.]

Clymer, R. Swinburne, MD. *The Natura Physician: Inculcating the* Natura *System of Therapeutics for the Prevention and Elimination of Disease.* 2 vols. Quakertown, PA: Philosophical Publishing Company, 1933.

Heinerman, John. *Heinerman's Encyclopedia of Fruits, Vegetables and Herbs.* Paramus, NJ: Prentice Hall, 1988.

_____. *Heinerman's Encyclopedia of Healing Juices.* Englewood Cliffs, NJ: Prentice Hall, 1994.

Jensen, Bernard, DC, ND. *Nature Has a Remedy.* Escondido, CA: Privately published, 1979.

HERBAL MATERIA MEDICA, BIOMEDICAL

Bisset, Norman Grainger, ed. and trans., and Max Wichtl, ed. *Herbal Drugs and Phytopharmaceuticals: A Handbook for Practice on a Scientific Basis.* Stuttgart: Medpharm Scientific Publishers, 1994. [Contains German E Commission reports.]

Hoffmann, David, FNIMH, AHG. *Medical Herbalism: The Science and Practice of Herbal Medicine.* Rochester, VT: Healing Arts Press, 2003.

Murray, Michael T., ND. *The Healing Power of Herbs.* Revised and expanded 2nd ed. Rocklin, CA: Prima Publishing, 1995. [A careful discussion of the most commonly used herbal remedies from a pharmacological perspective; limited to herbs of commerce.]

Sears, Barry. *Enter the Zone.* New York: HarperCollins, 1996.

HERBAL MATERIA MEDICA, GERMAN

Aloysius, Brother. *Comfort to the Sick.* Originally published in Holland, 1903. Reprint ed. New York: Samuel Weiser, 1992.

Gümbel, Dietrich, PhD. *Principles of Holistic Therapy with Herbal Essences.* 2nd revised and expanded English ed. Brussels: Haug, 1993.

Kneipp, Sebastian, Father. *The Kneipp Cure: An Absolutely Verbal and Literal Translation of "Meine Wasserkur."* Complete American ed., translated from the 50th German ed. New York: The Kneipp Cure Publishing Company, 1896.

Pahlow, Mannfried. *Das grosse Buch der Heilpflanzen.* Munich: Gräfe und Unzer, 1989.

Rademacher, Johann Gottfried, MD. *Rechtfertigung der von den Gelehrten misskannten, verstandesrechten Erfahrungsheillehre der alten scheidenkunstigen Geheimarzte und treue Mittheilung des Ergebnisses einer 25 jahrigen Erprobung dieser Lehre am Krankenbette.* 2 vols. Berlin: G. Reimer, 1841.

Treben, Maria. *Health through God's Pharmacy.* English translation. Steyr: Wilhelm Ennsthaler, 1984.

Weiss, Rudolf Fritz, MD. *Herbal Medicine.* Translation. Beaconsfield, England: Beaconsfield, 1988.

HERBAL MATERIA MEDICA, FRENCH

Kenner, Dan, and Yves Requena. *Botanical Medicine: A European Professional Perspective.* Brookline, MA: Paradigm Publications, 2001. [An attempt to analyze European and Western herbs in terms of traditional Chinese medicine.]

Mességué, Maurice. *Health Secrets of Plants and Herbs.* New York: William Morrow and Co., 1979.

_____. *Of Men and Plants: The Autobiography of the World's Most Famous Plant Healer.* French ed., 1970. New York: The Macmillan Company, 1972. [Entertaining reading. This was my first herbal.]

Palaiseul, Jean. *Grandmother's Secrets: Her Green Guide to Health from Plants.* French ed., 1972. Translated from the French by Pamela Swinglehurst. New York: G. P. Putnam's Sons, 1974.

HERBAL MATERIA MEDICA, EASTERN EUROPEAN

Hutchins, Alma R. *A Handbook of Native American Herbs.* Boston and London: Shambhala, 1991. [Despite the title, this book contains extensive information on Russian herbal research and experience with very little on American Indian usage.]

Talalaj, S., PhD, and A. S. Czechowicz. *Herbal Remedies: Harmful and Beneficial Effects.* Melbourne: Hill of Content, 1989.

Zevin, Igor Vilevich. *A Russian Herbal: Traditional Remedies for Health and Healing.* Rochester, VT: Healing Arts Press, 1996.

HERBAL MATERIA MEDICA, TRADITIONAL CHINESE MEDICINE

Bensky, Dan, and Andrew Gamble. *Chinese Herbal Medicine: Materia Medica.* Seattle: Eastland Press, 1986.

Lu, Henry C. *Chinese Natural Cures: Traditional Methods for Remedies and Preventions.* New York: Black Dog and Leventhal Publishers, 1994.

Zhongjing, Zhang. *Treatise on Febrile Disease Caused by Cold.* Translated by Luo Xiwen, PhD. Beijing: New World Press, 1985.

_____. *Synopsis of Prescriptions of the Golden Chamber: A Classic of Traditional Chinese Medicine.* Translated by Luo Xiwen, PhD. Beijing: New World Press, 1987.

HERBAL MATERIA MEDICA, AYURVEDIC

Kacera, Walter, DN, PhD. *Ayurvedic Tongue Diagnosis.* Twin Lakes, WI: Lotus Press, 2006.

Lad, Vasant, PhD, and David Frawley. *The Yoga of Herbs: An Ayurvedic Guide to Herbal Medicine.* Santa Fe, NM: Lotus Press, 1986.

Tirtha, Swami Sada Shiva. *The Ayurveda Encyclopedia: Natural Secrets to Healing, Prevention, & Longevity.* Technical editor, Dr. R. C. Uniyal; contributing editors, Dr. S. Sandhu and Dr. J. K. Chandhok. Bayville, NY: Ayurveda Holistic Center Press, 1998.

HOMEOPATHIC MATERIA MEDICA

The following authors are particularly appropriate for herbalists.

Anshutz, E. P. *New, Old and Forgotten Remedies.* Philadelphia: Boericke & Tafel, 1900.

Blackwood, Alexander L., MD. *A Manual of Materia Medica, Therapeutics, and Pharmacology, with Clinical Index.* Reprint of the 2nd ed. of 1922. New Delhi: B. Jain Publishers Pvt. Ltd., 2002.

Boericke, William, MD. *Pocket Manual of Homoeopathic Materia Medica.* 9th ed., revised and enlarged. Philadelphia: Boericke & Runyon, 1927.

Burnett, J. Compton, MD. *Best of Burnett.* Edited by Dr. H. L. Chitkara. New Delhi: B. Jain Publishers, Ltd., 1992. [This anthology unfortunately truncated Burnett, but is a good source for those not interested in collecting his numerous tomes individually. For a complete bibliography of his individual works, see Matthew Wood, *Vitalism* (1992).]

Clarke, John Henry, MD. *A Dictionary of Practical Materia Medica.* 3 vols. Originally published 1900–03. 3rd ed. Rustington, Sussex: Health Science Press, 1962.

Haehl, Richard. *Samuel Hahnemann: His Life and Work.* Translated into English by Marie L. Wheeler. Edited by J. H. Clarke and F. J. Wheeler. 2 vols. London: Homoeopathic Publishing Co., 1927.

Hale, Edwin M., MD. *Homoeopathic Materia Medica of the New Remedies: Their Botanical Description, Medical History, Pathogenetic Effects and Therapeutical Application in Homoeopathic Practice.* 1st ed., 1864. 2nd ed., revised and enlarged. Detroit: Edwin A. Lodge, Homoeopathic Pharmacy, 1867. [A very important source of information on folk medicine in America in the middle of the nineteenth century that is not well appreciated because of its homeopathic provenance. Hale was attempting to incorporate eclectic and folk medical agents into homeopathy.]

_____. *Materia Medica and Special Therapeutics of the New Remedies.* 2 vols. 4th ed., originally published 1875. Reprint. New Delhi: B. Jain Publishers Pvt. Ltd., 1999.

Millspaugh, Charles, MD. *American Medicinal Plants.* First published 1892. Reprint ed. New York: Dover Publications, 1974.

Sinha, Yadubir, MDS. *Miracles of Mother Tinctures, with Therapeutic Hints and Treatment of Diseases.* 1st ed., 1962. New Delhi: B. Jain Publishers, 1981.

Tetau, Max. *Gemmotherapy: A Clinical Guide*. French ed., 1987. Canada: Éditions du Détail, Inc., 1998.

Tumminello, Peter L. *Rhus glabra: A Homoeopathic Proving: A Portrait of Abuse*. Leichhardt, AU: Sydney College of Homoeopathic Medicine, 1997.

MATERIA MEDICA, FLOWER ESSENCES

Bach, Edward. *Collected Writings of Edward Bach*. Edited by Julian Barnard. Cheltenham: Bach Educational Programme, 1987.

Cowan, Eliot. *Plant Spirit Medicine*. Newberg, OR: Swan•Raven & Co., 1995.

Dalton, David. *Stars of the Meadow: Medicinal Herbs as Flower Essences*. Great Barrington, MA: Lindisfarne Books, 2006.

Katz, Richard, and Patricia Kaminski. *Flower Essence Repertory: A Comprehensive Guide to the Flower Essences Researched by Dr. Edward Bach and by the Flower Essence Society*. Special reprint ed. Nevada City, CA: Earth-Spirit, Inc., 2004.

MATERIA MEDICA, ANTHROPOSOPHIC

Bott, Victor. *Anthroposophical Medicine: An Extension of the Art of Healing*. 1st French ed., 1972. Translated by F. L. Weaton and G. Couch. London: Rudolf Steiner Press, 1978.

Husemann, Friedrich, and Otto Wolff. *The Anthroposophical Approach to Medicine: An Outline of a Spiritual Scientifically Oriented Medicine*. Translation of the 2nd German ed. by Peter Laborsky. Vol. 1. Spring Valley, NY: The Anthroposophic Press, 1982.

Pelikan, Wilhelm. *Healing Plants: Insights through Spiritual Science*. Vol. 1. German ed., 1988. Translated by A. R. Meuss. Spring Valley, NY: Mercury Press, 1997.

Steiner, Rudolf. *Spiritual Science and Medicine*. Lectures delivered in 1920. 1st English ed., 1948. London: Rudolf Steiner Press, 1975. [The original inspiration for anthroposophical medicine. One of Steiner's mentors was an old country herbalist.]

Wolff, Otto. *Home Remedies: Herbal and Homeopathic Treatments for Use at Home.* Translated by A. R. Meuss and J. Collis. New York: Anthroposophic Press, 1991.

LECTURE NOTES

Graf, Eva. *Herbs.* Privately published, 1978.

LeSassier, William. Lecture at Self-Heal School of Herbal Studies and Healing in San Diego, April 21–22, 1995.

_____. Lectures at Green Nations Gathering, Phoenicia, NY, 1994–5.

_____. [Notes from William LeSassier; not identified as such.] In *Nutrition & Your Health,* edited by Edward Bauman. Privately published, 1984, pp. 15–18.

_____. Personal conversations.

Red Elk, Paul, Yako Tahnahgah, and Matthew Wood. Lectures on Animal Medicines, St. Paul, 2003–5.

INDEX OF HERBS

INDEX OF CONDITIONS

Parasites, 205, 210
Pelvic congestion, 328
Pemphigus, 210
Peritonitis, 156
Pimples, 317
Pneumonia, 83–84
Poison ivy, 125, 261
Pregnancy, 134
Premenstrual syndrome (PMS),
    120, 354
Prostate problems, 107, 141, 142,
    302
Psoriasis, 318
Pulse, rapid, 232, 233
Pyelitis, 214
Pyelonephritis, 213

R
Rashes, 201, 210
Rattlesnake bites, 147–48, 149
Rectal fissure, 345
Respiratory conditions, 59, 73, 78,
    83–84, 146, 164, 231, 290
Restlessness, 325
Rheumatism, 120, 234
Ringworm, 157, 210
Rupia, 210

S
Scrofula, 321
Sexual neurosis, 353
Shingles, 210
Shoulder, frozen, 84
Sinusitis, 209
Skeletal conditions, 120, 134, 161,
    268
Skin conditions, 64, 66, 84–85, 88,
    120, 205, 210, 268, 318, 346
Small intestine, irritation of, 290

Smoking, conditions linked to, 231
Snake bites, 147–48, 149, 159–60
Spasms, 231
Spine, torn disks in, 197
Spleen complications, 104–5, 106
Strangury, 55
    Sweating
    excessive, 300
lack of, 88
Swellings, hard, 148, 149

T
Throat, sore, 267
Thyroid problems, 200, 208–9,
    210, 232, 233, 280
Timidity, 73
Tinnitus, 241
Toenail fungus, 368, 369
Tongue
    with coating, 236, 250
    enlarged, 106, 196
    unequal appearance of, 231
Tonsillitis, 267
Toxins, 216
Tracheitis, 59
Tumors, 210
Typhoid, 156

U
Ulcers, 196, 197, 247, 346
Uric acid buildup, 137, 213
Urinary tract infections, 347
Urination
    excess, 300
    painful, 369
    suppression of, 55
Uterus
    atony of, 186, 328, 340
    enlarged, 162